Studies in Disorders of Communication

General Editors:

Professor David Crystal
Honorary Professor of Linguistics, University College of North Wales, Bangor

Professor Ruth Lesser
University of Newcastle upon Tyne

Professor Margaret Snowling
University of Newcastle upon Tyne

Dedication

To the memory of my father.

Communication Skills in Hearing-impaired Children

R. JOHN BENCH

Department of Communication Disorders
Lincoln School of Health Sciences
La Trobe University
Bundoora, Victoria, Australia

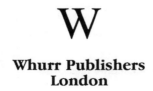

Whurr Publishers
London

© 1992 Whurr Publishers Ltd
19b Compton Terrace, London N1 2UN, England

British Library Cataloguing in Publication Data

A catalogue record for this book is available from the
British Library.

ISBN 1-870332-385

Photoset by Stephen Cary
Printed and bound in the UK by Athenaeum Press Ltd,
Newcastle upon Tyne

Preface

The topic of communication covers such a wide area that, even if limited to the hearing-impaired child, the potential coverage is very great. I am well aware that, using 'communication' in a general sense, one or more whole books could be written about the material summarised in each chapter of what follows. Thus, the present text can give the reader only a taste of, and hopefully for, the area. Nonetheless, it is surprising that in the narrower social sense of interpersonal communication the discussion of communication for hearing-impaired children is not well developed in the literature. The area of communication skills is even less well developed.

Two areas of endeavour which receive only passing attention in this book are the anatomical and linguistically oriented work of recent years. Although they are of abiding interest, I have not set apart a special section for them, as they have received extensive, expert and recent coverage elsewhere.

My brief was to write a book of around 125 000 words as an overview for the more senior undergraduate students in audiology, speech and language pathology, psychology, special education or related disciplines. The brief was also to update graduate students and practitioners. This book, then, assumes that the reader has a basic knowledge of psychology, acoustics and linguistics, and at least an elementary knowledge of work with hearing-impaired individuals. A glossary is included to help readers who may not be too familiar with the terminology, and where different terms are used in different countries. Mostly, I have chosen references which are accessible in the literature to make it easier for student readers to pursue points of interest, though this approach was not always possible.

The behaviour of hearing-impaired people, like that of human beings in general, presents as a seamless robe. Although it is possible to separate the facets of such behaviour conceptually, it is extremely difficult to design studies to isolate them at the empirical level, given the many practical constraints. The result is that salient variables are often confounded with one another, as the following pages clearly show. My approach has been generally to stick close to the published literature, giving enough detail for the reader to develop a feel for such difficulties, and limiting my own assessment and evaluation. In any case, the confounding of variables in investigative work, and the great diversity among hearing-impaired individuals, make it hard to be firmly prescriptive about methods of therapy or education. I myself make no such prescription, recalling Gallaudet's maxim of nearly 100 years ago: 'Nothing could be more unscientific, unprofessional, at variance with the testimony of experience, nor more cruel than to attempt to stretch all the deaf on the Procrustean bed of a single method' (British Deaf Mute, 1896, per National Union of the Deaf Steering Committee, 1982).

Not all authors have been specific about the hearing loss and other characteristics of their subjects. I have used the authors' terminology, however imprecise, in such cases. Elsewhere, I have avoided technical details in favour of commonly accepted terms whose meaning is clear and accurate enough. Thus I may refer to, say, 83 dB HTL in an original report as 'severely deaf'. Further, the term 'congenital' is used with two meanings in the literature. Some authors restrict the usage to issues occurring around birth, such as hypoxia, and exclude hereditary considerations. Others include both. I have generally followed the usage of the author. Also, I have tended to use the terms 'deaf' and 'hearing-impaired' as synonyms, thinking it a nonsense to restrict 'deaf' to those people, such as the 'stone deaf', whose numbers are vanishingly small, and declining to limit myself to the sometimes euphemistic 'hearing-impaired'. Where required, I have qualified either term with the relevant expression, such as 'moderately' or 'severely', to make the meaning clear.

Children whose hearing is within normal limits are referred to as 'hearing children' throughout. The terms 'preschool' and 'kindergarten' may have different meanings in different countries, or even in different states in the same country. Because it would have been tedious for the reader, I have not given the specific meaning for each instance.

This book played a part in a personal renaissance. Having spent most of the last 12 years or so in the gatekeeping role of an academic administrator, and having recently relinquished that role to return to teaching, clinical practice and research, I needed to bring myself up to date across the field. One thoroughgoing, if somewhat daunting, way of doing this was to write a book. The following pages are the result. I trust that, having perused the book, not too many readers will conclude that I should return to work in administration.

John Bench
Melbourne

General preface

This series focuses upon disorders of speech language and communication, bringing together the techniques of analysis, assessment and treatment which are pertinent to the area. It aims to cover cognitive, linguistic, social and education aspects of language disability, and therefore has relevance within a number of disciplines. These include speech therapy, the education of children and adults with special needs, teachers of the deaf, teachers of English as a second language and of foreign languages, and educational and clinical psychology. The research and clinical findings from these various areas can usefully inform one another and, therefore, we hope one of the main functions of this series will be to put people within one profession in touch with developments in another. Thus, it is our editorial policy to ask authors to consider the implications of their findings for professions outside their own and for fields with which they have not been primarily concerned. We hope to engender an integrated approach to theory and practice and to produce a much-needed emphasis on the description and analysis of language as such, as well as on the provision of specific techniques of therapy, remediation and rehabilitation

Whilst it has been our aim to restrict the series to the study of language disability, its scope goes considerably beyond this. Many previously neglected topics have been included where these seem to benefit from contemporary research in linguistics, psychology, medicine, sociology, education and English studies. Each volume puts its subject matter in perspective and provides an introductory slant to its presentation. In this way we hope to provide specialised studies which can be used as texts for components of teaching courses at undergraduate and postgraduate levels, as well as material directly applicable to the needs of professional workers.

David Crystal
Ruth Lesser
Margaret Snowling

Contents

Acknowledgements

My grateful thanks to Trish Collocott, Janet Doyle, Pierre Gorman, Jane Mulcahy, Elaine Saunders and Thein Tun for their advice on various sections of the text. Roslyn Doyle kindly allowed me to draw on some of her work in my discussion of pragmatics. Nicola Daly cheerfully helped with a multitude of details. The staff of the La Trobe University library, Carlton Campus, and Jane Mulcahy were invaluable in chasing up references. Heather Russell typed the draft manuscript with her customary zest. My deepest gratitude is due to my wife, Margaret, who had to put up with me as a semi-recluse during the preparation of the work. I owe her a great deal.

Chapter 1
The Nature of Human Communication

This introductory chapter considers the nature of human communication, its aims and goals, and communication as skilled behaviour. The discussion includes outlines of traditional approaches to communication from the referential and sociolinguistic viewpoints, the pragmatics of communication, and the biological and psychological features that affect the way in which communication is expressed. The chapter concludes with some remarks on the communication problems of hearing-impaired children, to set the context for the rest of the work.

Communication is about the transmission of information. Effective human communication relies heavily on language, a system of verbal and/or gestural symbols governed by rules in a sophisticated code, though some simple forms of communication, such as a handclap to attract attention, are non-linguistic. People communicate purposefully, but apparently without conscious effort. Yet the processes involved are among the most complex of human activities. As talkers, we choose from vocabularies of up to 50 000 words (Newell and Simon, 1972) at a rate approaching five selections each second. At the same time we draw on a knowledge of syntax which sets rules for ordering these lexical choices; semantics which links words to accepted meanings; prosody which shapes the rhythms and stresses of speech; and pragmatics which relates to usage and users. In addition, we may have to switch frequently from language to metalanguage, as in using English to talk about English structure or meaning, when we want to illustrate, emphasise, or explain points of interest. We also use gestures and change our facial expressions while talking (Kendon, 1981a, b). So we make use of language, paralanguage, and kinesics, involving semantics and grammar, modulation of pitch and volume, and facial expressions in what Poyatos (1983) called the basic triple structure of human communication. There is probably no other human activity which requires such a high decision rate or involves interactions of such intricacy (Levelt, 1989; Pitt and Samuel, 1990), except perhaps that our complex behaviour as talkers is mirrored by matching activities as listeners.

The situation is further complicated by the need to perform roles as turn-takers, from talker to listener, and back again. Sometimes we deliberately break the usual conversational conventions, as with ironic or sarcastic statements, often cued by unusual emphasis or intonation. As well, the processes involved are subtly changed by the conversation itself when, as listeners, we come across new phraseology or meanings. Even as we converse, we are developing our conversational experience, which in turn shapes our ongoing discourse.

Communication by conversation, then, involves a high rate of word selection and recognition, while maintaining grammatical, semantic, rhythmic and pragmatic conventions and a readiness to slip into alternative or complementary forms. This high rate strongly suggests that, although the sounds of speech occur in an identifiable serial order, much of the processing of speech and language, in both production and perception, occurs simultaneously rather than in series. Whether we are speaking or listening, there simply is not time to process all the material item by item, though some serial processing may occur. Hence, simultaneous or parallel processing models have been introduced in the study of speech production and perception. The extent to which speech processing takes place serially or in parallel is a formidable task currently occupying the energies of speech scientists, linguists, cognitive psychologists and some philosophers, among others. The reader is referred to Garman (1990) and Levelt (1989) for comprehensive coverage of the area.

Human communication allows people to describe events, to teach and learn, and to share experiences and ideas. It is related to our ability to think in the abstract. It permits knowledge to be passed from one generation to another. Communication in some form is a feature of every known society, even the least well developed.

Forms of communication

Communication through speech, with its great flexibility, efficiency and variety, clearly excels where people need to relate closely and immediately to one another. There is no known society whose hearing members have to rely on gestures rather than words (Farb, 1973). Only a minority of members do not have speech as their main mode of communication. The fingerspelling and sign or gestural languages of some profoundly deaf and intellectually disabled groups offer two well-known examples. Although there is good reason for certain groups not to use speech as their main vehicle for communication, there is no doubt that failure to communicate in everyday activities by speech is socially isolating. Whilst blind people usually manage to communicate very well in speech with their sighted fellows, profoundly deaf signers have very considerable difficulty in communicating with most hearing people. They are detached from society at large. 'Many of us are shocked at the thought of deaf being able to communicate only with deaf' (Conrad, 1976).

People also need to communicate across distances, a need conveniently met by telecommunications devices. Distance communication now plays an important part in the everyday lives of most people in both work and recreation. It is particularly purposeful and goal directed. It takes extra effort to initiate and maintain, is more limiting than face-to-face communication, and has a financial cost. Distance communication is not initiated or maintained as casually as many face-to-face exchanges. Thus, although we tend to see human communication in real time as a face-to-face activity, we need increasingly to communicate at a distance via telephones, teletypes and computer terminals. Teletypes for the deaf, perhaps more correctly called telecommunications devices (Rittenhouse and Kenyon, 1987), are now commonly used by hearing-impaired people who would have difficulty in using the telephone (Erber, 1985). This use of teletypes has encouraged hearing-impaired people to improve their keyboard abilities for real-time communication.

Developed civilisations also make widespread use of written communication, so that writing is taken as one of the principal marks of a developed society. Some people spend more of their time in writing and reading books and articles than in other kinds of communication. Writing further offers a means not only to communicate in the present, but also to convey information to future generations. Despite recent developments in electrical data storage, the written word is still the most enduring general means of communication.

Interpersonal communication

Human communication is interpersonal. It involves the sharing of thoughts, meanings and ideas between people. Hearing-impaired children will develop their own manual communication system without instruction (Heider and Heider, 1941; Mohay, 1982), showing how pressing is the need to communicate with others. One act of communication usually requires a reciprocal act. Even without reciprocity, communication aims to affect the recipient, to add to or change the recipient's perceptions. It is thus remiss to describe communication in terms solely of methods and techniques, or of instruments and devices. A full understanding of human communication requires comprehension of the thoughts, motives and intentions of the communicator, the relationships between communicator and recipient, and the organisational setting in which communication occurs (Haney, 1973).

Communication skills are bound up with social skills, as shown by frequent use of the phrase 'interpersonal communication skills'. Argyle (1972), and Bellack and Hersen (1979) have developed theoretical reviews of interpersonal communication with an emphasis on social skills, whereas Ellis and Whittington (1981) have reviewed a number of attempts to train individuals in these skills. In an informative book, Hargie et al. (1981) identified and discussed the nature of social skills in interpersonal communication with the needs of 'interpersonal professionals', whose work involves communication with other people, in mind. They reviewed nine main skill areas in terms of social skills. However, it is clear that the social skills they considered are essentially interpersonal communication skills. Their review illustrated the extensive range of skills involved in interpersonal communication, showing that such skills are goal-directed, interrelated, defined in terms of identifiable behaviour, learned, and under the control of the individual.

Extensive research in this field is relatively recent, with most of the salient work emerging in the last 25 years or so. As yet, however, little similar work has been done with hearing-impaired people.

Goals of interpersonal communication

In communicating we adopt recognised roles and follow conventions or rules. Communication skills are directed skills, whether we are transmitter or receiver, which are applied to attain communication goals. These goals are interdependent for transmitter and receiver (Higgins et al., 1981) because each person influences, and is influenced by, the other.

In any interchange the transmitter and receiver not only play different roles, but also have different aims and goals. The transmitter's goal is to convey a message clearly to the receiver, and thus the transmitter needs relatively organised, unified and differentiated cognitive processes (Zajonc, 1960). The receiver, on the other hand, has to be ready to receive a broad range of possible messages, at least to start with, and hence needs cognitive processes that are not overly organised, unified and differentiated. In reviewing Zajonc's and similar studies, Higgins et al. (1981) concluded that, because transmitters need to convey clear and concise messages, they tend to polarise and can distort stimulus information more than receivers, who have to anticipate a wide range of messages. It is thus not unexpected that research in communication has sometimes found that the effectiveness of talkers and listeners is unrelated, or even negatively related. Talkers and listeners need and use different kinds of information processing in a communication 'game' (Rommetveit, 1974).

As well as the social goals of initiating personal contact and developing and maintaining personal relationships, communication may aim to develop a shared goal of social reality, particularly if that reality is ambiguous or difficult to establish (Stamm and Pearce, 1971). Shared goals of social reality develop from the exchange of beliefs and indications of personal awareness about issues, and expressions of self-worth. These goals can be tested by speculation and imagination, by recall of past circumstances, and by predictions of future events and outcomes. Elsewhere, Collins and Raven (1969) discussed communication goals where a group works together to solve problems. Such communication activities not only involve simple association with other people to solve the problem in hand, but they may also aim to influence the behaviour of others in the group to obtain control or power, and may benefit from coalitions among group members to attain objectives. Again, Goffman (1967) described face goals in the rituals of face-to-face behaviour, where the interchange aims at self-presentation and the maintenance of self-esteem. Other goals of interpersonal exchange include seeking reassurance, sympathy and the like through the expression of emotions and anxieties; obtaining relief from boredom and pursuing entertainment by the reading and writing of poetry, drama and song; the exchange of information by identifying an attribute, object, action or idea from a set of alternatives in referential communication; and the sharing of opinions and advice.

This short review of human communication has outlined its great richness and diversity. As we shall see later, only some of this variety has been studied systematically in work with hearing-impaired people.

Communication Skills as Skills

What constitutes communication skills? Is there a definable set of such skills? Are they acquired in the same way as other skills of the perceptual–motor kind? To answer these questions, we first consider the nature of skills and then proceed to discuss what skills may be involved in communication.

Because we are all versed in communication and see ourselves as expert in the use of communication skills, we may envisage that the answers will come easily. Nothing could be further from the truth. The reader is advised that the area is most complex and difficult, as the following pages will show.

Skills have a practical reference, with a strong element of training. Historically they have been considered in the context of motor behaviour, often in work situations such as typewriting, and of cognition, as in clinical decision-making (Harvey, 1991). Hence, besides motor or, more properly, perceptual–motor skills, we find skills across the whole spectrum of human behaviour. Early work showed that skills involve precision, speed, strength and rhythm (Seashore, 1951), and are characterised by low energy cost. Wolfle (1951), who investigated how skills are acquired, identified six principles which could be manipulated under practical training conditions: knowledge of results; avoidance of habit interference; variety of practice materials; methods used in training; knowledge of the procedures involved; and effectiveness of guidance. It is of interest to note in passing that Bode and Oyer (1970) used such principles in auditory training for speech discrimination in noise, for 32 adults with a mild inner-ear hearing loss, in one of the few published studies involving hearing-impaired subjects to do so.

Clarke (1958), working on the abilities and trainability of imbeciles in motor skills, referred to the importance of well-motivated subjects, achieved by setting realistic goals; task breakdown to basic constituents in a series of steps, to be mastered sequentially; spaced learning with overlearning; and verbal reinforcement.

The principles of Wolfle (1951) and Clarke (1958) translate almost exactly for normally developing children who are acquiring communication skills. The elementary skills are effected without awareness. Young children acquire their first skills in communication and language without deliberately setting out to learn them. To consider Wolfle's list first, the environment in which communication and language develop is one in which knowledge of results is usually immediate; inappropriate habits are discouraged by the caregiver; the caregiver naturally provides a variety of practice situations and materials; and several means are employed, from use of naturally occurring events to communication 'lessons'. Explicit, thoroughgoing knowledge of the principles involved is not found in the young child. A capacity for language and ongoing guidance by the caregiver ensure that the principles are internalised as they are introduced. Later, the child receives formal training at school from teachers, when most of the requisite principles are expressly learned.

In the case of Clarke's principles, young children are strongly motivated to communicate to attain other goals; the communication 'task' is broken down to basic constituents, or a series of steps in the right direction, by the capacities of the children themselves to which caregivers are sensitive; the acquisition of language and communication abilities is spread over months and years, with ample opportunity for overlearning; and verbal reinforcement is provided by the very nature of the situation.

We think of skills as relatively discrete attributes (Ammon, 1981): using the telephone; sharpening a pencil; reading some notes; or delivering a speech, for instance. However, skills can or may need to be combined (Wilson et al., 1989). For example, it helps to be highly practised in the skill of reading from notes in developing the complex skill of delivering a speech. A complex skill, as in speech-making, hence relies on a number of subordinate skills, all or most of which are highly overlearned and are delivered smoothly and automatically. Some examples would be modulation of the voice, keeping an eye on the clock, and judging the reaction of the audience from time to time. Such subordinate skills may be relatively simple, or themselves quite complex, but all skills, even the most complex, can be reduced conceptually to a combination of individual skills. That such reduction is possible shows that all skills may be regarded as either unitary, or comprised of a number of unitary skills, even though it may be difficult to isolate individual skills in practice.

Work is now being done on general thinking skills and problem solving, particularly more complex problem solving (Chipman et al., 1985; Klahr and Kotovsky, 1989; Resnick, 1989). Sternberg (1983) outlined eight criteria for general intellectual skills training, which should: be based in the theory of information processing; be culturally relevant; offer direct instruction in the desired skills; consider the motivation of the subject and associated individual differences; relate to real-world behaviour; be effective through empirical test; be lasting over time; and transfer to related areas. Apart from the first criterion, the normal development of intellectual and communication skills progresses naturally from the young child's home and family environment according to these criteria, though this progression depends on the variety and sophistication of the experiences which that environment can offer. Several recent studies in the area of general intellectual and communication skills training have met many, if not all, of Sternberg's criteria (e.g. Larson et al. (1984) who studied transfer effects on verbal ability and cooperative learning, and Leinhardt and Greeno (1986) who explored the cognitive skills involved in teaching). Sternberg's list apparently omitted a feedback criterion. However, MacKay (1981, 1987) emphasised the need for external feedback, particularly during the early stages of skill acquisition, to ensure that an action has the desired effect. Without external feedback during the early stages, practice may strengthen the wrong associations. However, as the skill is developed, the strength of associations already formed can be further strengthened, without feedback, by mental practice.

There is recent and welcome emphasis on cognitive analyses of learning, performance and instruction, which has moved away from the study of training and learning processes themselves (Glaser and Bassok, 1989). Attention is now increasingly paid to the way in which knowledge is structured and to ecologically meaningful performance (Chi and Ceci, 1987; Greeno and Simon, 1988; Abkarian et al., 1990); the speed at which knowledge and skill are applied by experts and novices (Schneider, 1985); the translation of the content 'knowing what' into the procedural 'knowing how'; and ways in which knowledge is internalised through metacognitive processes (Bransford et al., 1986). So far, relatively little of this recent work has affected the management of hearing-impaired children, whether partially hearing or profoundly deaf. The view of the hearing-impaired child as a metasubject, for example, is rare in the literature.

Communication skills have frequently been considered in specific contexts, as in the work of King (1989) on Shulman's Test of Pragmatic Skills (Shulman, 1985), which covered ten conversational intentions in four scenarios for both listener and speaker roles. Nevertheless, the term 'communication skills' has often been used so generally and widely as to imply no more than communication behaviour. At times, it has been used to mean little more than 'social behaviour'. This global use of 'communication skills' confounds three important distinctions, conveniently separated by Ammon (1981): the distinction between skills and other forms of knowledge; the distinction between knowledge that is relevant only to communication and knowledge that is relevant to communication but not communication alone; and the distinction between knowledge and psychological factors other than knowledge that affect communicative performance.

Skills compared with other forms of knowledge

We have referred to 'knowing what' versus 'knowing how' – to content knowledge versus skill knowledge, respectively. Skill knowledge is practical, applied knowledge. When we use our skills we expect some result to follow. We employ our skills to achieve some desired end. As transmitters, we wish to influence the behaviour and/or the thinking of a receiver, and we shape our contribution to the communication to suit. As receivers, we may take notice of the communication or not. This situation does not hold in the same way for other kinds of knowledge. Content knowledge – knowing the names of the days of the week and the months of the year, for example – is not properly a skill in the practical sense. Such knowledge has practical consequences only when we employ it, as when, for example, we use the skills needed to set up the date of a meeting.

We may be able to recognise, and recognise the usefulness of, certain skills, but not be able to put them into practice. We may be able to state, from a study of the principles involved in communication, how a speaker should address a particular audience, but prove incompetent in the task ourselves. Thus factual knowledge about communication is not the same as possessing the practical skill.

Knowledge relevant to communication versus other knowledge

Communication skills could be defined as all those skills that are used from time to time in communication. Unfortunately, this definition includes a very large number of intellectual and social skills. As a result, it is of little practical use. Ammon (1981) pointed out that such a definition would be limited only by previous knowledge of the world. He argued that competence in communication should be restricted to those skills that arise only in communication tasks, thus forcing a focus on the competencies underlying communicative competence.

Knowledge compared with other psychological factors affecting communication

Skills that are used only in the observable aspects of communication are not enough to characterise communicative behaviour. Other skills, such as cognitive skills which are independent of communication, are clearly needed. This immediately raises problems for the analysis of any sample of communicative behaviour, since the social factors involved in communication will be tied up with other, psychological, factors. Further, although communication skills, narrowly defined, are needed for effective communication, they cannot account for individual variations in performance. Nor do they allow for the development of new communication skills in novel situations. This situation is so complex that few authors have attempted to grapple with it. Ammon (1981) is one of these few. He developed a rather complicated approach, which is not easy to follow, arguing for the analysis of communication skills into predicative and transformational schemas. His approach allows the educator to identify specific communication skills and to provide separate instruction for them, and for knowledge about communication.

Communication skills in hearing-impaired people

So far we have outlined some recent work on communication in hearing people. Only occasional reference has been made to findings related to hearing impairment. What, in more detail, have researchers into hearing impairment had to say about communication as a set of skills, and in the context of everyday communication?

Surprisingly little, for the most part. Although there are exceptions, most authors working with hearing-impaired people have not analysed in detail the communication skills of their patients or clients with an emphasis on skill as skill, despite the large literature with a pragmatic insistence on the abilities and attributes of hearing-impaired people (Prinz and Prinz, 1985). Reference to the contents list or subject index of books written about hearing-impaired people will rarely turn up the word 'skill(s)' or even the phrase 'communication skill(s)'. The approach to communication taken in such books may be full of analytical detail about hearing-impaired people, but not detail relating directly to the deployment, assessment and management of, or therapy for, skills as such.

On examining some well-known texts about hearing impairment and aural rehabilitation, we find, for example, that Clarke and Kendall (1976) referred to a number of areas (language, auditory training, speechreading and speech, fingerspelling and sign, and total communication) under the broad head of 'Language and communication skills', in training for methods of communication used in Canada. Schow and Nerbonne (1980a) discussed speechreading, auditory amplification procedures, aural rehabilitation, counselling, and psychosocial rehabilitation. They referred to the American Speech and Hearing Association description of the responsibilities of the audiologist (ASHA, 1974): '... evaluation of auditory disorders, development or remediation of communicative skills through training, use of devices to increase sensory input when indicated, guidance and counselling in terms of the auditory problem, re-evaluation of auditory function, and assessment of the effectiveness of the habilitative procedures.' Vernon and Ottinger (1980) remarked directly, if briefly, on communication skills in terms of assessment of both expressive and receptive skills, in addition to an audiological workup, as: ability with written language, evaluated through the use of school records, various educational and language tests, or sentence completion, with the verbal subtests of the Wechsler Intelligence Tests also yielding some information; speech and speechreading, which have relevance for the child at school and the adult at work; and evaluation of the clients' manual communication skills.

The justifiably well-regarded, but now somewhat dated, text *Deafness and Communication* (Sims et al., 1982) contains chapters more concerned with communication skills than most other such texts. Under the subhead 'Assessment of communication skills', the book describes hearing and speechreading assessment for the severely hearing-impaired child and for the deaf adult, speech assessment of the hearing-impaired adolescent, English skill assessment with the severely hearing-impaired, sign language assessment, and individual educational planning. Chapters on speech improvement by the deaf adult, the use of speech training aids, and functional speech therapy for the deaf child, follow under the subhead of 'Speech training'. In a section on receptive training, ensuing chapters deal with auditory training, speechreading, hearing-aid evaluation and cochlear implants. A subhead on English training covers English training for children of school age, and reading and writing instruction for young deaf adults. All these subheads are closely concerned with communication skills, as is much other material in the same text, but skills as skills were discussed relatively rarely.

Some of the chapters in Sims et al. (1982) emphasised the relevant skills, as skills, in those areas which may operate in roughly the same way in hearing and hearing-impaired people, such as interpreting. The use of skills was considered also where there is an extensive literature on the normal development or acquisition of the ability in question, such as acquisition of skills in English, and certain cognitive skills. On the other hand, skills in speech production and in hearing tended not to be considered specifically as issues of skill. The distinction perhaps occurred because authors working with the speech or voice production and hearing abilities of hearing-impaired people may be relatively less familiar with the literature on normal communication skills.

These conclusions are supported by contributions to Northcott's (1984) *Oral Interpreting*. In a discussion of speechreading in that book, Green and Green referred to vision and listening as skills. They also referred to the processes which underlie such skills, within a communication context which allows the receiver to 'size up' the communicative situation. They further remarked on inductive skills that affect a receiver's willingness to guess and/or form decisions on the basis of visual information. Siple, in the same text, mentioned the need to identify or analyse the precise skills needed to attain stated instructional goals, and the place of subordinate skills that can be shaped into a hierarchy of instructional events. Castle's chapter drew attention to the relationships between speechreading skills and education of the deaf, linguistics, phonetics, experimental psychology, audiology and speech and language pathology, as they bear on the role of the oral interpreter. She pointed to research (Berger, 1972) showing that speakers who are the easiest to speechread are also the most intelligible for a listener, concluding that precise articulation matters in understanding a message both through vision and listening. Careless, indistinct or exaggerated speech tends to interfere with speechreading. The relationship of these observations to communication skills is evident from work showing that better speech habits can be developed by training (Gonzalez, 1984).

In reviewing the relations between hearing impairment, auditory perception and language disability, Bamford and Saunders (1985) drew attention briefly to the dependence of linguistic abilities on cognitive skills in normal child development. Such skills allow the non-linguistic processing of experiences before language develops. Linguistic representations are thus 'mapped' onto meanings of events which have already been processed by non-linguistic cognitive skills, as a result of the desire to communicate (McAnnally et al., 1987). However, little is known about the extent to which these skills operate in hearing-impaired children.

Erber (1985, 1988) is one of the few workers in the field who has commented consistently on normal communication skills, and projected them to communication for hearing-impaired people. His views are well worth perusal. Erber (1985) summarised some of the work in children's referential communication skills. He showed that, in order to devise an adequately descriptive message and to succeed in communication, a child has to identify not only the critical attributes of the item concerned, but also the relevant characteristics of the receiver. Children come to realise that not everyone has the same knowledge or experience, and hence children need to learn the skills of shaping messages differently for different receivers. These skills form part of the talker's role. Alternatively, when children develop as listeners, they need to develop skills in the listener's role, which involves appreciation of the quality and completeness of the speaker's message. In time, children develop awareness that messages may often be fragmented, ambiguous or too complex for comprehension. Until such skills have developed, children are unaware of the limitations in their messages, and thus fail to give the required feedback to the talker. It seems, therefore, that hearing children need specific instruction or experience to develop good communication skills.

Since these skills are complex and hearing-impaired children have trouble in developing them, special techniques have been proposed to help their teachers and therapists (Brackett, 1983). The techniques that appear to be useful include role reversal, giving the child experience of both the talker's and the listener's viewpoints; confrontation training, which instructs the child directly about a spoken message and the listener's need; modelling relevant talker or listener behaviour; and active listening plans, to persuade and encourage the child to seek clarification when the message is unclear.

The 'talking heads' models of human communication, in which one hearing person converses with another, as when a teacher talks with a child, were seen by Erber (1988) as too restricted. He showed clearly and convincingly that conversations between two people can not only begin with either one of them, but that it can be difficult to identify the start of the conversation. Thus a teacher may appear to open a conversation, but in fact be responding to some non-verbal shift of a child's body position. Similarly, a mother may speak to her baby as a result of some bodily activity, other than vocalisation, on the baby's part. Erber saw verbal communication as a unitary skill with many components: a wish to communicate; recognition of the partner's interests; patterned communication activity, such as role-taking; non-verbal aspects, such as eye contact, posture, etc.; clear, intelligible speech; confirmation that the message has been received as intended; introduction of remedial strategies as needed, to keep the conversation going; judgement of success in attempts at clarification; and response to the partner's wish to change the topic of conversation. This list was developed especially with the needs of hearing-impaired partners in mind, but it is clear that the components are frequently found in conversations between hearing communicators.

A valuable account of developmental aspects in the assessment and enhancement of communication has been given by Moeller (1985). She commented on the difficulties of obtaining valid and reliable evaluations of communication skills in hearing-impaired children, especially when the children have additional handicapping conditions. Moeller argued that an adaptive approach is needed, in view of the marked individual differences shown by children with various kinds of disorder or disability. She also referred to a large number of formal tests covering social skills, communication strategies, and receptive and expressive language skills, many of which were developed on the basis of communication skills in hearing children. She remarked on the ways in which these may need to be adapted, especially when evaluating hearing-impaired developmentally disabled children.

Another valuable outline of the complex system that hearing children develop over their first few years of life, and which is important to communication and language development in deaf children, was provided by McAnnally et al. (1987). This outline included the need to communicate, which precedes the ability to communicate; the interaction which is essential to language development; the prosodic elements of language which can be more important initially than words; the form of adult input; feedback to children on how well they have represented their intended meanings; children's vocabularies, which grow rapidly and follow patterns; and children's syntax, which also grows rapidly and follows patterns.

McAnnally et al. were at pains to stress the very important point that language is learned through communication *for* communication. They were critical of the practice of teaching language through structured lessons, which stress patterning and imitation without reference to the underlying aim of communication. Language skills are to be learned or acquired as a subset of communication skills. Thus the teaching of language skills should make use of everyday experiences and events in the life of the child, about which the child is likely to want to communicate. McAnnally et al. would also stress that the teaching of language skills should follow the normal developmental sequence and structure of such skills. It should not, however, lose sight of the aim of promoting communicative competence, the ultimate goal of any language learning programme. McAnnally et al. further drew attention to inferencing skills, namely relationships between events that are not directly stated (Santrock, 1986), which play a significant part in human communication and which have attracted increasing interest (Wiig and Semel, 1984; Mason and Au, 1986).

Although this brief review of communication as a set of skills is incomplete, the various aspects are so many that to devise a catalogue of them all would be a very large and almost open-ended task. Whilst it is fair to say that most workers with hearing-impaired people have avoided detailed consideration of skills and skill hierarchies in communication, normal or otherwise, as a basis for their work, the magnitude of such a task, considered as a whole, is daunting. It seems only practical to consider those facets of communication skills which relate to particular communicative situations, to particular messages, and to particular communicative contexts (compare Hoemann, 1988). Henceforward, these aspects of communication are the ones we will consider.

Referential and Sociolinguistic Approaches to Communication

It has been traditional (Dickson, 1981) to consider research in the area under the two heads of referential communication and sociolinguistics. These two traditions have been highly influential in setting frameworks for the investigation of communication skills in hearing children, but they have not been nearly as influential in work with the hearing-impaired child.

The referential approach

The referential tradition, with its emphasis on the analysis of communication tasks involving the ability to give and understand specific information about objects or actions, stems from the work of Piaget (1926, 1929). Piaget believed that communication develops from the egocentricity of infants and young children to the socially orientated interchanges of adults. His studies were taken up by Flavell and colleagues (1968, 1977), who set out first to study the general skill area, especially its developmental aspects, seeking a general representation of what verbal communication skills and role-taking would imply. Secondly, they differentiated subskills in role-taking and verbal communication, proceeding from the general situation to specific role-taking or verbal communication activities. Thirdly, they sought tasks that measured the differentiated subskills. Data were then obtained from children of various ages who were attempting the tasks. Among his conclusions, Flavell (1968) specified five major attributes of communication for which a child has to develop knowledge or ability:

1. Existence – appreciating that different communication partners have different perspectives.
2. Need – realising that analysis of the partner's perspective in a given situation helps to obtain one's own goals.
3. Prediction – ability to undertake accurate analysis of the partner's perspective.
4. Maintenance – maintaining awareness of the predictions, namely, of the outcomes of the analysis of the partner's perspective.
5. Application – applying the awareness so developed and maintained to the communication in question.

These attributes have little to say about the causes of communication exchanges from which they are derived. They do not account for individual differences, nor do they explain the structure of role-taking, and so on. Nevertheless, they help to flesh-out Piaget's previous work. As children develop, they become increasingly aware of the needs of their communication partners. The egocentric speech of the young child, much of which occurs without reference to partners, gradually becomes attuned to partners' listening needs. Both Piaget and Flavell took the view that communication skills involve a developing ability to take communication partners' perspectives into consideration, with a gradual departure from the initial egocentrism.

More recent research, however, has shown that this view does not adequately explain the development of communication skills. For example, research now shows that very young children alter the nature of their communication behaviour, depending on the person to whom they are speaking. Children of preschool age address adults differently from young children (Shatz and Gelman, 1973; Sakata, 1989). Other research suggests that some of the egocentric speech of the young child is for the child's own passing use, perhaps as thinking aloud, since the speech may not only be largely meaningless to adults, but may not help the child to select referents (Asher and Oden, 1976).

Several reports have compared children's communication skills in role-taking with accuracy in communication. The general finding has been that correlations between abilities in these two areas are moderate or low, even though children improve in both areas as they grow older (Rubin, 1973; Johnson, 1977). The role-taking approach to the analysis of referential communication skills, then, does not explain the development of accuracy in communication. Asher and Wigfield (1981) observed that attempts to improve children's referential communication skills by training in role-taking had not been notably successful either. However, by observing a model verbalising the correct strategy, practising the strategy, and receiving feedback, communication accuracy in a verbal task was improved, with maintenance of the skills so trained, though there was no generalisation to other referential tasks.

Research in referential communication reviewed by Dickson and Mioskoff (1980), using meta-analysis techniques, showed that specific referential communication skills can be taught to children, as in the Asher and Wigfield study; children can be trained to realise that communication via referents is to appreciate and to describe differences; children can be trained to ask increasingly specific questions, yielding more accurate information exchange; and children can learn to understand that communication breakdown may be due to failure in the speaker's perspective, rather than in that of the listener. There was little evidence that referential communication performance is related to egocentrism or role-taking.

The area of referential communication skills was further reviewed by Bowman (1984), who considered listening plans, feedback and modelling. Referential tasks could be simple or complex, and should be relevant and stimulating. Bowman concluded that, although referential communication skills were seen to be important pragmatically between the ages of 2 and 9 years in normally developing children, little information was available on the referential skills of language-disordered populations, which would include hearing-impaired children, even though such children may have difficulty with this kind of communication.

Work on the normal development of referential communication has continued, notably in the researches of Sonnenschein and Whitehurst (1984) for skill hierarchies. The most recent review was published by Bunce (1991), who took up Bowman's call by offering some helpful guidelines for therapy.

The sociolinguistic approach

A tendency towards increasingly tightly controlled studies of hearing children's referential communication skills fell away somewhat in the 1970s, shifting towards more naturalistically oriented research with a sensible emphasis on the classroom and home environments. At the same time, there were developments in the complementary research tradition – the sociolinguistic approach. This tradition drew principally on the disciplines of linguistics, sociology and social psychology. The aim was to describe communication in a wide sense, in natural settings.

The sociolinguistic approach emphasises social and rhythmic rather than individual and cognitive aspects. Referential skills, it is argued, cannot be separated from social aspects of meaning (Erickson, 1981), though emphasis on the social aspects of communication may exclude referential exchange. The sociolinguistic stress is on ecological validity, on the grounds that communication exchanges are in part culturally determined. Communication exchanges have been analysed for interpretive cues, non-verbal communication and paralinguistic features – the 'how' of communicating as well as the referential content. The interpretation and misinterpretation of literal meaning has been a special area of study in the sociolinguistic tradition (Goody, 1978). The timing of aspects of communication can also be important, as role-taking alters at observable intervals in conversations (Erickson and Schultz, 1980), depending on the social relationship between conversational partners. Language can thus be used both to transmit information and to determine the social setting (Fasold, 1984). This dual function arises because a given message can be communicated linguistically in different ways. The form and the timing by which the information is transmitted are governed by the social situation.

Sociolinguistic analyses of the communication skills of hearing-impaired children have been few. Some interesting insights have been provided by Davis (1976), Montgomery (1976), Mitchell (1978), Scott (1978), and Hay (1978), but a thoroughgoing analysis of such skills in hearing-impaired people has yet to be done. However, an informative report on the sociolinguistic impact on its students of a residential school for the deaf has been provided by Evans and Falk (1986), and an instructive first book to define a range of sociolinguistic issues of concern to the deaf community has recently been published by Lucas (1989).

Contrasts between referential and sociolinguistic approaches

The contrast between the referential and the sociolinguistic traditions is highlighted in the sociolinguistic tradition by a more subjective, qualitative analysis, with emphasis on situational and social validity. Conversely, the research into referential skills emphasises quantitative and objective analysis, with the emphasis on reliability. Researchers adopting the sociolinguistic orientation have mostly used large numbers of observations, small numbers of subjects, realistic naturalistic tasks, broad competences in communication, social situations, and ecological contexts. A subjective approach has been accepted as unavoidable, and perhaps of special value. Research using the referential approach has made use of laboratory situations, specific and sometimes contrived tasks, small numbers of parameters or variables, large numbers of subjects, and cognitive explanations. Additionally, attempts to train subjects in communication skills have been made, often successfully, using the referential approach (Bunce, 1991). Training studies by researchers with a sociolinguistic orientation are relatively rare.

Despite the considerable influence of the referential and sociolinguistic traditions on the description and analysis of communication skills in hearing children, neither tradition has greatly affected the study of communication skills in the hearing-impaired child. Few texts in the field of hearing impairment even mention them. This is probably because the main problems in communication for hearing-impaired people have been seen as linguistic or cognitive. The focus for the education and rehabilitation of the hearing-impaired child has thus been on language, including sign language, and cognition. This focus is narrower than that on communication.

Notwithstanding these comments there is one area, associated with the sociolinguistic tradition and reflecting elements of the referential approach, which has made some impact on work with hearing-impaired people – the area of pragmatics.

Communication in Practical Contexts – Pragmatics

Pragmatics can be described (Moerk, 1977; Gallagher and Prutting, 1983; Prutting and Kirchner, 1983) as the use of syntax and semantics in the context of interactions between people. Recent research in pragmatics (Miller, 1981) has considered the unspoken rules people follow in conversing; the assumptions made by talkers about listeners in judging how to convey information, and how much to convey; and how the talker's intentions are expressed linguistically in different situations. Pragmatics therefore operates at a level above that of the words, phrases and clauses which form the immediate context of the message.

One of the more commonly cited definitions of pragmatics was stated by Morris (1946), who described its relationship to syntax and semantics as:

Syntactics – the relationships between signs.
Semantics – the relationships between signs and their referents.
Pragmatics – the relationships between signs and their users.

Bates (1976) criticised this definition, regarding it as too vague. It missed, she argued, an epistemological or recognisable difference between content and use, and a psychological distinction between objects and procedures. She related her preferred definition to the original work of Peirce (1932): pragmatics is the study of linguistic indices – signs that relate to what they stand for because they participate in or are part of the event or object for which they stand. Hence a ringing tone indexes a telephone, because both are part of the same phenomenon. Further, it is not possible to describe the meanings of indices, but only the rules for relating them to a context in which the meaning can be found. Nonetheless, Morris's definition remains the one most generally accepted.

The emerging, but relatively sparse, literature on the pragmatics of communication in hearing-impaired people is considered in Chapter 8.

Pragmatics contrasted with metalinguistics

Before leaving this brief introduction to pragmatics, it may be well to distinguish pragmatics as the skill of using language in a practical context, and metalinguistics as awareness and self-regulation of language. Van Kleeck (1984) remarked that, in conversing, neither talker nor listener particularly notices how the message is being communicated until some unexpected, pragmatically deviant, conversational event occurs, as when a particular word is used incorrectly. Then the talker and/or listener switch, if only momentarily, to a metalinguistic mode, shifting their attention from the meaning of what is being said to the language being used to say it. Thus a pragmatic slip in conversation produces a metalinguistic reaction in the conversants.

While metalinguistics refers to thinking about language, metapragmatics refers to bringing consciousness to bear on pragmatics, as when children make comments on the social use of language. Thus children may remark on what is being discussed in a conversation; on turn-taking ('Let me finish talking!'); and on the manner of the conversation ('Don't shout!'). Such remarks concern the social use of language, namely pragmatics, as compared with metalinguistic remarks about the grammar and meaning of the language itself.

Metaprocesses in connection with hearing-impaired children are discussed in Chapter 7.

Biological Abilities and Learned Accomplishments

Like other issues in human behaviour, communication skills do not escape discussion of the relative importance of biologically or genetically based factors as compared with learned factors. Even with skills that are heavily influenced by learning or other experiences, the so-called nature/nurture problem needs to be addressed. Prelingually profoundly deaf people have great difficulty in acquiring spoken language, and their cognition is usually very different from that of hearing people and those who are profoundly deafened postlingually. This situation shows that communication skills depend on systems or structures of the biological type. The communication difficulties associated with prelingual profound deafness cannot be fully overcome by special training or learning of communication skills, despite the remarkable achievements of some profoundly deaf individuals (Epstein, 1980). Although we are unable to separate the variables necessary to provide a definitive answer to the nature/nurture question by experiment, it seems that the biological aspects relate to the learned aspects on a continuum. Research with congenitally profoundly deaf people shows that, even with the complete loss from birth of one of the senses primary for communication (the nature end of the continuum), it is possible for them to develop skills (the nurture end) to assist in interaction with their hearing fellows, though not completely so.

A most informative discussion of the area has been offered by Rieber and Voyat (1983) who reported the answers of Chomsky, Osgood, Piaget, Neisser and Kinsbourne to the nature/nurture question as regards language and thought. These answers are now described in turn.

Chomsky proposed that the language system is very complex, but is essentially the same over a range of individuals. The basis of language is thus determined genetically, despite its different manifestations in various cultures. There is an intrinsic, genetically determined factor in the growth of language, a 'universal grammar', which characterises the human genotype.

Chomsky's markedly nativist view of language on the one hand, and the behaviourists' extreme emphasis on learning at the other, were both opposed by Osgood. He stressed a role for prelinguistic cognitive activity, believing that both a child's innate cognitive capacities and learning through prelinguistic experiences are universal in human beings, so that children can acquire any language.

An important role for cognition was also accepted by Piaget, who believed that the development of cognitive structures proceeds by replacing exogenous knowledge, derived from experience, with endogenous or internal reconstructions which incorporate the experiences into existing systems. However, all exogenous knowledge presupposes an endogenous framework because knowledge is assimilated into endogenous forms.

Neisser's contribution turned the discussion back towards nativism. The influence of genetic factors in resolving the nature/nurture question turned out, according to Neisser, to be more important than originally expected, though he favoured an interaction between nature and nurture in explaining language development. He argued that research with deaf children born to hearing parents, who were advised not to teach sign language to their children, showed that, nevertheless, the children developed a rudimentary sign language by themselves. Neisser thought that this signing indicated innate pressures towards language development, although we might see the development of the rudimentary sign system as primarily reflecting a need to communicate with deaf others in the environment. Conversely, and indicative of a nurture effect, attempts to teach language to chimpanzees had turned out to be less successful than they originally appeared to be, when studies with chimpanzees reared in isolation were considered.

An interaction of genetic and environmental factors was also favoured by Kinsbourne, who believed that the child's brain is innately preprogrammed to provide a set of responses, the probabilities of which are biased to particular contingencies which will release them. Thus the environment imposes adaptive modifications on the initial predisposition, depending on the circumstances. The more instructive the environment, the easier it is for the child to modify response probabilities. Kinsbourne illustrated his view with reference to echolalia. Normal young children echo words in a holistic way to pick up phrases without a reference before they can analyse them into their components. The relatively high prevalence of echolalia among autistic children suggests that they cannot map their phonological system onto their cognitive system, as the lack of reference disconnects the children's verbal behaviour from their cognitive processes, giving a 'free-floating phonology'. Such instances show that the speech system and the cognitive system can develop independently (Bartak et al., 1975; Cantwell et al., 1978).

The debate on the nature/nurture question continues, and we will not be so rash as to attempt to resolve it here. We note, however, that the nature/nurture question is associated with the issues of cerebral hemispheric specialisation and neural plasticity. It is generally held that the hemispheres are relatively unspecialised and the neural circuitry is relatively plastic at birth, but become progressively less so as a child develops, though Efron (1990) has recently issued a forceful challenge to much of the rationale for hemispheric specialisation. Witelson (1982, 1985) argued that neural plasticity does not logically require hemispheric specialisation; in fact these two neural characteristics may be independent. Thus cerebral lateralisation may be fixed from birth, while neural plasticity is progressively reduced as the child develops, at least for some cognitive functions. Witelson (1987) further expressed a view that hemispheric specialisation exists from birth, and is not subsequently changed in nature or degree. She interpreted the apparent increase in hemispheric specialisation during childhood as an epiphenomenon of the child's increasing cognitive and behavioural repertoire. What does increase, she suggested, is the amount of cognition available for asymmetric mediation by the hemispheres. The implications of Witelson's position for the acquisition of language skills by prelingually hearing-impaired children may lie with the extent to which language, generally regarded as a left-hemisphere specialism, is mediated by the right cerebral hemisphere, or shared between the two hemispheres. The capacity of the right hemisphere to mediate language is not fully known. However, studies of children who have sustained left-hemisphere damage from birth show that many of these children perform roughly within normal limits on verbal intelligence tests (Woods and Carey, 1979). There is also increasing evidence to show that affective language is mediated in the right hemisphere, while propositional language is left-hemisphere mediated (Gorelick and Ross, 1987).

Age effects have been emphasised, particularly in work related to hearing-impaired children, through the concept of critical periods in language development, to be examined in Chapter 2. For the present we note that the concept has often been proposed to support the view that the experience of auditory and other stimuli during certain stages in child, and especially infant, development has profound and lasting effects on later behaviour, especially language behaviour. Should such experiences be denied, the child will experience long-lasting deleterious effects in the acquisition of hearing and listening skills and the development of speech and language.

There is a conceptual difficulty with the critical period hypothesis, because an argument based on critical periods insists on an irreversibility of the effects (Riesen, 1961). If some means can be found to change the effects back to normal, thus reversing the apparently irreversible, then the so-called critical period is not critical after all. Since it is not possible to be sure that the effects of some 'critical period' stimulation are irreversible, the usefulness of the critical period concept is frustrated by its own specificity. It may be more reasonable to forgo the concept of critical period, and replace it with 'sensitive period', or some such expression, allowing that certain periods in development may be very important for later behaviour, without forcing the notion of irreversibility (Bench, 1971). We may then allow that a child's brain is programmed to provide the child with a set of responses to certain stimuli for which, following Kinsbourne (see above) the probabilities are biased, even strongly biased, to particular releasing contingencies. For example, the infant's exposure to speech sounds shapes for the child a modification of the predisposition to develop language. Further, the richer the exposure to speech over time, the easier it should be for the child to release the potential for verbal language development.

The Interplay of Perceptual Cognitive and Linguistic Processes

Perceptions of simple, common events, such as the wind whistling through the telephone wires, will normally not attract our interest. This type of perception is not far removed from simple sensation. At most we register the percept, and then go back to what we were doing. But where the event forms part of a pattern which has significance for our activities, our perceptions are different. We bring our attention to bear on the relationship between the event and its context, as when we hear an ambulance siren while we are driving a car, and process the combination through pattern perception.

The perception of complex patterns allows us to recognise the relationships between external events and then to arrive at some hypothesis as to what is likely to happen next. To perceive complex patterns is to form conjectures (Gregory, 1974), in which we develop an internal running commentary about the status of the outside world, and our place in it. Perception, especially pattern perception, is thus central to cognition, to knowing and thinking about our circumstances. How we perceive complex patterns and associations and how, in response, we develop patterns of behaviour are thus at the core of the processes of cognition (Holland et al., 1986; Lakoff, 1987). Since we have language, we can mull over the complex pattern we have perceived and make judgements or calculations about it through a reasoning process. If we rehearse the situation to ourselves, we can also commit the complex percept and our cognitive response to our long-term memory.

To take an example from the hearing of speech, we know that the speech we perceive is a pattern of interrelated speech sounds or phonemes, which produces a pattern of sensations depending on differences of timing, frequency and intensity (Margolis, 1986). The meaning of a word, however, depends on the larger pattern the words in which it is embedded. The cognitive and linguistic processes of the listener then play an integral role in defining the semantic context of the word, as when the listener makes inferences about a talker's intentions, expectations and beliefs (Verbrugge, 1977). Thus, in using hearing to perceive speech, we bring our cognitive and linguistic processes to interpret the complex pattern percepts which are generated by the speech stimuli.

Oracy and Literacy

Human communication can be conveniently separated into oracy and literacy. Oracy involves the skills of speaking and listening. Literacy refers to reading and writing. There is a mutual relationship between each pair. To speak is to imply that somebody will listen to what is spoken, while listening in the context of human communication involves attending to speech. To write is to assume that somebody, if only the writer – as in the preparation of shopping lists, for example – will read what has been written, whereas reading requires that the substrate is written material. Whether the concern is for oracy or literacy, for speaking and listening, or for reading and writing, language is the foundation. Aspects of language, both expressive and receptive, are common to each pair. Skilled communicators, then, are skilled in language as a result of skills in at least one of these pairs, and usually in both. Whether we choose to speak, listen, write or read will differ with the need and context, but all deliver communication through language. Although the differences between good and bad readers, for example, can be due to differences in abilities in visual perception or visual memory, research has shown that the differences are related more to variation in the ability to process the material as linguistic material (Liberman et al., 1982; Vellutino, 1983).

Because of the common link through language, it helps to view oracy and literacy on a continuum rather than as opposites (Tannen, 1980; Westby, 1984). At one end of this continuum are found the pragmatic, participant (oracy) aspects of communication; at the other end are the deliberative, meditative (literacy) features. In reflecting these differences of function, oracy and literacy have rather different subject matter. Oracy aids direct understanding of immediate material affairs and the sharing of opinions. Oracy is particularly effective in communicating prosodic information and emotion (Olson, 1977) when the communication partners are together in space and time. Literacy lacks this aspect of mutuality. In order to avoid misunderstandings which cannot be put right at once, as with oracy, literacy relies on a more specific, formal and exact style of communication. Literacy excels in producing formal definitions and in making assumptions explicit, and therefore aids theorising of the more abstract kind. However, some oral styles, as in giving and listening to a lecture, seem analogous to literacy, and some written communications, like diary entries, are akin to oracy. Such instances fall towards the centre of the oracy–literacy continuum.

For most children, the main symbolic system is that of oracy. Children acquire their abilities in language by speaking and listening. Beginning with clause structures of the 'single word sentence' type where 'mama', for example, may mean 'I see mama', 'I want mama to pick me up', and so on, children elaborate their knowledge and use of language from the clause, phrase and word level up to clause coordination and subordination and the passive voice by about 4;6 years of age (Crystal et al., 1976), well before they begin to read and write. Hence hearing children base their literacy on their oracy. They draw on their abilities in speaking and listening to develop skills in reading and writing. Children who have poor oracy skills are likely to have problems with literacy, whatever the underlying disability. Since literacy, especially reading, helps children to develop their knowledge of the world, and to think about issues and events apart from context, children who are weak in oracy are doubly disadvantaged. First, their communication is impoverished by poor speaking and/or listening skills. Secondly their reading and/or writing abilities are impoverished because their language base, developed through oracy, is impaired. Such children need to develop special strategies to overcome their linguistic handicap in order to make sense of their environment.

Both oracy and literacy are facilitated if children develop that awareness of language known as metalinguistic awareness. Some metalinguistic skill is needed before children can manipulate their language to complement their perception of its immediate meaning (Liles et al., 1977; Donaldson, 1978; Robinson and Robinson, 1983). To be able to do things with words and phrases, to separate and integrate the individual sounds of a word or phrase beyond their actual meaning, seems to be possible only after extensive familiarity with the literal meaning. Thus this level of linguistic operation, too, is reduced for children whose oracy and literacy skills are poor.

Communication Problems of Hearing-impaired Children

At first thought hearing-impaired children seem to experience problems in communication simply because their hearing loss either prevents them from hearing speech at all, or enables them only to hear speech which is attenuated and/or distorted. Thus hearing-impaired children have difficulties in acquiring communication skills because they cannot hear, or find it difficult to hear, the sounds of speech. The relationship of speech sounds to hearing level is shown in Figure 1.1 (after Ballantyne, 1977), from which it is clear that children with mild to moderate hearing losses will experience some difficulty in hearing speech, while children with severe or greater deafness cannot perceive speech without amplification. However, this is only part of the problem.

Hearing children use their hearing for speech to acquire language. They subsequently employ their developing language base not only to elaborate the forms of their own talking and listening skills, but also to develop skills in reading and writing. There is also interplay between perception, language and cognition, which is important for the appreciation of the meanings of words and phrases and for thinking about language (metalinguistics). Hearing children learn to fit their communicative style to the context (pragmatics) and to deliberate about the appropriateness of such style (metapragmatics), as well as learn about other communication skills which suit interactions between people.

Depending on the degree and type of hearing loss, hearing-impaired children clearly have impaired speech perception. However, the problem does not stop here. Impaired speech perception leads to problems with language acquisition and cognition, which become evident in their communication. Then they

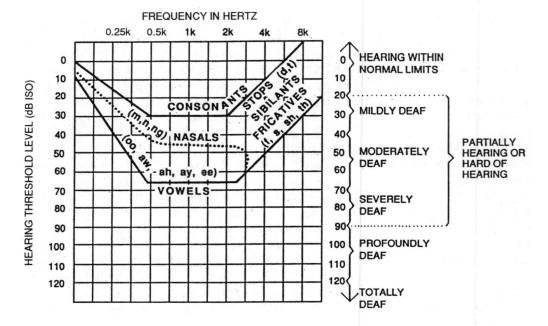

Figure 1.1 Pure-tone audiogram. (Source: Boole (1974), copyright *Perceptual and Motor Skills*, 1974.)

encounter difficulties in learning to read and write, since literacy skills depend on language and cognition. Their knowledge of affairs is reduced, also because of linguistic and cognitive factors. Such factors further deny them the normal range of the relevant metaskills. Again, hearing-impaired children come up against difficulties of a sociolinguistic kind. They have a lessened appreciation of the multi-faceted nature of communication in a variety of social settings. They also have difficulties in acquiring the usual pragmatic skills.

It would be wrong, however, to imply that there is a simple additive relationship between hearing loss and/or these other features. For instance, some children with a given hearing loss perform linguistically and cognitively very much better than others with the same loss, because of their experiences, or because they can compensate with their intelligence or other forms of communication (Liben, 1978). Hence, characterisation by hearing loss alone can be very misleading.

Subsequent chapters explore the diversity in accomplishments of hearing-impaired children, the extent to which they experience communication problems, and to what extent they make use of compensating forms of communication.

Chapter 2
Early Assessment and Intervention

It is generally believed that for verbal language to develop adequately, children must be exposed to speech in their first 2 years or so of life. Congenitally deaf children will lack this exposure unless their hearing impairment is identified early and suitable treatment and therapy are begun without delay. This chapter presents the background to this view and considers the evidence for the effects of early auditory and linguistic deprivation on later communication ability. It also considers the effectiveness of early auditory remediation programmes for hearing-impaired children.

Children need to develop a language and cognitive base if they are to progress with communication, and such developments begin from an early age in hearing children. Babies are responsive to sounds from birth, and even earlier (Bench and Mentz, 1975; Kisilevsky and Muir, 1991). They can discriminate between phonemes at 3 months of age (Eimas et al., 1971), though their frequency discrimination as shown by psychophysical tuning curves is not then fully mature for the higher audiofrequencies (Spetner and Olsho, 1990). They produce their first words from 9 to 12 months. Babies also interact with their mothers at a very early age in games of the 'peek-a-boo' kind (Schaffer, 1977), their first experiences of communication involving turn-taking. By 3;6 years of age children have acquired the essentials of grammar, with virtually all grammatical skills achieved by 4;6 years (Crystal et al., 1976).

Sensitive Periods

Early experiences of communication, especially via speech, are important for the development of language. They may even be crucial. The latter view stems from the critical-period hypothesis, developed from the animal work of ethologists by Lenneberg (1967) and others, and influenced by the psychoanalytic school (Freud, 1915). Lenneberg argued for a critical period for human language development, seeing language development as associated with the maturation of the brain. The development would occur from exposure to a language environment from the age of about 2 years up to puberty.

Lenneberg thought that, below 2 years of age, the brain is not sufficiently mature for a critical period to start. In early life, the brain is characterised by a 'plasticity' which allows it to receive a variety of language inputs. The brain is then undifferentiated for the locus and degree of specialisation of function. Thus, the argument goes, the plasticity of neuronal function is greatest at birth, and in the months immediately following. Thereafter the plasticity gradually decreases and ends at puberty. As the plasticity declines, there is increasing specialisation of brain function and increasing localisation within the central nervous system for processing environmental stimulation. Beyond puberty, the brain loses the plasticity which previously allowed a dynamic interaction between children and their verbal environments.

Children who are prelingually profoundly deaf, that is, deaf at birth or soon after, will not experience verbal environments over the language-critical years unless their hearing loss is improved by amplification or otherwise. Hence they will be linguistically impoverished for life, because to miss out on the relevant experiences during a critical period causes irreversible damage. That all children born profoundly or severely deaf do have major problems with verbal language acquisition is frequently cited as evidence for the critical-period hypothesis (Tervoort, 1965; Downs, 1976; Bochner, 1982; Fisch, 1983; Anastasiow, 1990). Similar arguments have been advanced about second language learning (Davies, 1991; Scovel, 1981) and the use of pidgin (Anderson, 1983a).

As noted, Lenneberg (1967) postulated critical years from the age of about 2 years up to puberty for language acquisition. However, we know that the inner-ear structures are well developed before birth and that the human fetus in the last trimester of gestation is exposed to relatively intense low-frequency sounds from the maternal vascular system and borborygmi (Bench, 1968; Walker et al., 1971; Henshall, 1972). The fetus is responsive to audiofrequency stimulation (Johansson et al., 1964; Grimwade et al., 1971; Bench and Mentz, 1975; Kisilevsky and Muir, 1991), and many studies attest to the responsivity of the neonate and older babies to sound stimuli (Kagan and Lewis, 1965; Downs, 1967; Eimas et al., 1971; Bench et al., 1976a, b, c). We may therefore ask if early auditory, if not language, input is needed if children are to avoid retardation in language.

A firm answer to this question is virtually impossible to achieve for human beings. A definitive study would require well-controlled auditory deprivation experiments, which are not possible, for obvious ethical and social reasons. Hence recourse has been made to work with animals and to careful observations, in a few cases, of 'natural experiments' in which children have been raised in severe social isolation, though these instances provide evidence for deprivation which is linguistic rather than auditory.

Deprivation in animals

The clearest evidence on the effects of auditory or other sensory deprivation comes from work with animals. There is not only definite evidence (Kyle, 1978,

1980a; Webster and Webster, 1979; Fisch, 1990) that sensory deprivation from birth over several stimulus modalities has significant effects on cortical and behavioural development, but animal studies of auditory deprivation have shown damage to cortical structures associated with later auditory behaviour. It is difficult, even with animals, to show the effects of complete auditory deprivation, because it is virtually impossible to reduce ambient noise below threshold. However, work by Batkin et al. (1970), in which rats were raised in a sound-reduced environment, showed that they experienced later behavioural problems when auditory stimulation was reinstated. Evidence is also available at the molecular level. Aoki and Siekevits (1985) studied the effects in the cat of cyclic adenosine monophosphate, which transmits signals received at the nerve-cell boundary to specific sites within the cell. They found that phosphorylation was different before and after early periods in brain development, related to the presence or absence of sensory stimuli, both visual and auditory. However, whether the central auditory connections are complete in animals at an early age is not known.

Although there is thus clear evidence that auditory deprivation affects neural structures and behaviour in animals, we have reservations about the immediate relevance of findings from creatures who do not have speech. Animal work may lead us to presume that auditory deprivation will have similar effects on people, but does not prove it.

Auditory deprivation in children

The effects of either complete auditory deprivation or reduced auditory stimulation on human infants are less certain than for infant animals. In any case it has been argued (Bench, 1979) that for human infants the issue is more one of linguistic than of auditory deprivation, and that this issue has been confused by ascribing to sensory deprivation what should more importantly be attributed to linguistic deprivation (compare Conrad, 1980). This view was indirectly supported by Mayberry and Eichen (1991) who found that the age at acquisition of sign language was significant for all levels of linguistic structure in 49 prelingually deaf signers who acquired sign at ages from birth to 13 years. Hence we should not be so much concerned with the intrinsic problem of reduced auditory experience for the hearing-impaired child, apart from those born without any usable hearing. We should rather concentrate on the extrinsic aspect of developing more adequate aural rehabilitation programmes in the preschool years for infants with residual hearing. However, the results of such programmes at present are not generally grounds for great optimism (Conrad, 1979; Northern and Downs, 1984; Bamford and Saunders, 1985), perhaps because of insufficient emphasis on the use of residual hearing in natural social interaction, namely, in everyday communication (Wells, 1981). While hearing children acquire language and communication by natural interactive dialogue, deaf children have to be taught (Gregory and Mogford, 1981).

Hearing infants produce babble, which begins to assume the inflections of the spoken language of the culture into which the child has been born from about 5–6 months of age (Tervoort, 1965; Weir, 1966). Infants aged 6 months can identify phonemes which are not found in their native language, but seem to lose this ability by 1 year of age (Werker and Tees, 1984). Thus we might suppose that a 'critical period' for some aspects of language development begins by at least 6 months of age, and that the experience of spoken language becomes increasingly important over the next few months. If so, this argument is at variance with Lenneberg's (1967) position that the language-critical period begins around 2 years of age. Nevertheless, it could help us to understand the achievements of Helen Keller, who became deaf and blind at the age of 2 years following an attack of meningitis, since she would have had considerable, though not full, experience of aspects of spoken language before becoming deaf.

There is no firm agreement as to which months or years constitute the critical period as far as hearing in children is concerned. Such lack of agreement is illustrated by comparing a 'crucial' period posited by Pollack (1967) over the first year of life, and a critical period over the first 2 years by Northern and Downs (1984) and Welsh et al. (1983). Griffiths (1988) argued for a critical age of hearing from birth to 8 months, during which hearing-impaired infants are presumed to be responsive to auditory therapy. Griffiths (1967) further specified a maturation period for learning to listen and talk over the first 3 years, without specifying crucial or critical periods, though she assumed that the relevant maturation was complete by 3 years. Mischook and Cole (1986) also argued for the importance of the first 3 years of life. Kyle (1980a) accepted that the critical period is not easy to define in terms of time intervals, and cited evidence from Witelson and Paillie (1973) and Krashen (1973) that lateralisation of language function may not be complete until 5 years of age. Bench (1970) preferred a hierarchy or system of periods which may overlap in time (compare Ruben, 1986; Wood et al., 1986; Hoemann, 1988), thinking that a singular critical period is not a very sophisticated idea. Such a hierarchy or system is in keeping with knowledge that the auditory pathways are functional before birth and their myelinisation takes place between about 7 months and 4 years of age (Lecours, 1975). The pathways thus mature slowly (Aslin, 1981), extending the critical period over several years, during which children normally acquire most of their phonology and grammar (Anastasiow, 1986) though some aspects of language, such as vocabulary, continue to grow well into the adult years.

Instances of Extreme Deprivation

The undoubted problems of prelingually deaf children in acquiring verbal language give face validity to some kind of critical period hypothesis. What, then, of the findings of the few available 'natural experiments', in which children have been raised in gross social and/or linguistic deprivation which has denied them exposure to verbal language in their early years? Does such denial impose a handicap which stops them catching up on language once they have been discovered and treatment begun?

The results are not clear-cut. Some well-documented cases which yield somewhat conflicting findings are outlined below. Fromkin et al. (1974) and Skuse

(1984a, b) have cited other instances of sensory or social isolation which are not considered here because they are less relevant or less well documented.

Isabelle

Mason (1942) and Davis (1947) studied the same case of a 6-year-old girl, 'Isabelle'. They reported independently on Isabelle, and their accounts were not discrepant. At discovery, aged 6;6 years, Isabelle had no speech as a result of extreme isolation. Many of her actions resembled those of deaf children. However, following intensive therapy, she rapidly progressed through all the usual stages to full development of speech and language. Isabelle had spent most of her time with her mother in a dark room shut off from the rest of the mother's family. The mother was a deaf-mute, could not talk, read or write, was blind in one eye from the age of 2 years, and communicated with her family and Isabelle by crude gestures. Hence Isabelle had no opportunity to develop speech. Isabelle's remedial programme seemed hopeless at first. It took one week of intensive effort before she made her first attempt to vocalise. However, once she had begun to respond, she passed through the usual stages of learning typical of the years from 1 to 6, in the proper order, and remarkably quickly. Just after 2 months from her first vocalisation, Isabelle could produce simple sentences. After a further 9 months she could identify words and sentences in print, could write well, and could count to ten. She could also retell a story after hearing it. She attained a normal educational level by 8;6 years of age. Thus in 2 years she achieved the educational development which usually took about 6, and appeared to have been unaffected by any critical period over her first 6 years as far as language and educational development were concerned.

Koluchova's twins study

Koluchova (1972, 1976) reported on twin boys raised from the age of 1.5 to 7 years in severe social isolation by a psychopathic stepmother and an inadequate father. The twins were kept in a closet and a cellar. They grew up in almost total isolation. They were subjected to physical abuse and extreme neglect. Following discovery at age 7 years, the twins could barely walk, reacted with surprise and horror to everyday events and objects, and were very shy with people. Their spontaneous speech was very poor and they communicated with each other by gestures characteristic of younger children. They tried to repeat the speech of adults, but could manage only two or three words at a time with poor articulation, and could not answer questions. Further, they could not understand the meaning or function of pictures.

With care first in a children's home and then placement with an accepting family, and with education in a preschool, their intellectual and speech abilities increased markedly. At 8;4 years their full scale WISC scores were 80 and 72, with verbal IQs slightly lower than performance IQs. By 11 years of age, the full scale scores were 95 and 93, with verbal IQs slightly higher than performance IQs. Thus the twins made very rapid progress over a period of almost 4 years, towards normal WISC scores. Koluchova also remarked on the twins' remarkable improvement in writing, drawing and ability to concentrate, but could not predict how their intelligence might develop or what the course of their further development might be.

Commenting on Koluchova's (1972) paper and reports by others, Clarke (1972) remarked on the inadequacy of theories which stressed the overriding importance of early experience in forming later characteristics. Although Koluchova's case of the twins showed that, for their first 18 months, they would probably have developed the bases for later perceptual and linguistic development, following discovery they showed a responsiveness to remediation which underscored a natural resilience, with an obvious bearing on hypotheses concerning critical periods in development. Clarke further remarked that the pessimism surrounding the area may itself have contributed to passive approaches to the treatment of deprived children.

Genie

Fromkin et al. (1974) reported the case of Genie, a girl who had been isolated from the age of about 1;8 to 13;9 years. She was confined in a small room, with the door kept closed and the window covered. Genie was hurriedly fed and minimally cared for by her mother, who was almost blind. There was no radio or television in the house, and any sound stimulation which she could have received behind the closed door was minimal, as her father was intolerant of noise of any kind. She was punished physically if she made any sounds. Apparently her father and older brother never spoke to her although they barked at her like dogs.

On discovery, Genie was mute and socially unresponsive. Four weeks later she showed adequate hearing, visual and emotional responses, and good eye–hand coordination. She also showed much stimulus hunger. She did not appear to be mentally retarded or autistic. Within a few days Genie began to respond to speech and to imitate single words. Eleven months after her emergence, when she was able to cooperate in comprehension testing, Genie could understand individual words which she could not speak herself, but otherwise had little, if any, understanding of grammatical structures. She had physical difficulties in speaking, ascribed to her earlier repression of all vocalisations. Over time, her linguistic development became in many ways parallel to that observed in normal children, but with some differences. For example, her vocabulary was large in relation to her level of syntactic development. Her cognitive growth rate exceeded that of her linguistic growth. Fromkin et al. considered that, while Genie's language acquisition at age 16 years differed from that of normal children, she was continuing to learn language, and therefore at least some degree of language acquisition appeared possible past the critical period.

Alice and Beth

Douglas and Sutton (1978) described the case of twin girls, Alice and Beth, who were cared for by a variety of people during their first year of life. Then their mother, who was separated from their father, took the twins back and lived with them in a house due for demolition. She suffered from social isolation and depression requiring medical help. The twins received very little stimulation. They walked at the usual time but at discovery, when nearly 5 years old and about to attend school, they could not talk intelligibly except in a limited private language to each other. They thus had very limited language, although they had a friendly outlook towards others. Following discovery, the twins attended an infants' school. At the age of 6;4 years their language comprehension was between 5;1 and 6;0 years, with language expression between 5;3 and 6;0 years. They also scored 108 and 92 points (performance) and 102 and 85 points (verbal) in IQ. Thus their language and intellectual performance was at, or not far below, normally expected levels only 17 months after discovery.

Louise and Mary

The final cases considered here are those of Louise and Mary (Skuse, 1984a,b). These sisters, whose father could not be traced, spent their early years in the UK. They lived in a very deprived environment as their mother was intellectually retarded (IQ 55), microcephalic, and possibly psychiatrically disturbed. Louise and Mary were discovered at ages 3;6 and 2;4 years respectively. They took no notice of anybody, except to scamper up to and sniff strangers, while making animal-like noises. Louise had normal very early experiences, but Mary was deprived from birth, as her mother became very withdrawn after Mary was born. Mary had no speech and no hearing reactions at discovery, but made a few high-pitched sounds. Louise had the language abilities of an infant aged about 1 year. At the age of 13 years, Mary had a language comprehension score of 4 years, and a language expression score of 3;5 years. Her performance IQ was 94 at age 8;11 years. Louise, at 10;1 years, had a performance IQ of 80 and a verbal IQ of 77. At 14;5 years, she had appropriate language for her age. Thus, Louise had attained relatively normal ability, but Mary was linguistically very retarded.

Interim summary of outcomes

All the children described above had very limited verbal language abilities at discovery, having received much reduced or no exposure to language, although, apart possibly from Mary, they would have received some auditory stimulation. Subsequently, and with treatment, their language and cognitive abilities improved remarkably. Only Genie and Mary remained retarded in speech at the time of the latest reports, but Genie was not discovered till around the age of puberty, and there was known severe intellectual retardation in Mary's family history. Clarke and Clarke (1976) commented that the evidence was clear that in an improved environment, from the middle to the late childhood years, the speech of severely deprived children showed major gains.

Of the cases described, apparently only Isabelle and Mary were deprived of language from birth. Mary remained severely linguistically retarded, which may have been associated with her family history of severe intellectual retardation, but

Isabelle acquired language very quickly. It is possible that Isabelle's limited gestural communication with her mother may have been of some help here. However, Isabelle's case shows that deprivation of spoken language from birth to 6;6 years did not prevent her from making remarkable gains in spoken language by the age of 8;6 years.

Further observations of Genie

Curtiss (1977) reported extensively on continued work with Genie, making Genie's case very well known. Sometimes, Genie's case has been the only case of its kind to be cited in reference to critical periods, with potentially misleading conclusions (see below). Curtiss showed that Genie's language development continued to improve, but was by no means fully developed. Her language production and comprehension continued to be abnormally disparate. She showed unpredictable variability in the use of grammar, stereotypic speech, gaps in acquisition of syntax, and a generally retarded rate of linguistic development. However, Curtiss expressed the hope that Genie might develop far beyond what was described in the 1977 report.

Curtiss observed that Genie's language performance was in some ways similar to that of righthemisphere language learners. For example, Genie showed word-order discrimination problems similar to those found in child left hemispherectomies. Dichotic listening and other tests also suggested that her language was right-hemisphere based. These results may indicate that, after a 'critical period' for language acquisition, the left hemisphere cannot further control language acquisition. The right hemisphere then assumes this function, for which it is less appropriately 'wired', although Curtiss did not present evidence confirming normal left hemisphere functioning in Genie (Skuse, 1984b). However, the extent to which the right-hemisphere can mediate language is controversial. Work suggesting that language cannot develop as well in the right as in the left hemisphere is suspect (Bishop, 1988), as is the view that the special function of the left hemisphere is uniquely associated with language (Kimura, 1990). While Genie's case disproves the critical period hypothesis in a 'strong' form, namely, that children cannot acquire verbal language after puberty, it may support a weaker version of the hypothesis, that verbal language acquisition cannot occur fully beyond puberty.

In comparing the above cases it is, however, clear that Genie's case is unlike those of the others. First, Genie's language acquisition occurred around the menarche and subsequent years, namely around and post puberty. There was only limited exposure to language in the first, more 'plastic', years which are of interest for the early detection and remediation of hearing loss. Secondly, Genie was physically and emotionally punished in attempts at communication, whereas for the other cases, attempts at communication were not so treated, or at least to nothing like the same extent. The effects of this treatment were observed by Curtiss to have retarded at least Genie's speech development. The family environment accompanying her early attempts at communication were the very opposite of the encouragement which is given to hearing-impaired children. Thirdly, Genie was malnourished, which may have affected her neurophysiological development. Although we have no hesitation in agreeing with Kyle (1980a) that Genie's case is the most comprehensively documented, we cannot also agree that it is the one which allows meaningful evaluation in the context of congenital, or early-acquired hearing impairment (compare Mayberry and Eichen, 1991). More relevant cases are those outlined above, other than Genie, where the children were less harshly treated and were discovered at a younger age. Skuse (1984b) concluded that, in the absence of genetic or congenital anomalies and gross malnourishment, children experiencing severe environmental deprivation have an excellent prognosis. Although aspects of language may be more at risk than other factors as a result of some critical period effect, these cases suggest rather convincingly that all is not lost for young deaf children, even if they do not receive speech until school age, provided that they obtain suitable remediation.

We conclude that early linguistic deprivation may, but will not always, have lasting deleterious effects on the development of communication in some situations (compare Rutter, 1981). The dimensions of any critical period are not sufficiently well known for us to be more definite (Ruben, 1986).

Sam – a deprived deaf child treated in early middle age

Wolff (1973) described the case of 'Sam', a deaf–mute aged 43 years, and therefore well past puberty. Sam was born with a severe to profound hearing loss. He spent a short period in a school for the deaf and resided in a hospital for the mentally subnormal from the age of 12. Non-verbal intelligence tests showed Sam to be of about normal intelligence. At the start of treatment, Sam could say his own name indistinctly and 'shut the door' very indistinctly. He had no other speech and no comprehension of speech through hearing or speechreading. He knew the written alphabet almost completely in capital letters. He could write lower case letters, presumably learned in the school for the deaf, but was less happy with these, because of poor eyesight. He knew about three-quarters of the Standard Manual Alphabet used in the UK. His sister had taught him to write a few simple words, but his vocabulary was minimal. He had no knowledge of sentence structure.

With gestural communication, Sam would seek the words for pictures of objects of his own accord. His concepts and conceptual groupings of common objects, in object matching tests, were similar to those of normal people, although he had no spoken or written language. After a few months' teaching, Sam rapidly learned new names of objects, reflecting the 'naming explosion' of normal children. He was also taught syntax and semantics. Although at the time of Wolff's report Sam's language ability was limited and not fully productive in the linguistic sense (Chomsky, 1971), it seemed possible that he would make further progress. Wolff concluded that if Sam's efforts were accepted as rudimentary language, then that part of the language critical period which postulates that language learning is not possible after childhood, was disproved. The universality of the critical period concept was likewise disproved.

Congenitally profoundly deaf children

Recent studies show that verbal language can be acquired by at least a minority of congenitally profoundly deaf children, possibly through lipreading and/or the tactile sense. For example, Conrad (1979) found that five children in a group of 218 school leavers with severe to profound hearing losses had normal reading ability for their age, and possessed inner speech. Wood et al. (1986) showed that competence in reading and writing is associated with abilities in receptive and expressive speech in profoundly deaf primary school children. Thus work at literacy facilitates the development of listening to and expressing speech. Geers and Moog (1987, 1989) have shown that more than a small proportion of congenitally profoundly deaf children can learn verbal language. Hence some profoundly deaf children escape many of the effects ascribed to missing out on the 'critical period', and others can improve their verbal communication skills when they have missed out. We will return to these studies later. Meanwhile we observe that the issues, of course, are whether the improvement is adequate to some criterion, and how, and how far, it can be developed.

Early and Late Assessment of Hearing Impairment

A focus on the sequelae of auditory deprivation takes emphasis away from the development of improved approaches to aural rehabilitation, especially for language learning (Bench, 1978, 1979). Such a position is supported by the work of Williams (1970) who observed, in a study of maladjusted deaf children which is a lesson to us all, that early assessment of hearing loss had harmful effects on the later acquisition of speech. Williams found that early assessment of deafness was associated with a lower incidence of speech than when the assessment was not made till age 2 years. He studied 51 children aged 5–14 (mean 10) years, with severe to profound mainly prelingual losses, and neurotic, developmental and kinetic problems. Williams set aside five children with late-acquired deafness, expecting to find for the remainder that the earlier the assessment, the higher would be the incidence of children with speech. But the opposite was found. This result seemed so improbable that the data were reviewed. Cases showing educational subnormality and psychosis were discounted, whereupon the failure of early assessment of deafness to increase the incidence of children with speech became even higher. Those children assessed as deaf before their second birthday achieved speech in 27% of cases. Those assessed after their second birthday achieved speech in 80% of cases. There was no evidence to indicate that early assessment of deafness was associated with the severity of hearing loss, psychiatric disorder or social class.

Williams offered three reasons for these results. First, his early-assessed group could have contained a high proportion of children with central speech and language disorders. However, there was no evidence to support this argument. Secondly, some of the early-assessed children may have been fitted with unsuitable hearing aids, but this seemed unlikely as most of the aids would have had similar gain and frequency responses. Thirdly, early assessment which was not followed by appropriate rehabilitation and counselling may have led to parental indecision, depriving the child of affection unfettered by anxiety. The figures suggested, stated Williams, that to rely on early assessment and the fitting of a hearing aid is not enough. Intensive counselling and guidance are needed for all hearing-impaired children and their families. Although not directly considered by Williams, other factors may be at work. Children's linguistic competence reflects the language communicated to them by more experienced language users (Bruner, 1983; Wells, 1984). If parents are informed early that their infant has a hearing problem, they may modify their speech and other forms of communication, making it more difficult for the infant to experience natural language.

Features of parent–infant interaction

Generally, adult speech addressed to young children is characterised by simplicity, consistency, redundancy and exaggerated prosody (Snow, 1972; Gleason, 1975; Nienhuys and Tikotin, 1985), a 'motherese' which facilitates the child's acquisition of language. There are similarities between the speech of mothers and fathers to infants in mean length of utterance (MLU), though mothers use a simpler vocabulary and speak more than do fathers (Golinkoff and Ames, 1979), and mothers interrupt conversations more than children (Bedrosian et al., 1988). The child's abilities also influence adults' speech (Cross, 1977; Cross and Morris, 1980).

Similar findings have been found for hearing-impaired infants and their hearing parents, even though the poor intelligibility of the infants' speech and their reliance on idiosyncratic non-verbal cues makes parent–infant communication difficult (Kenworthy, 1986). Thus Tucker et al. (1983) reported similarities between mothers' and fathers' speech with 10 preschool children aged 1–4 years, who had severe or greater hearing losses, with fathers talking less, and using shorter and more variable MLUs, often employing single words to gain the children's attention. Blennerhassett (1984) described the communicative styles of a 13-month-old hearing-impaired infant, with a sloping mild to profound hearing loss, finding that both parents approached their child as a conversational partner and engaged in turn-taking exchanges. Both parents were seen as sensitive to feedback from the infant. Both adjusted their MLUs. The mother was more sensitive than the father in responding to the infant's topic shifts. Differences between the infant's style with her father and mother suggested that, even at 13 months of age, she adjusted to different communication situations, such as the more challenging demands of her father. Matey and Kretschmer (1985) compared mothers' speech to Down's syndrome, hearing-impaired and hearing children. In each of these three groups, children were studied at ages 18 months and 3 years. Mothers modified their speech to both Down's syndrome and hearing-impaired children, based on the perceived language level of the child. The 18-month-old Down's syndrome and hearing-impaired children received more direct imperatives than the hearing age-matched children. The 18-month and three-year-old hearing-impaired children were offered shorter MLUs, and the 3-year-old hearing-impaired children also received fewer questions. Similar results were reported for communication addressed to a hearing and a hearing-impaired child by Seewald and Brackett (1984). Likewise, Lartz and McCollum (1990) reported that a mother of 3-year-old twins addressed twice as many questions to the hearing as to the deaf twin.

Nevertheless, parental adaptations to interactions with their hearing-impaired infants may not necessarily be appropriate. Reduced syntactic and cognitive complexity of utterances, reduced use of expansions, more imperatives and different turn-taking aspects have been found in mothers' speech to hearing-impaired infants (Nienhuys et al., 1984, 1985). A pattern of reduced complexity and reduced variability in mothers' speech indicates that this speech may not be properly adaptive and could impede the infants' development of communication skills (Pratt, 1988; Power et al., 1990). Interestingly, women without experience of deaf people also tend to take a leading role in initiating interactions with unfamiliar deaf children (Lederberg, 1984).

Nienhuys and Tikotin (1985) further investigated the relative roles of vocalisation, hearing and gaze in maintaining mother–baby communication and the effects of babies' deafness on mother–infant interaction with infants aged 39–44 weeks. They concluded that hearing-impaired babies were less likely to be active in meaningful social and play interactions with their mothers than hearing babies. The hearing-impaired babies attended to their mothers or to objects, rather than playing with them. They did not engage in rhythmic periods of social involvement and play with their mothers, even though the mothers provided the opportunities. In similar vein, Spencer and Gutfreund (1990) suggested that mothers of hearing-impaired infants are as responsive in 'dialogues' with their infants as mothers of hearing infants, but since hearing-impaired infants produce less topic-initiating behaviour, their mothers come to dominate the interactions. We should, however, note that although hearing impairment will affect the nature of communication between infant and parents, it need not affect the quality of social attachment (Lederberg and Mobley, 1990).

In conclusion, we have seen that parents adjust their communicative style towards the linguistic and intellectual development of their hearing-impaired and hearing children. There is a nice, but important, distinction to be drawn between adjusting parental speech appropriately to suit the abilities of the child and reduction of speech because of pessimism or otherwise ('Why should I talk so much to my child if he can't hear properly?'). Unfortunately, published reports seldom allow the reader to appreciate this distinction. Although parents may be sensitive to the linguistic levels of their hearing-impaired child, only careful monitoring will show whether this sensitivity is appropriate, or results in non-optimal opportunities for the child to develop linguistically and cognitively. The astute therapist will monitor the mother–infant dyad carefully, and check that the parent is providing appropriate opportunities for the child.

Given these caveats, it is generally agreed that the earlier hearing loss is identified and therapy begun, the better for the development of communication. The effects of early intervention programmes on communication by hearing-impaired children are thus of particular interest (see below).

Some further technical considerations

It is increasingly possible to identify a large proportion of hearing-impaired babies within their first weeks or up to 1 year of age, and to fit them with hearing aids.

The introduction of behavioural hearing screening tests, as conducted by health visitors in the UK, maternal and child nurses in Australia, and public health nurses in Malaysia, for example, has led to the identification of many, though not all, instances of hearing impairment around 8 months of age. Recent technical developments, such as evoked auditory brain-stem responses (Stockard and Curran, 1990; Gorga and Thornton, 1990) and oto-acoustic emissions (Kemp et al., 1986) are used most cost-effectively in neonatal intensive care units in paediatric hospitals, where the numbers of babies with hearing impairment may be up to ten times the figure in the general population (McCormick et al., 1984).

Where a hearing-impaired baby is identified early and fitted with a hearing aid there are a number of practical problems to be overcome in following a successful communication programme. Parents are usually eager to learn how hearing aids will help their infant (Rushmer and Schuyler, 1984), but should be advised that the infant will probably not behave like a hearing child when the aids are first fitted. Parents also need advice and practice in the operation and maintenance of the aids and earmoulds. Where an infant spends much time lying down, it is often difficult to keep a behind-the-ear aid in place. A body-worn aid in a harness may be more suitable, though this can cause problems of noise from clothes-rub. Earmoulds can drop out of the ears of small children, in which case the mould and aid may be taped to the pinna or mastoid process. Some infants may pull on or pick at the aid or cord. Downs (1966) has outlined a familiarisation programme for such cases, which gradually increases the time in which the aid is in situ. Otherwise (Ross, 1975) it is probably best to fit the aid and mould, and leave them on.

Other technical issues complicate this situation further. Although parents may try to communicate normally with an infant assessed early as hearing-impaired and fitted with hearing aids, there will still be difficulties with speech and language acquisition. Speech perception via hearing aids may not reach the loudness which hearing children experience. Hearing aids introduce distortion to the speech signal, and amplify the background noise as much as the speech. Also, sensorineural hearing loss often involves poor frequency resolution (Wightman, 1981; Turner and Nelson, 1982). Thus the impaired ear causes distorted as well as attenuated hearing. Hearing aids and speechreading do not sufficiently redress the most severe and profound hearing losses (Erber, 1983).

Early intervention for the development of communication

Early intervention concerns the management of a hearing-handicapped child before the primary school years, and especially before 2 years of age. Late intervention generally refers to intervention after spoken language is normally acquired – say, after 3–4 years of age.

Although it is generally thought that early intervention programmes for the development of communication in hearing-impaired children are well-nigh essential (Northern and Downs, 1984; Riko et al., 1985), and although the advent of cochlear implants for young children has increased interest in early intervention, well-designed studies in the area are the exception. There are many descriptive comments and papers from teachers and therapists, but most papers have been concerned with an empirical rather than experimental approach to intervention, from which it is difficult to identify cause and effect. There is a dearth of quantitative studies, of specific hypotheses and of identifiable criteria by which to select children for, and to estimate the effects of, the intervention. Controls are often lacking, even same-subject controls. However, it would be hasty to discount this material. Although most of the evidence for early intervention is weak, this does not necessarily mean that early intervention does not work (see below).

As a result of such design flaws, the methods of therapy adopted in early intervention programmes are the subject of continuing debate. Liden and Kankkunen (1973) suggested that the decision as to what kind of educational or therapeutic method should be used in intervention would be helped by considering the difference between aided and unaided pure-tone thresholds. A large difference between these thresholds across the frequencies used in speech-hearing implies good candidacy for an aural–oral approach, namely the use of hearing and speechreading. Most children with moderate to severe hearing losses would be so suited. A large difference between aided and unaided thresholds at frequencies up to 1 kHz, and little or no difference thereafter, also implies candidacy for an aural–oral approach, as there is usable residual hearing. However, language development is likely to be slower and the eventual outcome questionable. Little or no difference between aided and unaided thresholds, with apparent hearing for low-frequency sounds ascribed to responses to vibrotactile sensation, implies candidacy for a manual approach from the beginning. Although Liden and Kankunnen's approach is relatively objective, it assumes a strong correlation between aidable, usable residual hearing, hearing for speech, and language development. However, the correspondence may not be very strong (Erber, 1974; Bamford et al., 1981). Further, Liden and Kankunnen's approach does not take into account motivational, cognitive and parental support variables. It emphasises the audiological status, rather than the 'educability' of the child.

Downs (1974) included both audiological and non-audiological factors in the Deafness Management Quotient (DMQ). This is a 100-point scale based on five items:

1. residual hearing (30 points);
2. central intactness – brain damage, perceptual dysfunction, intact central processing, etc. (30 points);
3. intellectual factors (20 points);
4. family constellation – support/no support (10 points);
5. socioeconomic status (10 points).

This scale was validated by post hoc data on young adults, showing that a DMQ of 81 or more was needed for success in aural–oral education.

The DMQ goes a long way towards meeting the criticisms of Liden and Kankunnen (1973) outlined above. Whereas Liden and Kankunnen weighted audiological factors at 100%, Downs weighted them only up to 30%. However, the DMQ is more difficult to apply to infants and young children than Liden and

Kankunnen's approach, because some factors such as intellectual level are hard to assess in infancy, and because the family constellation may change over time. Further, some DMQ factors need subjective judgement, which may be difficult to make. For example, estimates of family constellation would require considerable experience with the family to gauge familial support.

In a similar approach to that of Downs, Geers and Moog (1987) restated the need for objective data on which to base recommendations for oral communication, manual communication, or some combination of these two. They sought objectivity both at the initial placement stage and after the child had been enrolled in an educational programme. Geers and Moog developed the Spoken Language Predictor (SLP) Index in an attempt to overcome the perceived problems of the DMQ by: choosing factors which better predicted a hearing-impaired child's potential for spoken language acquisition; specifying more precisely the methods for assigning weights to the factors; and providing a category for those children for whom intensive instruction and periodic re-evaluations were needed. Five factors were chosen as affecting a child's success with oral teaching, and which could be estimated reliably in clinical evaluations from 3 years of age. Points were allotted to each factor by clinical judgement and a trial application to actual cases:

1. hearing capacity, 30 points;
2. language competence, 25 points;
3. non-verbal intelligence, 20 points;
4. family support, 15 points;
5. speech communication attitude, 10 points.

Total scores of 80–100 suggested a speech emphasis; 60–75 a provisional speech emphasis; and 0–55, a manual emphasis. The SLP procedures were validated concurrently against three teachers' estimates of oral language skills on a three-point (poor/fair/good) spoken language ability rating scale. All children ($n = 66$) aged 11–15 years enrolled in the Central Institute for the Deaf (CID) were assigned points from data and descriptive comments in the children's files, yielding a contingency coefficient of 0.71, and suggesting good validity. The SLP procedure was also validated retrospectively on 51 CID children aged 11–16 years, with complete information in their files before 6 years of age, again with a contingency coefficient of 0.71. A third study compared the reliabilities of the SLP over time on 51 children for preschool data and information obtained from 11 years of age, yielding a contingency coefficient of 0.74. Given that language competence may vary with different kinds of educational intervention, and that the estimate of family support seems rather subjective, as does that for speech communication attitude, the results are fairly impressive. However, even given the respectable contingency coefficients, a large amount of variation in spoken language was not 'explained' by the selected variables. As Geers and Moog accepted, more research is needed. Further, since it was designed for use with children aged 3 years or more, the SLP is of value only for children who will already have progressed some way in their cognitive and linguistic development.

As we have seen, there are moderate correlations between pure-tone thresholds and hearing for speech (Erber, 1974; Bamford et al., 1981), and it is possible to estimate pure-tone thresholds with fair to good accuracy in young children and infants with modern electro-acoustic methods. Therefore infants and young children with average pure-tone thresholds lower than, say, 85 dB HTL (hearing threshold level) may be fitted with hearing aids and instructed with aural–oral methods to begin with, and until other, non-audiological information becomes available to complement the measures of their hearing. The acoustic information in speech signals should be useful to most such children, and they should, for example, be able to use manner, nasal and place information from perceived speech (Davis and Hardick, 1981). If they can discriminate phonemes successfully, they may not require later manual supplements. Infants and young children with hearing losses of greater than about 85 dB, who will have difficulty in perceiving manner and place information, should probably be treated to both speech and sign simultaneously (Wolff, 1973; Conrad, 1980; Davis and Hardick, 1981) until it is clear if they will continue to require a combined method of communication, or if they will develop communication best with either speech or sign alone (see Chapter 9).

Early versus Late Intervention

Increasingly, early intervention programmes have emphasised a role for home-based treatment, and the involvement of parents (Schaefer, 1976; Meisels and Shonkoff, 1990). Training centres may model themselves on a home environment and encourage the involvement of parents in the child's training, not only as primary care-givers, but also as those with a primary responsibility for training, with the centre offering advice.

Design problems

Notwithstanding such precepts, it is difficult to establish unambiguous and easily defensible prescriptions for early intervention to develop communication skills for hearing-impaired children (Kretschmer and Kretschmer, 1978; Simeonsson et al., 1982; Greenberg and Calderon, 1984; Greenberg et al., 1984). On examining published work, the type of hearing loss has often been ambiguous. Although the severity of the hearing impairment and ensuing difficulties with spoken language and cognitive development are likely to have major influences on the effectiveness of early intervention, they have seldom been well described. Some important areas, such as cognition, may not have been considered at all. Most hearing-impaired children enrolled in early intervention programmes will be fitted with a hearing aid, but different aids are fitted to different children. Even if they were all fitted with similar aids, the child–aid interactions would be different. Therapist–child or teacher–child interactions are equally problematical. Ethical issues complicate the situation, because each child needs to receive treatment and such considerations make it difficult to design thoroughgoing research studies which withhold treatment from a control group. Prospective designs are difficult to implement as 'blind' studies. As Guralnick and Bennett (1987a) remarked, it is easy to reject much of the existing early intervention research outright and select data to fit one's own biases, or make unreliable generalisations through an uncritical acceptance of findings.

Although design problems bedevil research in early intervention, the area is too important to be ignored. Therefore, while maintaining a critical attitude, we now consider the effectiveness of early intervention with hearing-impaired children. Such intervention can only involve oral, aural or gestural aspects, or combinations thereof. The children are too young to read or write.

Selected studies

Meadow-Orlans (1987) did a major service in presenting a review of eight reports which compared early with late intervention – all that could be located at the time. These reports on early versus late intervention are now considered, with some additional data.

Craig (1964) described a programme in which 151 residential and day-school hearing-impaired children, with hearing losses of 60 dB or more, the experimental group, received oral preschool training between 2;10 and 4;6 years of age. The programme consisted of individual tutorials and group activities in two residential schools for the deaf. The parental role was not reported, but appears to have been minimal or nil. The experimental group was compared with a control group, which had no preschool training, of 92 hearing-impaired children who enrolled in the two schools between 5 and 7 years of age. Testing was completed between the ages of 6;8 and 16;6 years via speechreading and reading tests. Retrospective data analysis found no significant differences between the scores of the children with and without preschool training.

Early amplification and intensive treatment were emphasised by Horton and others (Horton, 1975, 1976). They compared the performance of an early intervention group of six children assessed as hearing-impaired (median loss 87 dB) and fitted with a hearing aid before 3 years of age (median age 2;3 years) with a late intervention group of five hearing-impaired children (median loss 84 dB) assessed and fitted after 3 years (median age 4;0 years). The parents of the early, but not the late, intervention group were involved in the treatment. A third group consisted of six hearing children, judged by teachers to be average achievers in the same second-grade classes as those of the early intervention group. The intervention consisted of visits to a demonstration home, working with the teacher, and weekly checks of hearing aids. Practice at home with parents was encouraged to develop the use of language in familiar, everyday situations. Children in all three groups were assessed in the second grade with Lee's (1966) Developmental Sentence Types, when the linguistic competence of the early intervention group was found to be similar to that of the hearing group. Statistically significant differences arose only in comparisons of the late intervention group with either the hearing or early intervention groups. The results thus suggested that early intervention with parental involvement allowed the early intervention group to express themselves in spoken language at a level comparable to that of the hearing children. The same suggestion would not apply for the late intervention group. However, the late intervention children were enrolled in a class for hearing-impaired children, rather than in regular classes, because their language was inadequate. This difference in class of enrolment was a confounding factor, leaving the interpretation of the results open to question. The testing was post-intervention only, with no allowance for uneven abilities of the children allocated to the two hearing-impaired groups.

An evaluation of early and late intervention with hearing-impaired infants in a strongly oral programme with an emphasis on parental support was reported by Greenstein et al. (1975). The mean ages at first enrolment for two groups of children who had hearing parents was 13 months ($n = 9$) and 21 months ($n = 10$). The mean enrolment age for another group with deaf parents ($n = 11$) was 7 months. The mean hearing losses for all groups were comparable (96–105 dB unaided; 42–54 dB aided). The intervention consisted of 90-minute weekly sessions with a teacher in an auditory training programme, plus weekly workshops for parent groups in which parents were instructed in the cognitive, linguistic and affective development of infants and young children, until the infants were aged 40 months. Assessments were made of language performance, mother–child interactions via videotape, and teacher ratings of communication skills by repeated comparisons of performance. The early-admitted children, whether of hearing or deaf parents, scored significantly higher on language performance at 24, 36 and 40 months of age, than the late-admitted group. In the early-admitted group the infants looked at, vocalised to, and moved to the mother more than the late-admitted infants. Also, teachers gave the mothers of early-admitted infants significantly higher communication ratings than the mothers of late-admitted infants. There were no significant differences between infants with hearing and deaf parents in the early-admitted groups. These results seem rather impressive. However, the infants were not randomly assigned to different groups and the hearing/deaf parents variable for the early-admission groups was confounded with admission age.

A retrospective analysis of reading and other academic achievements, from data in school files over 16 years from 1956 to 1971, was described by Balow and Brill (1975) for graduates of a residential school for the deaf. The intervention was oral-only preschool treatment with parental involvement. The children were considered in four groups: Group 1 ($n = 36$) attended a 6 week summer preschool with their parents at the John Tracy Clinic; Group 2 ($n = 15$) had attended preschool programmes at the clinic for 1 or 2 years; Group 3 ($n = 21$) had attended such programmes for 3 or 4 years; and Group 4 ($n = 240$) had access to the clinic programme via a parental correspondence course. With controls for IQ, Group 3 (3–4 years of clinic preschool programme) achieved the highest Stanford Achievement Test (SAT) battery scores (Gentile and Di Francesca, 1969) at high-school graduation. All groups achieved higher scores than students who had no contact with the clinic preschool programme. This study is of interest, but there were problems with the allocation of children to groups, which was non-random. Further, the extent of contact with the clinic preschool programme may have been affected by unknown but relevant variables.

In a comparison of North American programmes, Brasel and Quigley (1977) retrospectively reviewed several oral-only preschool interventions for children with hearing parents and manual interventions for children with deaf parents. The children with hearing parents were split into two groups: those who had experienced intensive oral training begun before 2 years of age; and those who experienced less intensive oral training begun between 2 and 4 years. The children with hearing-impaired parents were separated into those whose parents routinely used American Sign Language and those who used Manual English. Each group contained 18 children with a mean age of 14;8 years, mean performance IQ ≥ 90, and mean hearing loss > 90 dB. Deafness was confirmed before 1;3 years. The socioeconomic status was higher for the intensive early oral intervention than for the other groups. Parents were involved with the intensive early oral intervention group, and minimally involved for the less intensive oral intervention group. The involvement of the parents who were deaf was not stated. All children were tested with the SAT battery and the Test of Syntactic Ability (Quigley and Power, 1971). Those children who began intensive training before the age of 2 years attained higher levels of achievement than the children who partook of less intensive training begun between 2 and 4 years of age, with the latter scoring lowest of all four groups. The children whose parents used Manual English obtained the highest score of all groups, significantly so for the four language subtests of the SAT, with the children whose parents used American Sign Language scoring higher than the early intensive oral group. However, for the orally trained groups, although the group which began training before 2 years obtained higher scores than the group which began training between 2 and 4 years of age, the results were confounded by intensity of training, differences in parental involvement, and differences in parental socioeconomic status, besides the non-random allocation of children to groups because of the retrospectivity of the design.

Berg (1975, 1976a) and Watkins (1984) described the early intervention Ski-Hi programme developed between 1972 and 1975. The main features of this programme included baseline and periodic measures of hearing obtained until thresholds were established; two hearing aids often fitted soon after an estimate of the hearing loss was made; parents oriented to and provided with group counselling and instruction in adjustment to hearing loss in their child, and aspects of parent–home intervention; preparation of parents by home managers who were specialists in communication disorders and listening and language programming; and individual evaluation for each child regarding demographic information, significant dates, audiometric data, speech input, hearing aid data, and longitudinal data on measures of child and parental progress. Parents were given the options of oral-only or total communication training. Watkins compared four groups of children (each of $n = 23$) with comparable severe to profound hearing losses: a group experiencing home-based intervention before age 2;6 years; a group experiencing the same intervention after age 2;6 years; a group receiving centre-based (not Ski-Hi) rather than home-based training after 2;6 years of age; and a group with no training before enrolling in kindergarten at 5 years of age. The socioeconomic status of parents in the last group was lower than that of the parents for the other three groups. At testing, in the age range of 105–133 months, with Carrow's (1974) Elicited Language Inventory, the Peabody Picture Vocabulary Test

(Dunn, 1965), Lee's (1966) Developmental Sentence Types, and other tests, there were few differences between the early and late home intervention groups, or between the group with centre-based training and the group with no intervention before 5 years of age. However, the home intervention groups combined obtained a higher level of proficiency in 22 of the 24 test comparisons than the other two groups combined. The design weaknesses of this study were that the testing was post-testing only, and the children were not allocated to groups at random.

An oral-only intervention programme was reported by White and White (1987), which provided for strong parental involvement with spoken language training as the main emphasis. Teachers gave weekly 90-minute sessions of auditory training, and parent workshops were provided. Forty-six infants, with severe to profound hearing losses, were studied in four groups: group 1 ($n = 5$) had deaf parents and began the programme before 18 months of age; group 2 ($n = 4$) also had deaf parents and entered the programme after age 18 months; group 3 ($n = 9$) with hearing parents enrolled before age 18 months; and group 4 with hearing parents enrolled after 18 months of age. On testing by post-test, the hearing-impaired infants of deaf parents attained faster language development, on parts of speech and combinations of words and sounds, than the hearing-impaired infants of hearing parents, but not on all measures of a Revised Receptive and Expressive Emergent Language Test (Bzoch and League, 1971). However, infants with hearing parents scored higher than those with deaf parents for babble and jargon. Infants of hearing parents who enrolled before age 18 months scored higher than infants of hearing parents who enrolled after 18 months on 9 out of 10 comparisons, with no difference for one comparison. This finding was reversed for the infants of deaf parents. Here the early-enrolling group performed less well than the group which entered later. The design of this study, like some others above, allocated the infants to groups non-randomly, and the evaluation was done by post-testing. Also, the numbers of infants in the groups were small, especially for infants of deaf parents. It is therefore difficult to explain the differences between the groups.

In a comprehensive and well-conducted study of its kind, Levitt et al. (1987) identified all hearing-impaired children who were enrolled in US state special education schools or programmes, probably oral-only, in 1972, and who had been born in 1962. These children were tested in four successive years when the children were 10–14 years of age. Besides hearing impairment, data were collected on other variables, including hearing-aid use, IQ and socioeconomic status. The children were assessed with the Test of Syntactic Abilities (Quigley et al., 1978) and otherwise to obtain data for spoken and written expression, reading, speech perception, and speech intelligibility. Levitt et al. found that the age at which hearing aids were fitted was correlated with the age at which special education began. In turn, this age was correlated with high reading scores and high speech and language skills, when early intervention was begun at 3 years or younger. The correlation between early intervention and later speech and language development was particularly high in the oldest group of children, suggesting that early gains were maintained throughout the child's life. This investigation involved the use of sophisticated statistical techniques to unravel some important factors. It benefited, too, from repeated longitudinal testing, which was, however, post-test.

Conclusion

We are happy to conclude with Meadow-Orlans (1987) that, despite the problems of design and sometimes conflicting results, the balance of the evidence from these studies supported the case that early intervention increased the later achievements of hearing-impaired children, especially those achievements concerned with speech and language development. However, given some contradictory results, the situation was not clear, which could argue that any critical period effects were weak. In considering the above studies, and five others in which methods of early intervention were compared, Meadow-Orlans also concluded that early intervention programmes were likely to be successful if they had a strong emphasis on parent counselling, and access to experienced staff including audiologists to check and maintain hearing-aid performance. Although the evidence to support the distinction could be stronger, our own impression is that parental attitudes, and parental support and counselling, are probably more important for the success of early intervention than other differences in approach (compare Moores, 1989).

Our most important general conclusion concerns the plethora of poorly designed empirical work, not reviewed here, as compared with the scarcity of better designed studies which we have considered. Despite the practical and ethical difficulties, it is truly surprising that more of the better work has not been done in view of the great interest in, and the undoubted significance of, the area.

A further note

Very recently, Rittenhouse et al. (1990) presented the framework of an ongoing longitudinal study enquiring into the costs and benefits of early intervention for severely hearing-impaired infants. The programme includes a comparison of age at start of intervention, with one group of infants started before age 9 months and a second group started at age 18 months. Other important aspects are comparisons of different amounts of intervention, and a comparison of signed communication and oral approaches. Preliminary findings are available for the latter comparison only, for which no statistically significant differences were obtained across the several psychological domains assessed. The full results of this study, and especially for the effects of age at start of intervention, are awaited with interest. Meantime, and despite the authors' concern for reliable and valid work, we note that in starting the 18-month-old intervention group before the children were 3 years old (apparently because of a legal requirement) this study partly begs the question of early versus late intervention.

Chapter 3
The Speech Reception of Hearing-impaired Children

Speech reception involves both hearing and vision, requiring a discussion of both auditory speech reception and speechreading (lipreading). This chapter introduces the aural/oral area and discusses some important features of work with hearing aids, cochlear implants, and vibrotactile and electrotactile aids. There follows an account of speech perception by hearing-impaired children, with remarks on clinical applications. Finally, an outline is given of the processes involved in speechreading, and the extent to which it may be trained.

Although they use mainly their hearing to receive speech, communication by hearing children usually involves speech reception both by hearing and by vision – by hearing the talker's voice, and seeing the talker's lip movements, facial expressions and gestures. Speech reception is thus aural and oral. The oral features of speech are particularly helpful when listening to speech in a noisy background (Miller, 1947; Hawkins and Stevens, 1950; Festen and Plomp, 1990). For hearing-impaired children who communicate via residual hearing and speechreading (lipreading), the oral features are increasingly helpful as severity of hearing loss increases. For the greater hearing losses, the communication method is known simply as oral communication, or oralism, since stress is laid on the speechreading component. Reliance on speechreading alone is known as pure oralism. Thus oralism has no concern with manual communication. It disregards gesture, sign language and the like.

The hearing-impaired children who are expected to succeed best with the oral approach are those who have a significant degree of residual hearing, are fitted early with hearing aids, and are given early and ongoing training in speechreading and aural rehabilitation (Paterson, 1986; ASHA, 1990; Osberger, 1990; Smith and Richards, 1990).

Children with profound to total hearing loss who do not so succeed are sometimes referred to as 'oral failures'. Recent developments in cochlear implants and tactile devices offer to make speech perception more accessible to such children, and present a new impetus for the oral approach. We begin our review of speech reception in hearing-impaired children by briefly describing the use of hearing aids, cochlear implants and tactile instruments.

Hearing Aids, Cochlear Implants and Tactile Aids

There are few hearing-impaired children who are so deaf that they cannot receive some help from conventional hearing aids. However, they need training if they are to use the hearing aids to best effect. Even with training the benefit may amount to little more than perception of the suprasegmental stresses and rhythms of speech for children with profound losses. Further, there is a small proportion of profoundly to totally deaf children, whose deafness is such that they achieve little or no help from a hearing aid. Until recently these children would have relied on speechreading alone, or on manual communication, or on a combination of the two.

Conventional hearing aids

Electric amplifying hearing aids became available in the early 1900s. They soon stimulated work in aural/oral communication for children with usable residual hearing (Lou, 1988). The rationale is that, as soon as a significant hearing loss is determined, a child should have speech made accessible by a suitable hearing aid, with encouragement to use speechreading, thus increasing exposure to verbal language.

Technical progress with hearing aids progressed steadily. Electronic hearing aids were developed in the 1930s and 1940s, which saw the introduction of the first wearable hearing aids. Transistors permitted the miniaturisation of aids and the reduction of battery size in the 1950s. There followed further developments in solid-state electronics and the introduction of the microprocessor to develop signal processing aids, which shape the incoming signal to facilitate perception of speech. Microphones have been miniaturised and made directional. Amplification (gain) is now available up to 60–80 dB. Hearing aids have also developed cosmetically. Miniature hearing aids are now commonly fitted behind the ear or in the ear itself, and are made of inconspicuous flesh-tinted plastics. Yet the most sophisticated modern hearing aids, even those containing peak clipping, automatic gain control and/or noise-suppression circuits are only moderately successful in restoring hearing to normal, except for uncomplicated cases of conductive hearing loss. Hearing aids do not restore normal hearing as spectacles restore impaired vision to normal, not even the latest FM radio, speech coding, or digital noise suppressing hearing aids (Byrne and Walker, 1982; Flexer and Wood, 1984; Harris et al., 1988; Montgomery and Edge, 1988; McAlister, 1990; Thibodeau, 1990). The reasons are several. First, competing background noise intrudes on the speech signal (Chazan et al., 1987; McAlister, 1990). Secondly, the speech source will alter from one instant to another in distance or orientation from the hearing-aid wearer and hence is variously affected by background noise. Thirdly, most hearing aids are basically amplifying devices that weakly address the poor frequency resolution often found in inner-ear hearing loss (Turner et al., 1987). The best way to deal with background noise is to remove it at source. Unfortunately, however, in schools and other places where learning occurs few steps are taken to reduce background noise. As regards the third point, probably the most promising approach will be to undertake more detailed research into the characteristics of impaired hearing rather than to continue with the present technology-driven thrust in the design of hearing aids.

Selection of a hearing aid is a relatively complex procedure nowadays, but it was not always so. Just after World World II, prescriptive approaches were recommended by Davis et al. (1947) in the USA and the Committee on Electroacoustics, Medical Research Council (1947) in the UK. These approaches, developed independently in each country, recommended that the frequency response of hearing aids should be flat or increasing with audiofrequency, and that one frequency response would suit most hearing-impaired people. This resulted in a limited range of off-the-shelf hearing aids. It was criticised by Robbins and Gauger (1982) because many subjects in both studies had flat conductive losses. This criticism is fair, but hearing aids with frequency responses increasing with frequency, as most do, emphasise the middle to higher frequencies, notwithstanding that the ear-mould reduces the 2–4 kHz gain from the resonance of the open ear canal (Guelke, 1985). Such middle to high frequencies are important for understanding speech because salient speech information is carried by those same frequencies.

More recently, hearing aids have been selected to suit the individual's communication needs, as determined by psychoacoustic measurements. One commonly used method for sensorineurally impaired listeners (Byrne and Tonisson, 1976; Byrne and Cotton, 1988) involves selection of the in-the-ear frequency response of an aid such that the patient will hear all speech frequencies equally loudly, and with control of maximum power output. Preferred listening levels for aided speech occur typically between 1/3 and 2/3 of the interval between the hearing threshold and the level at which the speech is uncomfortably loud (Byrne and Cotton, 1987). This finding shows that it is better to amplify speech to comfortable listening levels, rather than seeking to restore hearing thresholds to normal. Ross (1975) has described a similar approach for preverbal children.

A child with measurable auditory responses up to about 500 Hz may be aided to perceive the first formant frequencies of most vowels, voicing and nasality cues, and the transitions of front plosive consonants, besides suprasegmental features. Auditory responses up to 1 kHz further allow access to the first formant frequencies of mid-vowels, the second formants of back and mid-vowels and the second formants of several voiced consonants (Stone and Adam, 1986). Hence, provided that they also get suitable guidance and instruction, even children with 'corner' or 'ski-slope' audiograms can use hearing aids to assist speech perception.

Despite such developments, there are often doubts that children are appropriately fitted with hearing aids (Matkin, 1981; Flexer and Wood, 1984; Diefendorf and Arthur, 1987), especially when the child has little or no speech with which to test the fitting. The emphasis has been on the electroacoustic functions of hearing aids, on technical aspects of selection and fitting, and on design features. It is disappointing that recent studies concerned especially with training in the everyday skills of using and maintaining hearing aids are few (Flexer and Wood, 1984; Stone and Adam, 1986), apart from instruction in simple maintenance (Diefendorf and Arthur, 1987). It is also of concern that little work has been published on the cosmetic or other psychological reasons why a child or parents may reject a hearing aid, even when properly fitted.

A small proportion of hearing-impaired children obtain no useful hearing for speech, even when fitted with the most powerful hearing aids. They perceive only grossly distorted speech or uncomfortable vibration. For these children the alternatives for speech perception, apart from speechreading, are cochlear implants or tactile devices.

Cochlear implants

Following earlier reports (Djourno and Eyries, 1957; Simmons, 1966; Michelson, 1971), but mainly since House (1976), those patients with an inner-ear hearing loss too great for them to be helped by conventional hearing aids have increasingly had the option of the cochlear implant prosthesis. The rationale is to bypass damaged hair cells in the cochlea and to stimulate the auditory nerve neurons (Parkins and Houde, 1982). Thus cochlear implants are designed to convert sounds into electrical energy to stimulate the auditory nerve fibres directly. The reader is referred to Northern (1984) for excellent descriptions of the relevant anatomy of the ear.

Work on cochlear implants developed fast. The ASHA Ad Hoc Committee on Cochlear Implants reported in 1986 that there were then more than 1000 cochlear implantees throughout the world (Ad Hoc Committee on Cochlear Implants, 1986). In the same year, House and Berliner (1986) considered that the House/37 cochlear implant system was no longer investigational and had become clinically feasible. Since then many more implants have been fitted, as teams of surgeons, engineers, speech and language scientists, audiologists and therapists have followed up the original advances. A small proportion of implantees can conduct a normal conversation without speechreading and some now use the telephone (Cohen et al., 1989). Reports on the management of communication for cochlear implantees are now appearing in quantity.

Cochlear implants can be grouped according to whether they are single-channel, with one active and one indifferent electrode, or multichannel devices, with up to 24 electrodes. House (1976) developed a single-channel device employing a carrier signal modulated by an analogue of the sound stimulus. Sounds relayed by this device appeared more natural than when the acoustic analogue was directly applied to the electrode placed in the scala tympani, but the device did not produce good speech perception without visual cues. Bilger et al. (1977) evaluated a number of single-channel implantees in the USA. These patients could identify some environmental sounds such as door-knocks, were assisted in speechreading because of intensity and timing information, improved their voice quality, and obtained some psychological benefits. All had good frequency discrimination up to 200 Hz, and a few up to 1 kHz. However, none had speech discrimination above chance level without visual cues. It is noteworthy that comparable results were obtained in the UK by Fourcin et al. (1979), using the much less invasive technique of an electrode on the promontory, within the middle ear.

Single-channel implants have been criticised for not operating according to the tonotopic structure of the organ of Corti, which functions as a series of bandpass filters, with low frequencies at the apex, towards the helicotrema, and high frequencies at the base, towards the oval and round windows. Thus, while single-channel work continued, other groups pursued multichannel devices, in which the active electrodes were distributed along the scala tympani, and hence along the organ of Corti. By the early to mid-1980s, patients fitted with multichannel devices were scoring above chance level on open-set word and sentence lists without visual information (Tyler et al., 1984; Dowell et al., 1985a). Subsequently, it has become accepted that multichannel implants offer more advantages for speech discrimination than single-channel types (Gantz et al., 1988; Spillman and Dillier, 1989).

Besides the number of channels and electrodes to be used, other important factors involve the design of the speech processor. This receives the sound signal, converts it to electrical form and then analyses and shapes it according to bandwidth, formant identification and selection output limitation, noise suppression, etc., before relaying it to the electrodes. This is a complex topic, beyond our present scope, but here, too, rapid advances are being made (Dowell et al., 1987; Wilson et al., 1988; Dorman et al., 1989; Skinner et al., 1991).

The performance of cochlear implantees was reviewed by Tyler et al. (1989) across five types of prostheses, with different numbers of channels and different processors, in France, Germany and the USA. Tyler et al. observed that all but one of the implant groups contained some patients who scored better than 10% on open-set words. They also remarked that the patients were selected as the better implantees in each clinic, so their results should not be seen as typical or average. Overall, performance on speech perception tests was modest, given that it was obtained from the better patients. Greater improvements can be attained with the addition of speechreading, though speechreading can be much improved with simple information such as speech envelope signals (Dorman et al., 1991).

Selection of patients for cochlear implantation

The earlier cochlear implant work was done with adults, especially bilaterally post-lingually profoundly deaf adults, but some work was soon done with prelingually profoundly deaf adults (Eisenberg, 1982; Fugain et al., 1985). Eisenberg reported responses to gross sounds and music, with changes in voice quality, but not speech perception. Fugain et al. found similar results with postlingually and prelingually profoundly deaf adults. Generally, the amount of benefit that prelingually deaf adults can acquire from cochlear implantation is not certain. Ling and Nienhuys (1983) thought that at least three kinds of profoundly deaf patients were eligible for cochlear implantation: infants who were congenitally or prelingually deaf; adolescent or adult prelingually deaf people; and adults deafened post-lingually through disease or injury. Each kind of patient would need a different kind of rehabilitation programme after implantation.

Experiments on the effects of cochlear damage in young animals (Trune, 1982; Chouard et al.,1983) led to suggestions for cochlear implantation at the earliest possible age. At present, the children most suited to cochlear implantation are those known to be bilaterally totally deaf. Even children born profoundly but not totally deaf may be more suited to conventional hearing aids. To assess definite bilateral total deafness before the age of 2 years is at present somewhat optimistic. Few children are considered for implanattion at so young an age. However, the number of reports showing improvements in life style, speech perception and speech production with cochlear implantation is increasing for children implanted at age 2 years and upwards (Bouse, 1987; Cunningham, 1990; Waltzman et al., 1990). Dawson et al. (1990) reported that of 21 implantees aged 3–20 years, five achieved significant scores on open-set speech perception tests using hearing without speechreading. Phoneme scores for monosyllabic words ranged from 30% to 72% correct. Word scores for sentences ranged from 26% to 74%. Four of these five patients were implanted before, and the fifth during, adolescence. Eight children, aged 3–11 years, could use auditory inputs in closed-set speech perception or vowel imitation tasks. The remaining implantees, aged 13–20 years, did not achieve open-set recognition but were all full-time implant users. It is likely that very young children will be candidates for implantation in the near future. The interest in early intervention for communication in hearing-impaired children suggests that this development will be a priority.

The remarkable feature of the advent of clinically viable and routinely available, if costly, cochlear implant programmes is that a prospect is in view in which most cases of total deafness may be eliminated. Many cases of profound deafness may be assisted to a handicap no greater than that sustained in severe hearing impairment. Even though there continue to be reports of patients who received minimal or limited benefit from the prosthesis (Abel and Tse, 1987) and the outcomes can be very variable (National Institutes of Health, 1988), such instances will decrease over time as surgical techniques become more apposite, the prostheses become more effective in converting speech sounds into appropriate electrical stimuli, and rehabilitation techniques become more sophisticated. In turn, this implies that over the coming years it will be increasingly possible for the profoundly to totally deaf to communicate via the auditory modality and, perhaps more significantly, for the prelingually hearing-impaired infant to receive therapy and education more effectively through aural methods.

So rapid have been developments in cochlear implantation that deaf people who communicate manually have seen cochlear implants as a threat to their existence as a separate culture within society. In some instances they have reacted negatively (Chapter 9). There is little doubt that this debate will become more acute in the next few years.

Vibrotactile and electrotactile aids

The use of vibrotactile stimulation was investigated long ago by Gault (1924) and Knudsen (1928). More recently, Oller et al. (1986) remarked that hearing individuals, with their hearing masked by noise, can learn to recognise a vocabulary of up to 150 words following 40–80 hours of practice on multichannel vibrotactile devices.

Such stimulation was not widely pursued as an aid to communication for hearing-impaired people until the advent of cochlear implants. Tactile stimulation now enjoys a new lease of life, especially as a supplement to speechreading (Oller et al., 1986; Terrio and Haas, 1986; Boothroyd and Hnath-Chisholm, 1988; Eilers et al., 1988a,b; Boothroyd, 1989). It offers both an alternative to implantation and a more exacting comparison or control for implant-assisted speech perception than conventional hearing aids, when patients are so deaf that they cannot perceive conventionally aided speech. Vibrotactile devices, using the sense of touch or vibration, can compete with cochlear implants if they are developed as wearable communication aids (Ling and Nienhuys, 1983; Blamey et al., 1988; Cowan et al., 1989).

The sense of touch has long been used with deaf–blind people, as the Tadoma method, to allow them to perceive aspects of speech and to develop some facility in language (Alcorn, 1932). In this method the subject places a hand on the talker's face to register mouth, lip and jaw movements, flow of air from the mouth and nostrils, and vibrations of the larynx (Reed et al., 1985; Chomsky, 1986; Leotta et al., 1988). The ASHA Ad Hoc Committee on Cochlear Implants (1986) observed that speech perception using the Tadoma method is similar to that of normal listeners for speech in noise, at signal-to-noise ratios of $-6\,\mathrm{dB}$, and offers a standard for the comparison of tactile instruments. Proficiency in the method requires lengthy training and physical contact between talker and listener.

Plant et al. (1984a) reported on a single-channel vibrotactile aid, which provided additional information on duration of voicing and intensity in speechreading for an experienced subject. They found significant improvements at the phonemic, word and sentence levels when using the aid to supplement the visual signals, and in aided tracking of discourse. Other tests showed that the aid helped in perceiving word syllable numbers and types, stress and syllabic structure of sentences, and final consonant contrasts. In addition, the aid facilitated the identification of several environmental sounds.

Some people use a 'tactual phonology' to identify words by analogy with familiar ones (Frost and Brooks, 1983). Eilers et al. (1988a) have argued further that the close correspondence between tactile and auditory discrimination and identification of some vowels and consonants is evidence that aspects of speech are amodal.

Collins and Hurtig (1985) suggested that the maximum usefulness of tactile instruments in reducing ambiguities in speechreading cues could depend on phonemic recognition by tactile signals alone. They observed that the boundary for the voiced–voiceless distinction in hearing subjects occurred at longer voice-onset times (VOTs) for tactile than for auditory perception. Their results could explain the findings of Johnson et al. (1984) who explored the categorical perception of hearing-impaired children on a VOT continuum. Johnson et al. found normal VOT boundaries in some children. Other children, however, with longer than normal VOTs and who tended to be profoundly deaf, showed results similar to those for tactile stimulation in the Collins and Hurtig work. The similarity between their categorisations of speech sounds, and the categorisations of speech sounds presented to the finger tip in the Collins and Hurtig study, suggests that their responses were to tactile stimulation, as Collins and Hurtig pointed out. This conclusion is consistent with clinical suspicions that the audiometric responses of profoundly deaf children may be to tactile rather than hearing sensations for lower to middle audiofrequency stimuli.

Training in tactile representation of speech was illustrated well by Brooks et al. (1987) with an 18-channel tactile vocoder which presented stimuli via solenoids on the arm. Two prelingually profoundly deaf teenagers, with some skills in sign language and speechreading, attained 80% correct identifications for a 50-word vocabulary in 24 and 28.5 hours of training. Notably, the faster learning rate was achieved by the teenager with the better language skills. Next they were asked to place 400 random presentations of 16 CVs into five phonemic categories (voiced and unvoiced stops, voiced and unvoiced fricatives, and approximants), for which their mean accuracy was 84.5%. Then they were asked to place 400 random presentations of 12 VCs into four phonemic categories (unvoiced stops, nasals, unvoiced fricatives, and voiced stops), for which their mean accuracy was 89.6%. The mostly successful placing of the CVs and VCs into phonemic categories, shown on a stimulus list, indicated that the teenagers had acquired general rules about speech features with this multichannel device.

It is to be expected that results with different tactile devices will vary for different applications. Plant (1988) compared the performance of five commercially available tactile aids using a closed-set test of speech contrasts with five profoundly deaf subjects. Four of the devices were single-channel and the fifth was multichannel. Plant found marked task-to-task variation in the use of individual aids for speech contrasts. For example, one of the single-channel devices was best for suprasegmental contrasts, while the multichannel instrument performed best for segmental contrasts. The implication is that single-channel devices suit perception of the more unitary features whereas multichannel devices are needed to discriminate features which vary multidimensionally.

The sensation of vibration can also be elicited by electrocutaneous stimulation, where the signal stimulates the skin electrically (Blamey et al., 1988; Cowan et al., 1989; Blamey, 1990). Oller et al. (1986) described an elementary and preschool programme using vibrotactile and electrocutaneous vocoders in speech reception and production training with 13 profoundly deaf children aged 3–6 years. These children used an auditory training device at the same time. Their training included presentation of speech through touch (vocoders), vision (speechreading), and hearing (FM auditory trainer), in combination and isolation. Phonetic training was based on normal phonological development patterns, speech error patterns of the hearing-impaired, and the relative salience of the tactual speech features of the two vocoders. Further training was given with syllables, words and simple sentences. After training over an academic year, there were gains in speech production and reception, with rapid progress by most children, and generalisation of speech learning to situations that did not involve tactual aids. Those children who progressed the least were multiply handicapped, but even they showed measurable gains. Overall, the children progressed in speech learning in ways not found prior to training with tactual vocoders, and their results look impressive. However, adequate controls were not included for progress which might have been attained by conventional methods alone, or for 'halo' effects from the wearing of the vocoder devices. No differences were reported for comparisons of vibrotactile and electrocutaneous stimulation. Alcantara et al. (1990), however, found that the electrical stimulation of nerves under the skin was more reliable and comfortable than stimulation of tactile receptors and nerve endings in the skin itself, suggesting that subcutaneous electrotactile stimulation is a technique well worth pursuing.

To conclude, this brief review of work with tactile aids shows they can be used to distinguish speech feature contrasts, especially at the segmental level, by both hearing and hearing-impaired adults and children. Some speech features can be distinguished categorically with tactile stimulation, as with hearing, and some people can use a 'tactual phonology' in processing new words. It also seems that single-channel devices may be better for suprasegmental recognition, whereas multichannel instruments are better at the segmental level, but more work is needed before firmer conclusions can be reached.

Tactile devices versus cochlear implants

We suggested earlier that tactile devices could be an alternative to cochlear implantation for hearing-impaired individuals who obtain no usable benefit from conventional hearing aids. We also suggested that tactile devices offer a comparison or control when considering cochlear implantation. Further, tactile devices might be considered for very young children, until their hearing levels and other characteristics can be assessed sufficiently accurately for cochlear implantation to be contemplated. So, how does the use of tactile aids compare with the results of cochlear implantation?

This question was considered by Pickett and McFarland (1985) in a review of data on speech perception with implanted electrodes and with tactile aids. Pickett and McFarland compared speech reception data with a multichannel electrotactile aid (Sparks et al., 1979) with data from a Melbourne multichannel speech processor implant (Clark and Tong, 1982; Dowell et al., 1985a, b). They concluded that, despite difficulties in data comparison, speech reception via implants, even with a processor specially designed to transmit speech information, was not much better than tactile reception of speech. The main reason was probably that both devices conveyed the spectral information of speech very grossly. There was spread of electrical stimulation by the implant and poor spatial (frequency) resolution on the skin by the tactile device. In comparing other sets of multichannel implants and tactile instruments, their general conclusion was that the speech perception of implantees was not substantially better than that of subjects well-practised with tactile-devices. Perhaps their most significant conclusion was that neither implants nor tactile devices, either then or in the near future, could provide more than a modest aid to speechreading.

More recently, Skinner et al. (1988) reported different conclusions. They presented a comparison of the results from three different vibrotactile aids and cochlear implants (Nucleus 22 Electrode) for postlingually deaf adults. Four such adults were assessed with a 1- or 2-channel vibrotactile aid and, following surgery, with the multichannel cochlear implant. Skinner et al. concluded that the speech perception using the multichannel cochlear implant, a later model than that used in the review by Pickett and McFarland (1985), far surpassed that of the vibrotactile aids. A similar conclusion was drawn by Staller et al. (1991), who observed a clear trend towards continued improvements with longer-term use of multi-channel implants. More studies of this kind, with multichannel devices of both types and with controls for practice, are needed before the findings can be generally accepted as conclusive.

There is a theoretical consideration suggesting that cochlear implants may be preferred to tactile devices. Hearing people process speech through a phonological code. Cochlear implantation, designed to stimulate the hearing structures, is likely to bring these phonological coding mechanisms into play in processing spoken material. Although (Frost and Brooks, 1983; Eilers et al., 1988a) some people can use a 'tactual phonology' to process new words, and although Collins and Hurtig (1985) found a close correspondence between tactile and auditory perception of several speech features, there is some doubt as to whether tactile devices can take full advantage of such coding. There is much work to be done before this issue can be resolved.

Training in the use of cochlear implants and tactile devices

Since our interest is in communication skills, we should ask for more information on how users of cochlear implants and tactile devices have been trained in their use. The literature suggests that most studies have relied on a kind of guided practice. According to the ASHA Ad Hoc Committee on Cochlear Implants (1986), most centres involved with implants use a mix of analytic and synthetic approaches, with auditory-alone and auditory–visual practice to assist in the understanding of speech through the implant.

Speech perception via cochlear implants is believed to be only approximately speech-like. The advice is therefore to expose the implantee to a variety of speech and non-speech sounds, so that key features of both can be recognised. Even so, improved performance takes a long time for many implantees, suggesting that much practice is needed. The speech tracking procedure of DeFilippo and Scott (1978) is used for training and assessment in many implant programmes. In this procedure, a talker reads text phrase by phrase while the listener repeats each word. If the listener's response is incorrect, the talker repeats the phrase, or parts of it, until it is perceived correctly. Robbins et al. (1985) have described the use of this technique, finding that implantees who were previous hearing-aid users achieved a higher tracking rate than implantees with no previous experience of amplification. The technique can be quantified by measuring a 'communication rate', where the number of words in the text is divided by the amount of time needed to convey it. The procedure enables therapist and implantee to monitor progress, with instant knowledge of the results, but is more like guided practice than a training programme with predetermined goals.

Eisenberg (1985) is one of the few to have published specifically on training methods for implantees. Eisenberg recommended the use of tape recordings of both open- and closed-set stimuli, with the therapist directing the implantee's attention to time and intensity cues, together with cues from context. A set of responses ('yes-yes', 'no', 'please repeat') was offered by Castle (1984) to help an implantee in the use of the telephone, but only simple telephone communication is possible in this way, and only a few implantees appear to achieve success with it.

Tyler et al. (1986) found that previous experience with one type of implant could have a confounding effect on performance with another type later on. This study also provided evidence for generalisation of training, or experience, for the implantee investigated, though Tyler et al. saw it as a source of confounding.

Similar comments can be made about communication with tactile devices. Much of the training seems to have been based on guided practice. The work by Oller et al. (1986), outlined above, is an exception. In this study, which used tactile devices in a multisensory programme, training both speech production and reception, profoundly deaf children focused on tactile, auditory or visual speech features for syllables in articulation training, followed by a greater emphasis on word perception as phonological skills developed. They also focused initially on speech sounds as maximally contrasting pairs, progressing to word recognition in open sets in speech reception training. The training was hence based on normal phonological developmental sequences. Proctor (1990) followed the same kind of approach to tactile training with three hearing-aided profoundly deaf children who received multimodality experience in listening to and feeling sound while looking at the speaker. She found that the rate of progress in understanding oral language exceeded that expected of hearing children, though her small-scale study clearly needs replication with suitable controls and more subjects.

Auditory Perception of Speech by Hearing-impaired Children

Description of the communication skills of hearing-impaired children requires consideration of their speech perception at the level of the phoneme, word, phrase and clause. It also needs discussion in terms of the stress and intonation patterns of speech, which can vary within a single word or syllable ('Oh!' versus 'Oh?'), or across a sequence of connected speech, as when a sentence is changed from a statement to a question ('You caught the bus.' versus 'You caught the bus?').

Phonemic (segmental) aspects

The range of audio frequencies available to a hearing child is 20 Hz–20 kHz, but only the range from about 100 Hz–8 kHz is used in communication by speech. The first (F_1) and second (F_2) formants, the frequency bands of high energy associated with resonances of the vocal tract, which are needed for the recognition of vowels and voiced consonants, and the spectral energy of the voiceless consonants, fall in this range. However, the latter tend to have most of their energy distributed at higher frequencies than the vowel sounds. Hence children with high-frequency hearing losses have problems in perceiving the voiceless consonants characterised by place of articulation.

The consonants have less acoustic energy than the vowels as well as having their spectral energy concentrated at the higher end of the frequency range for speech-hearing. They are therefore more readily affected than vowels by a decrease in signal intensity or an increase in environmental noise.

Fortunately, neither vowels nor consonants usually have to be recognised alone. They are embedded in a context of syllables, words and sentences, which offer additional cues to their recognition. For the more easily lost or masked consonants it is often the transition component of the respective syllable, rather than the accompanying vowel in coarticulation, that aids consonant recognition. Transitions, like vowels, contain greater energy than consonants, and so the consonants can be recognised not only by the vowel but by the transition (Fletcher, 1953; Ladefoged, 1962).

Speech perception ability at the phonemic level is conveniently evaluated by lists of words spoken under controlled listening conditions. Error scores on such lists provide useful information as to where the child experiences phonemic confusions, and hence give pointers for training or therapy. A large variety of such word lists is available (Lyregaard et al., 1976; Keith, 1984; Martin, 1987). Some lists have been designed to meet special needs or purposes, but among those most commonly used are the open-response-set phonemically balanced word lists, designed to represent the phoneme balance used in the community. Examples are the isophonemic word lists of Boothroyd (1968) used in the UK and Australia, and the CID-W22 monosyllable word lists used in the USA (Hirsh, 1952; Hirsh et al., 1952; Studebaker and Sherbecoe, 1991). For young children the Wepman Test (1958) is used commonly in many English-speaking countries, though the Word Intelligibility by Picture Identification Test (Ross and Lerman, 1970) has many adherents.

The Boothroyd and CID-W22 word lists serve as 'general purpose' lists (Martin and Forbis, 1978; Evans, 1987). They are quick and convenient to administer, and have face validity as more 'natural' than nonsense syllables or synthetic word lists. However, they have been criticised when used in diagnostic audiometry to discriminate among individuals with differing degrees of sensorineural hearing loss, or as site-of-lesion tests (Geffner and Donovan, 1974; Lyregaard et al., 1976). Moreover, they are not particularly suited to testing for phoneme confusions, for which other tests are more informative. We shall return to this matter after considering impaired phoneme perception in more detail.

In a classic study, Miller and Nicely (1955) showed that hearing listeners used the articulatory and acoustical features of place of articulation, voicing and manner of articulation to identify phonemes. This work was later developed for both hearing and hearing-impaired listeners (Walden and Montgomery, 1975). For low-pass speech material, with middle and high frequencies missing, for example, hearing listeners confused place of articulation, whereas they perceived voicing and nasal manner correctly. As we have seen, hearing-impaired listeners who suffer from high-frequency hearing loss tend to present with the same confusions. Thus information is obtained on how the problem may be alleviated – by fitting a hearing aid with a high frequency emphasis, for example.

As stated, hearing-impaired listeners generally recognise vowels more satisfactorily than consonants. We now describe selected studies to give the reader some idea of the type of work involved.

Perception of vowels

A study of the vowels /i, u, ɪ, ɑ, ʌ, ɔ, æ/ as recognised by 99 hard-of-hearing Gallaudet College students, was reported by Pickett et al. (1972). The students were in four groups with mean hearing losses of 67, 73, 82 and 88 dB HL. Allocation to these groups was made not by hearing loss but by scores on a version of the Modified Rhyme Test (MRT) (Fairbanks, 1958), with 50 monosyllabic words in a closed-set format presented to the better ear at 6 dB above each listener's most comfortable listening level.

Results were obtained for 20 initial and 20 final consonants, and 10 vowels. The respective vowel recognition for these groups was 91%, 76%, 62% and 48% correct. The group with the least severe mean hearing loss (67 dB), with 91% of vowels recognised correctly, produced minimal vowel confusions. For the 73 and 82 dB mean hearing loss groups the vowel confusions occurred mainly between vowels of similar F_1. Vowels with low frequency F_1 values were more readily confused than vowels which had F_1 values at the higher frequencies. For the 88 dB mean hearing loss group, vowels tended to be confused where their F_1 values were in the same frequency area, though vowels with low frequency F_1 values were the most confusable.

Vowel formant transitions, arising from the coarticulation of consonants and vowels, were investigated with a vowel synthesiser in three listeners with moderately severe, flat, sensorineural hearing losses by Martin et al. (1972). They found that, whilst this kind of hearing loss did not seem to impede the listener's abilities to use brief, small transitions in formant frequency as discrimination cues, it appeared to impede the ability to find such cues in listening to speech-like material, where the low-frequency formants masked the discrimination of transition cues in formants with higher frequencies. The effects were reduced by auditory training for some subjects.

The more severely hearing-impaired people can confuse vowels even when their formant frequencies differ considerably, as shown by Risberg (1976). He used a rhyme test with moderately to profoundly deaf Swedish children and young adults, aged 10–21 years, required to identify vowels in monosyllabic Swedish words. The vowels /u/, /o/ and /a/, which had frequency differences for F_1 and F_2 but had similar frequencies for F_3 and F_4, were used to determine hearing for formant frequencies below 1500 Hz. Hearing for frequencies above 1500 Hz was assessed by comparing /u/ and /i/, and /a/ and /æ/, for both of which pairs F_1 was similar but F_2 was different. Listeners with hearing losses between 60 dB and 69 dB showed the best recognition of vowels, though above 1500 Hz they partly confused vowels with different formants. Listeners with losses between 70 dB and 79 dB obtained recognition scores around 90% correct for vowels with different formants below 1500 Hz, and around 70% for vowels with different formants above 1500 Hz. A third group of listeners with losses of 80–89 dB obtained recognition scores of about 70% for vowels with different formants below 1500 Hz, and scores of only 40% for vowels with different formants above 1500 Hz. Risberg thus showed that listeners with the more severe to profound hearing losses tended to confuse vowels even when the vowels differed in formant frequencies. Listeners with moderate to severe losses, however, made confusions for mainly those vowels which were distinguishable by formants above 1500 Hz.

In similar work, Fourcin (1976) investigated vowel perception in hearing-impaired children with two-formant synthesised vowels /i/, /a/ and /u/, of which /i/ and /u/ had the same F_1 values but were distinguishable by the amplitude of F_2. The more severely hearing-impaired children were confused in recognising /i/ and /u/, but were able to recognise /a/ correctly. As with Risberg (1976), the children with the least severe hearing losses were able to recognise the vowels without great difficulty. More recent work (Pickett et al., 1983) has continued to show that, as hearing loss increases, it is more difficult to discriminate between vowels where the distinguishing acoustic features are of higher audiofrequency.

A different approach to vowel perception was taken by Bochner et al. (1988), who compared the perception of hearing and hearing-impaired listeners for changes in length of vowels and tonal complexes (filled intervals). Both hearing and hearing-impaired subjects showed greater acuity for the duration of filled as compared with unfilled intervals. The mean thresholds for filled, but not unfilled, intervals from the hearing listeners were significantly smaller than those from the hearing-impaired subjects, though a few of the latter showed acuity comparable to that of the hearing listeners under several listening conditions.

In an interesting twist, the usual experimental arrangement, in which perception of a given set of vowels is compared across various groups of subjects, was changed by Turner and Henn (1989) to allow for individual differences. They obtained measures of frequency resolution from individual hearing-impaired subjects to predict each subject's vowel recognition ability. Input filter patterns were obtained at six test frequencies from hearing and hearing-impaired listeners. These patterns were then used to compare frequency resolution with vowel recognition in the same listeners, to find the relationship between impaired frequency resolution and vowel recognition. This study therefore provided a link between individual differences in vowel perception by hearing-impaired subjects and the underlying problems of hearing loss and impaired frequency resolution. Taken with Bochner et al. (1988), it provides an increasingly complex, but increasingly complete, picture of the dimensions in which the vowel recognition of hearing-impaired listeners differs from that of hearing people.

Perception of consonants

There has been considerable research into consonant perception by hearing listeners (Pickett, 1980). However, research into consonant perception by hearing-impaired listeners is comparatively recent. It is generally agreed that moderately to profoundly deaf listeners have reduced access to speech contrasts and spectral cues, for example, in consonant distinctions (Boothroyd, 1984; Revoile et al., 1991a, b), and where frequency selectivity is impaired (Preminger and Wiley, 1985) or otherwise.

We now consider consonant perception by selecting from work on voiced and unvoiced consonants, and on the perception of consonants characterised by place of articulation. Space does not allow us to give more attention to this important area, but the outline which follows should give the reader an overview of salient aspects.

Voiced consonants

Perception of initial stop consonants was studied by Bennett and Ling (1973) for CV monosyllables by hearing and severely hearing-impaired children. The stimuli, with six stops, were prepared for systematic variations in voice onset time (VOT), the period after the initial stop before the onset of the following vowel. The CV stimuli, with varying VOTs, which are relatively short for voiced stops and longer for unvoiced stops, were presented binaurally at comfortable listening levels to ten children with severe or greater hearing losses. Whereas hearing children make the distinction between voiced and unvoiced stops at VOTs of between 20 and 40 ms, similar to hearing adults, the hearing-impaired children showed inconsistent performance. They tended to identify more unvoiced than voiced stops at VOTs of 60 ms or more.

An additional cue was introduced by Fourcin (1976) in a second test as part of the synthetic vowel perception study described earlier. He varied the cut-back of F_1, so that for some trials the F_1 cue did not coincide with the initial VOT cue as it would in natural speech. He concluded that hearing-impaired children needed both cues for correct phoneme identification. The children with the more severe hearing losses could not perceive the VOT contrast at all. This finding is generally consistent with that of Bennett and Ling (1973) – see above – and a study by Parady et al. (1981), which used synthetic /da/–/ta/ stimuli generated along the VOT continuum.

The upward spread of masking, in which the lower speech frequencies mask the higher ones, has long been suspected of causing, at least in part, the poor speech perception of the more severely hearing-impaired listeners (Martin et al., 1972; Pickett and Danaher, 1975; Wightman et al., 1977). To test this hypothesis, Dorman et al. (1985) eliminated F_1 entirely from the speech stimulus. They found, nevertheless, that removing the first formant did not improve the stimulus intelligibility for listeners with sloping mild to moderate hearing losses for levels above, at, or below the level of maximum intelligibility. In particular, they concluded that this and similar results (Trinder et al., 1980; Kaplan and Pickett, 1982) showed that spread of masking from the first formant was not a significant factor in the identification of voiced stop consonants.

The use of cues by moderately to severely hearing-impaired and hearing listeners in voicing perception of initial stop consonants was explored by Revoile et al. (1987). They prepared tests in which different parts of syllable onsets were either deleted or changed for syllables of cognate voicing, and they flattened the F_0 contour for syllable pairs. Twenty hearing-impaired subjects with mild to severe hearing losses, and six hearing Gallaudet College students were the listeners. The results confirmed that VOT was a strong voicing cue for both hearing and hearing-impaired listeners, supporting the findings of Parady et al. (1981) in that the moderately, and some severely, hearing-impaired students showed relatively normal use of the VOT cue. The results did not, however, support Bennett and Ling (1973), where VOT cues were not perceived by the children tested, though these latter children generally had greater hearing losses than the Gallaudet students (compare Fourcin, 1976).

Perception of place

Some consonants characterised by place of articulation can be distinguished by means of the rate of change in transition frequency in the formants of the preceding and/or the following vowels ('by' versus 'die'). In these instances the consonants are both voiced and articulated in a plosive manner, but differ in place (bilabial and alveolar respectively). The acoustic cue is a fast change in the higher part of the acoustic spectrum, which causes problems for many hearing-impaired people (Sher and Owens, 1974; Reed, 1975), unless they supplement perception of the acoustic feature distinction by speechreading.

For instance, Godfrey and Millay (1978) asked listeners with mild and moderate sensorineural hearing impairment to report on synthetically produced /bɛ/ and /wɛ/ sounds across a range of frequency transition durations from 10 to 120 ms, in 10 ms stages. Nine listeners identified /bɛ/ and /wɛ/ normally, by ascribing /bɛ/ to transitions of 40 ms or less and /wɛ/ to transitions of 80 ms or more. The remaining six listeners showed a variable response, both among listeners and within individual listeners, depending on the stimulus presentation level. Some of the listeners identified all transition durations as /bɛ/ or as /wɛ/, while some produced nearly random identifications of /bɛ/ and /wɛ/ across the range.

Ochs et al. (1989) examined place of articulation in the synthesised syllables /bi/, /di/ and /gi/ in a group of subjects with a high-frequency hearing loss and two groups of hearing subjects, one listening with, and one without, masking noise. Stimuli with a moving F_2 formant transition ('moving F_2 stimuli') were compared with stimuli in which F_2 was constant ('straight F_2 stimuli') to assess the F_2 transition in perceiving stop consonants. For both moving and straight F_2 stimuli, the performance of the three groups was similar in identifying /di/ and /gi/. However, performance of the hearing-impaired and noise-masked hearing listeners was below that of the unmasked hearing group for /bi/ for moving F_2 and especially for straight F_2. Errors with /bi/ most commonly involved confusions with /di/. Among possible explanations, Ochs et al. noted that Dubno et al. (1987) had observed that both /b/ and /d/ were harder to perceive than /g/ for listeners with a sloping high-frequency hearing loss. Such a loss may distort the onset of /b/ and /d/ more than the more compact onset of /g/.

The general conclusion from this selection of reports is that the vowel and consonant perception of hearing-impaired listeners is far from a simple attenuation or other modification of speech as perceived by hearing listeners, and controlled stimuli are needed to explore it. The reports also show that hearing-impaired listeners differ from each other in phoneme perception, depending on the type and degree of hearing loss. Hence it is important to have information about phoneme perception by hearing-impaired individuals in devising aural rehabilitation programmes to improve communication skills. Although, as expected, misperceptions of speech commonly occur in noisy situations, a hearing-impaired child can fail to understand speech because of inability to discriminate phonemes in the quiet. Fortunately the facility to synthesise speech sounds has considerably sharpened our ability to test the phonemic features which cause difficulty for a given hearing-impaired child (Damper, 1982; Kangas and Allen, 1990). We will consider the place of such tests shortly, but first some mention must be made of perception of the suprasegmental phonemes.

Perception of suprasegmentals

Little work has been done on the perception of prosody by hearing-impaired children, apart perhaps from the use of prosody as a supplement to speechreading (Grant, 1987a, b). Erber and Alencewicz (1976) have, however, developed the CID-CAT test, available in expanded form as the CID-MONSTER, which consists of four words to be presented in three different prosodic forms, as in monosyllables, trochees and spondees. The test is then scored in two ways, first by the percentage of words identified correctly and secondly by the percentage of correct stress patterns correctly identified. So, when a monosyllable is presented and the child responds with a monosyllable the response is scored once for reporting its phonetic form and also once for its prosodic feature. This test recognises that a child with a profound hearing loss, say, may be able to perceive the prosodic information in the word although the phonetic feature is elusive. Merklein (1981) also prepared a test related to perception of prosody in his short speech perception test for severely and profoundly deaf children. His time pattern item, involving the ability to perceive and count syllable pulses, as monosyllabic versus multisyllabic utterances, underscores the perception of rhythm and disjuncture.

A further test, designed to assess prosodic information in connected speech, is the Stress Pattern Recognition in Sentence (SPRIS) test of Jackson and Kerry-Ballweber (1979). This test contains four repetitions of 12 simple sentences, each of which consists of four monosyllabic words. A different word is stressed on each presentation of each sentence. The test is scored in the same way as that of Erber and Alencewicz (1976), with scoring both for identification of the sentence and for identification of the stress pattern of the sentence. Interestingly, the authors found that young adults with severe to profound hearing losses showed a wide range of performances on the SPRIS test which could not be predicted from audiograms. They suggested that individuals with relatively good auditory skills who relied on spectral cues could be given training based on word recognition, whereas individuals with poor auditory skills who relied on prosodic information should receive training in word pattern recognition.

Clinical and Practical Applications

The recent work in perception of acoustic features, or speech patterns, by hearing-impaired listeners presents a challenge to conventional speech audiometric assessment with phonemically balanced word lists of the type mentioned earlier. So far, however, this challenge has not been particularly well recognised in the clinic.

Phonemically balanced word lists versus 'speech pattern' tests

Merklein (1981) thought it puzzling that phonemically balanced word list testing persisted in the light of work on speech pattern tests. He criticised phonemically balanced word lists for their large, inappropriate vocabularies, open-response format and learning effects (see Byrne (1983) and Walker et al. (1982) for some examples and further comment). Merklein sought tests of speech-hearing which would produce more precise and valuable information for selecting hearing aids, assisting in educational placement, and for auditory training and speech therapy. He pointed to tests and observations such as those of Boothroyd (1972a), Erber (1974, 1978) and Erber and Alencewicz (1976), which considered spectral or speech envelope information for testing speech-hearing, as a way forward. He himself presented a short test for severely and profoundly deaf children, which assessed perception of speech-envelope versus spectral patterns, together with suprasegmental (prosodic) versus segmental (phonemic) aspects.

The routine clinical use of conventional phonemically balanced word lists probably endures because clinical audiologists, pressed for time, choose a procedure that will quickly give them an overview of their patient's phoneme perception via tests that are well known and widely used, facilitating communication of patient data. It may also be due to concern to identify peripheral neural lesions, which result in disproportionately poor speech recognition (Evans, 1987), particularly for vowels (Hannley and Jerger, 1985).

The research on acoustic features has generally shown that the greater the hearing loss, the greater is the difficulty in discriminating differences in vowel formants, especially in the higher audio frequencies. Children with severe to profound sensorineural losses have poor discrimination of F_2 transitions, perhaps more so in the presence of F_1, as occurs in natural speech. They also show poor discrimination of the rate of frequency transitions. As regards final consonants, some hearing-impaired subjects show poor perception when the preceding vowel-duration cue is removed, while others can use the remaining spectral cues (King, 1987). Perception of differences associated with VOT is difficult for severely to profound deaf children, as we saw.

King (1987) proposed sound pattern tests based on differences in acoustic features and reflecting also the sound patterns related to the prosodic aspects of speech. Other recent approaches which make use of spectral and similar pattern information have been suggested by Fourcin (1976), Erber (1980), Plant (1984), Hutchinson (1990), Hazan et al. (1991). The FAAF test (Foster and Haggard, 1979, 1984) further aimed to assess word identification scores rather precisely in the region of the maximum score as a function of spectral parameters. The PLOTT test (Plant, 1984) was also developed to assess the ability of hearing-impaired children to use spectral or time–intensity cues. It consists of nine subtests: Subtest 1 measures the ability to detect vowels and consonants; Subtests 2 and 3 measure the ability to use spectral versus time–intensity cues; Subtest 4 is a test of discrimination for very familiar non-confusable words; and Subtests 5–9 assess perception of vowel length, vowel discrimination, consonant voicing, consonant manner and consonant place, using a picture-pointing response. The results from the PLOTT test provide very useful data about a child's speech perception in hearing-aid use, but the test takes a long time to administer.

It may have occurred to the reader that techniques now available for the computer manipulation of speech features could provide selective enhancement of aspects of speech, making the speech more intelligible to hearing-impaired listeners. For example, it might be advantageous to increase the silent intervals in speech to reduce the possibility of forward masking (Cazals and Palis, 1991). It could also be helpful to amplify consonants, whose acoustic energy is usually below that of vowels, so that the energy of the consonants approximates that of the vowels. Montgomery and Edge (1988) have done this kind of study with adults. They amplified the consonants by computer enhancement to produce near-zero consonant/vowel intensity ratios. The duration of consonants was also increased to provide an additional 30 ms of sound, with compensatory vowel shortening to maintain the original overall duration. A word stimulus set so manipulated was presented at 65 dB SPL(sound pressure level) to one group of 20 adult listeners with a moderate sensorineural loss, and at 95 dB SPL to a second, similar group of 10 listeners. The amplitude processing gave an increase of 10–12% in intelligibility for the 65 dB SPL stimuli, but there was no significant effect for the 95 dB SPL stimuli. Increase of consonant duration gave no benefit at 65 dB SPL, but resulted in a 5% improvement at 95 dB SPL. The effects of speech stimulus enhancement therefore appear to be relatively small and differ for different stimulus presentation levels. More research is needed in this area, especially with subjects who have different types and degrees of hearing loss.

Perception of Connected Speech

Children appear to perceive speech on the basis of sentences, not words alone (Houston, 1972). They learn about the functions of morphemes, syntax and vocabulary in the context of sentence perception (Streng et al., 1978). Further, the suprasegmental characteristics of connected speech, in the forms of stress, intonation, rhythm and phrasing directly affect the meaning of the speech, and thus inform the child further about the functions of the segmental aspects.

We saw that practitioners prefer phonemically balanced lists of words to other types of speech material for assessing the speech-hearing of hearing-impaired children. Such word lists are commonly used in routine clinical practice when connected speech material might be used to advantage. One of the main reasons is undoubtedly the extra time taken for sentence test administration unless a reduced number of test items (sentences) per list is provided but, for statistical reasons, reduction in the number of items leads to lower reliability in response measures.

Sentence tests estimate speech perception in daily communication with a much higher naturally appearing face validity than word tests. The case for the use of connected speech material for clinical testing and rehabilitation is persuasive when, for example, natural sentences – namely sentences with commonly occurring vocabulary, familiar syntax and semantics – are considered as an alternative to phonemic balancing in word lists. The main case for using sentences is that perception of words alone does not necessarily predict the perception of sentences, because it cannot estimate the grammar and semantics in sentences. Such aspects constrain words in sentences, but not isolated words. Sentences also permit systematic studies of the time domain, since they are usually sufficiently long to allow variations in the temporal properties of speech (Speaks and Jerger, 1965). It is likely that most of the time we operate on the basis of the largest speech or language units, and only use smaller units to resolve ambiguities or to accommodate the unexpected. It is also likely that we ignore a large part of the more detailed acoustic and linguistic information in speech in order to achieve high speed and accuracy in processing it (Boothroyd, 1978).

In what follows, we consider connected speech mainly in the form of sentences. Of course, not all connected speech consists of sentences, particularly single sentences. There is a role for continuous discourse, as in discourse tracking, currently popular in assessing the use of cochlear implants (see above), though discourse tracking is broken up into phrases because of the memory load. It may also be objected that, in conversations between people who know one another fairly well, natural speech is markedly context-bound, seems rather unconnected, is heavily pragmatic, and is more like a set of loosely connected phrases than sentences. This kind of conversation is characterised as much by short, phrase-like interruptions, interjections or questions ('So what?', 'Ridiculous!', 'Can't follow') as by sentences. These objections are recognised, but in the following material we choose to concentrate on the perception of sentences as the standard form of connected speech.

Hearing for speech in sentences by hearing-impaired people differs from their hearing for words. Niemeyer (1972) presented a study of dissociated hearing loss in which a zone of normal hearing, or mild hearing impairment, is juxtaposed with a zone of severe or profound hearing loss (the ski-slope audiogram). He argued that what is redundant in sentence material for hearing people is essential for communication in the hearing-impaired, allowing them to close the gaps in speech perception. Thus the contextual association between words in a sentence makes it easier to perceive words in sentences than the same words presented in isolation. This difference can be measured as an 'informational reserve'. Niemeyer proposed a sentence-specific informational reserve as: $X = (SD - WD)/SD \times 100\%$, where SD is the discrimination score of words in sentences and WD is the discrimination score of the words presented in isolation. For German speech material, the informational reserve was about 54% for hearing people. Hence, about half of the information in the sentences was due to context.

Being dissatisfied with sentence list tests then available for child speech audiometry in the UK and the USA (see below), which were lengthy and contained unfamiliar vocabulary, Bench and Bamford (1979) devised new sentence lists from a detailed linguistic analysis of spoken language samples of 208 hearing-impaired children. The resulting BKB Sentence Lists were deemed suitable for testing the speech-hearing of hearing-impaired children aged 8 years or more. These lists were available in picture-related and standard non-picture-related forms. Only the latter is considered here.

Bench et al. (1979) compared the speech-hearing abilities on these BKB sentence lists with other sentence list tests (Fry, 1961; Watson, 1967) and word list tests (Boothroyd, 1968; BKB word lists) on 129 partially hearing children, with losses mainly of prelingual sensorineural origin. They found that the BKB standard sentence lists gave steeper slopes for performance-intensity functions, lower speech reception thresholds and higher discrimination scores than the other sentence lists and, relevant to the present discussion, the Boothroyd Word Lists and the BKB words. A similar study, with similar outcomes, was reported by Bench et al. (1987), on the BKB sentence lists adapted for use in Australia (BKB/A lists). Consistently better speech-hearing was shown in tests with the BKB/A sentences than for other sentence lists and, importantly, than for word lists. It follows that to assess a hearing-impaired child's ability for speech-hearing in an everyday communication context with word lists will generally underestimate such ability, and sometimes markedly so.

The implications for aural rehabilitation are clear, though individual examples vary depending on linguistic competence, as further work showed. Thus Bench et al. (1987) also presented data from three individual children, all of whom had similar pure-tone hearing losses (62–69 dB three-frequency averages) and similarly shaped audiograms. Near-perfect scores were obtained for one child at 90 dB relative speech level for sentences, whereas the child obtained only about 63% for word lists at the same level. The second child obtained a score of 86% for sentences, but only about 18% for word lists, showing a large effect associated with the contextual aspect of the sentences. The third child obtained about 40% with the sentences and about 26% with the word lists in the range of 70–80 dB relative speech level, thus obtaining relatively little information from the contextual information in the sentences and suggesting poor linguistic competence, with the words in sentences perceived perhaps as strings of unconnected or loosely connected words.

The CID or CHABA sentences (Silverman and Hirsch, 1955) have been the sentence list material most widely used in the USA, particularly with adults. They are especially helpful in assessing postlingually hearing-impaired patients of more mature years, especially geriatric patients, who are unable to communicate adequately. However, they are too difficult for most children, and even for some young adults with severe to profound hearing losses (Webster, 1984), as the vocabulary is suited to adults and the sentences are rather long.

Speaks and Jerger (1965) developed the Synthetic Sentence Identification Test, in which the test materials do not form natural-seeming sentences. They are statistical approximations to English connected speech, and have found acceptance in aural rehabilitation, in the assessment of central auditory dysfunction, and may be used in assessing the use of hearing aids. Dubno and Dirks (1983) suggested ways in which their reliability may be optimised. They are not generally suitable for work with hearing-impaired children, especially young children, but rather with the postlingually deafened adult.

The North American Speech Perception In Noise (SPIN) test (Kalikow et al., 1977), adapted for use in Australia by Upfold and Smither (1981), has taken the use of context further. Half of the sentences, presented in speech babble, contain high-predictability, and half contain low-predictability, test items. The subject is asked to identify the final word in each sentence. The score is obtained from differences between the tallies on high- and low-predictability items. The SPIN test finds its main applications in aural rehabilitation, hearing-aid fitting, and assessing central auditory dysfunction, since the speech information is degraded by the babble, with a decrease in redundancy and consequently increased perceptual difficulty for the central auditory system.

Children do not discriminate speech in noise as well as adults (Mills, 1975), and the use of a signal-to-noise ratio of +9 dB was suggested by Keith (1981b) for standardised speech material, such as the WIPI or other word list tests, with children. Somewhat surprisingly at first thought, performance-intensity functions can be obtained for words and short sentences from children as young as 2 years of age. The Pediatric Speech Intelligibility Test (PSI – Jerger et al., 1981; Jerger et al., 1983; Jerger and Jerger, 1984) was developed with a restricted message set and concrete target words, allowing performance-intensity functions to be assessed for the perception of sentences and words in the quiet and at varying message-to-competition ratios.

Conclusion: Need for Clarification of Objectives

From overviews of recent work on the perception of speech by hearing-impaired children, such as those by Dermody and Mackie (1987) and Markides (1987), it is clear that speech perception tests are recognised as an essential part of the assessment of the child's hearing abilities. However, the plethora of available tests shows a lack of clarity about the use and purpose of techniques for measuring speech perception. A clarification of objectives is needed to put speech perception tests on a sound basis for regular clinical and educational use. To give one example of what might be done, research with hearing children (Bever, 1970; Strohner and Nelson, 1974) has indicated that in developing sentence comprehension strategies in English, young children tend to rely on pragmatic and semantic strategies, whereas older children rely mainly on word order to decide on the basic grammatical relations. However, following a cross-linguistic study, Bates et al. (1984) expressed caution about the existence of universal hypotheses of language structure. They felt that young children aged 2–5 years may not be able to make full use of some interpretative cues for sentence comprehension because they cannot appreciate the discourse functions of the cues.

Generally, the writer believes that for routine clinical work the most promising information about a child's hearing for speech will be obtained from speech pattern tests for phoneme perception and from sentence materials for perception of connected speech. As with Merklein (1981), it is difficult to see a continuing role for word lists.

Enhancement of the Intelligibility of Perceived Speech

On a different but related topic, work on speech perception in hearing-impaired children can suggest to teachers and therapists ways of enhancing their own speech to make it more intelligible to the children. There are many publications on the linguistic styles used by teachers and others to classes and groups of hearing-impaired children (Craig and Collins, 1970; Hutton and Whatton, 1981; Kyle and Allsop, 1982; Wood et al., 1986; Wood, 1991). There is also a long history of research on the characteristics of clear speech (Snidecor et al., 1944; Tolhurst, 1957; Nooteboom, 1973; Gay, 1978). However, studies of speech characteristics that affect the intelligibility of speech to hearing-impaired listeners are relatively recent.

Picheny et al. (1985) presented a set of nonsense sentences ('Their pail bails my tone') spoken by three male talkers to five adult listeners who had moderate to severe inner-ear hearing losses, increasing with frequency. The talkers recorded 40 'conversational sentences' alternating with 40 'clear sentences'. For conversational sentences, the talker was asked to recite the sentences in the way he spoke in ordinary conversation. For clear sentences he was asked to speak as clearly as possible, as if trying to communicate in a noisy environment or with a hearing-impaired listener. He had also to enunciate consonants more carefully and with greater vocal effort than in conversational speech, and to avoid slurring words together. Talkers were asked to stress nouns, adjectives and verbs in both types of sentence.

The results gave a 17% advantage overall in perception of clear versus conversational speech. The difference depended on the listener and talker to only a small extent, and was independent of presentation level and frequency-gain characteristics. Analysis of segmental-level errors showed that the increase in intelligibility with clear sentences occurred across all phoneme classes.

In a second study, Picheny et al. (1986) reported acoustic analyses of conversational and clear speech. They found that speaking rate decreased substantially for clear speech, and was achieved by inserting pauses between words and lengthening the durations of individual speech sounds. Also, while the vowels were modified or reduced and word-final stop bursts were often not released in conversational speech, the vowels were modified to a lesser extent and the stop bursts, as well as almost all word-final consonants, were released in clear speech. Further, the intensities for plosives, especially stop consonants, were greater in clear than in conversational speech. Interestingly, since the listeners were hearing-impaired with poorer hearing at the higher frequencies, the changes in the long-term spectrum were small, so that speaking clearly was not equivalent to giving the speech a high-frequency emphasis, though it would be of practical interest to try such an experiment.

Speechreading

Watching a talker's lips is like hearing speech by eye instead of by ear. Hearing speech by eye in speechreading shares the attributes of hearing written words by eye in reading (Williams, 1982), where inner speech serves a mediating role for most hearing people (Conrad, 1972a, b, 1979; Moores, 1970).

Speechreading assists hearing individuals in speech perception but, for most of the time, speech can be understood perfectly well without speechreading. The situation is quite different for profoundly and the more severely deaf individuals. If they wish to understand speech, if only imperfectly, they need to speechread. The use of residual hearing by itself seldom offers a full alternative.

Speechreading and hearing

A very useful test of primary modality for speech perception in hearing and hearing-impaired children was described by Seewald et al. (1985). The test material consisted of the four 25-item lists of the Word Intelligibility by Picture Identification (WIPI) test, which were video-recorded. Lists 1 and 2 were prepared for an auditory/visual conflict condition by pairing, for example, the visual production of the word 'school' from list 1 with the acoustic production of 'broom' from list 2, and so on, with the vowels matched but not the consonants. List 3 was used for auditory-alone, and list 4 for vision-alone testing. Responses from conflict lists were scored twice, once for accuracy for video-presented, and once for audio-presented, stimuli. Subtracting the visual from the auditory performance score gave the primary modality for speech perception (PMSP).

Results from 15 hearing and 69 mildly to profoundly deaf children aged 7;5 to 14;8 years, with known or suspected congenital hearing impairment, showed the PMSP score decreasing through the auditory portion of the PMSP continuum into the visual part, as hearing loss increased ($r^2 = 0.84$). All hearing children had PMSP scores which were strongly auditory, and all children with hearing losses greater than 90 dB HL were strongly visual. All children with losses of more than 95 dB HL had scores within the visual part, even with their auditory amplification functioning properly. The shift from auditory to visual speech perception as the primary modality occurred between 80 and 90 dB HL. Hearing loss and auditory word identification performance accounted for about 90% of the PMSP variance. The authors thus concluded that the relative use of hearing or vision in speechreading of words was almost entirely related to the children's hearing level and aided speech reception. Such clear-cut results are not often found for congenitally hearing-impaired children. It would therefore be of interest to replicate this study.

Although speechreading is like hearing by eye, speechreading is not as effective as hearing by ear in perceiving speech. Even highly skilled speechreaders have difficulty in perceiving some parts of speech. Many phonemes and words, such as the homophenous words 'man' and 'ban', look very similar on the lips. A large proportion of speech sounds cannot be seen on the lips, as they are produced in the rear of the mouth. Thus some of the vowels can be distinguished only with difficulty in speechreading, as their articulation is barely reflected in lip position contrasts. Also, vowel intelligibility may be poorer for CVCs with highly visible consonants, especially fricatives and labiodentals (Montgomery et al., 1987). Only about 40% of speech sounds in English are visible on the lips (Bode et al., 1982).

Hence speechreading skills depend heavily on filling the gaps between the visually apparent phonemes, or visemes, by drawing on linguistic and other contextual information. Skilled speechreaders are linguistically highly able. They are also practised 'gamblers' – or perhaps 'informed guessers' would be a better way to describe them (Lyxell and Ronnberg, 1987). For the profoundly deaf speechreader the knowledge of vocabulary and syntax, which informs the guessing of phonemes which do not have visemic counterparts, has to be learned via residual hearing and poor visual information to begin with. Such an impoverished cycle implies a difficult and protracted learning process for obtaining skills in speechreading, even though normal human vision, like hearing, has a wide dynamic range and can resolve fine time differences down to 20ms (Geldard, 1972).

Hearing people can increase their speech perception in noisy situations considerably if they can see the talker's face. The advantage is equivalent to increasing the signal-to-noise ratio by about 15 dB (Sumby and Pollack, 1954). Seeing the talker's face increases speech perception from minimal to 80% correct or more for sentences presented at about 10 dB below the noise level, for noise of uniform spectrum from 100 to 7000 Hz (Miller et al., 1951). The reasons seem to be fourfold. First, acoustic cues for place of articulation, unlike the cues for voicing and nasality, are of low amplitude, are mainly above 1 kHz, and are defined by narrow, often transient, spectral features (Kryter, 1970). Conversely, speechreading is particularly effective for the visual perception of place (Binnie et al., 1976; Boothroyd, 1978). Secondly, seeing the lips of the talker provides additional reinforcing information to hearing speech at the segmental level. This redundancy of speechreading on hearing helps to reinforce perception of consonants, particularly the voiced consonants. It also aids perception of some vowels. Hence, when the auditory segmental information is masked by noise, it can be seen visually on the lips of the talker (MacLeod and Summerfield, 1987, 1990). Thirdly, speechreading allows the hearer to concentrate on the talker rather than the noise, by providing visual cues on the timing of the speech signal, and fourthly it provides paralinguistic information about the broader context, such as the communication environment and characteristics of the talker.

While the use of vision in speechreading assists the perception of speech in noise by hearing people, the use of hearing can help the speechreader. A number of studies (Utley, 1946; O'Neill, 1954; Brannon, 1961; Hull and Alpiner, 1976; Erber, 1979) found that vision alone permits the attainment of about 50% of speech intelligibility, which would be 100% in the auditory modality. Hearing, even at minimal levels, adds considerably to the comprehension of visible speech (Hull and Alpiner, 1976). Even auditory information limited to voice intensity cues, F_o or to low-pass (200 Hz) speech can lead to significant improvements in speech perception (Plant et al., 1984b; Grant, 1987b; Rosen et al., 1987), especially for listeners with no auditory frequency selectivity or who have narrow dynamic ranges above 500 Hz. Other work (Faulkner et al., 1990) suggests that profoundly deaf listeners who can use information from the manner of articulation are aided more in speechreading by selected speech pattern combinations than by exposure to whole speech.

Processing of speechread information

In a famous study, McGurk and MacDonald (1976) reported that hearing 'ba' while watching a video-recorded 'ga' on the talker's lips gave rise to the illusion of perceiving 'da'. This finding has been confirmed and extended by others, producing fusions, as in the above 'ba' + 'ga' = 'da', where the percept shares phonological features of the phoneme and viseme but results in the perception of a new consonant, and blends where both consonants are perceived, as in 'ba' (seen) + 'ga' (heard) = 'bda' or 'bga' (MacDonald and McGurk, 1978; Summerfield, 1979). Audiovisual fusions have also been reported for vowels (Summerfield and McGrath, 1984). Subjectively, the subject has the experience of hearing the illusory syllable. Even when told to report only the acoustic component, the subject reports the illusory compromise (Summerfield and McGrath, 1984).

This finding suggests strongly that both the heard and the seen syllables are processed at some stage by the same perceptual mechanism. What sort of process might this be? Both share a common source in articulation. It might therefore be that the speechreader refers both visual and auditory speech inputs to an articulatory processor. The modification of the auditory input by incompatible visual input in the audiovisual fusions supports such a view. However, such fusions are heard and not seen, and not some heard and some seen, which may raise problems for an explanation based only on an articulatory processor.

Audiovisual fusions have forced researchers in speech perception to take account of visual information besides the auditory input. That fusions or blends are obtained, rather than that either the visual or the auditory input is dominant, suggests that speech perception is to some degree amodal, and not as acoustically special as some would have it (Diehl et al., 1991; Fowler, 1991). Further, it raises the question of whether speechreading plays only a gap-filling function when speech is difficult to hear, or whether vision is of use in speech perception even when the speech sounds are heard clearly.

We know from our earlier discussion that speechreading serves to fill at least some of the gaps when speech is imperfectly heard. Further Reisberg (1978) reported that, when the speech is clearly heard, hearing subjects' performance in shadowing speech improved with vision, even when the visual information was only a loudspeaker grille. Thus, one function of vision while perceiving speech is to keep attention on the speech source. Reisberg et al. (1981) also showed that their subjects' auditory attention was associated with where they were looking. If they looked at a loudspeaker presenting the speech, their recall of the speech material was better than if they looked at a loudspeaker which produced irrelevant material. The conclusion is that we can better attend auditorily to speech while we are looking at the source than if we look at the source of alternative material. This conclusion confirms our everyday experience. It is of practical relevance for speechreading the teacher in noisy classrooms, where there are many possible competing speech sources from chattering children (compare Markides, 1989a).

In subsequent experiments Reisberg et al. (1987) showed that speechreading improved speech perception by 15% when shadowing a foreign language, when the speech material was hard to understand rather than hard to hear. Similar findings were obtained when shadowing complex speech material in English, the subject's native language. Thus speechreading added to the understanding of the speech, even when the acoustic signal was heard clearly. Together, these findings suggest that speechreading and hearing share the same perceptual processing system at some level. Tactile representations of speech can be perceived phonologically, as we have seen. There is thus a sense in which speech perception is amodal.

Costello (1957), Myklebust (1964) and Fry (1966) were among the first to develop the insight that speechreading, which monitors speech articulation, could be processed by a phonological code, based on hearing, which allows thinking to be done in words as inner speech. This view gathered adherents in subsequent years, covering reading and writing also (Morton, 1970; Locke, 1978). It is of interest to review the literature on speechreading and auditory speech perception from infancy, to assess to what extent speech perception develops synchronously in the two modalities.

We noted that the fetus is responsive to audiofrequency stimuli, that newborn babies are responsive to sounds, particularly complex sounds rather than tones, and that young infants of a few months old can make phonemic distinctions. Newborn babies and young infants show a preference for looking at human faces in a variety of test situations (e.g. Wilcox, 1969). According to Kuhl (1980), 4-month-old infants can distinguish all, or almost all, the acoustic cues at the segmental level of speech, while Spelke (1976) found that infants of the same age could associate sight with sound. With these findings in place, suggesting the potential in young infants for associating lip movements with speech, Dodd (1979) studied attention to speech by 12 hearing infants aged 10–16 weeks, when the speech and lip movements were in and out of synchrony. She found that the infants attended significantly more to the in-synchrony presentations, a result congruent with the view that the visual and auditory inputs are mediated by a single code, which is not specific to either modality. A similar conclusion can be drawn from Dodd (1972), who reported that the babbling patterns of 9- to 12-month-old infants were affected by auditory/visual stimulation, in the form of 'babbling' by the experimenter, and eye contact, probably including watching of lip movements, with the experimenter, but not by auditory or social (play) stimulation alone.

Although these studies suggested that infants can associate lip movements with hearing for speech in their first year of life, they did not show that the infants were speechreading. Therefore Dodd (1987) further studied a group of 18–36-month-old infants to test their ability to speechread known words presented in a carrier sentence ('Show me the _____') in a picture identification task. The target word was spoken by the experimenter in a pre-test and silently mouthed in the test condition. Although performance was poorer in the test (speechreading) condition than in the pre-test (heard) condition, the speechread task was completed significantly above chance level, showing that the infants could speechread familiar words. Interestingly, the infants understood easily that a speechread stimulus corresponded to a word.

These results indicate that speechreading and hearing for speech develop synchronously in infancy, and that speech stimuli in the auditory and visual modalities are processed together, suggesting that the processing is amodal. Infants combine the two speech-information inputs, rather than treating them separately.

Nevertheless, the correlation between scores on auditory-only and speechreading-only performance for the same test material may be low, or statistically non-significant. For instance, Raney et al. (1984) found no significant correlation between auditory and visual performances on CID Everyday Sentences for 30 normally hearing and sighted, or vision-corrected, young adults, implying that the ability to perceive speech in one modality provided little information about speech perception in the other. However, only one speaker was used, as was the case with most of the studies described above. The perception of speech can differ markedly between auditory and visual perception of different speakers (Lesner, 1988).

Speechreading and hearing impairment

Vision can play an important part in the perception of those consonants, vowels and diphthongs which are articulated on the lips and from the middle to the front of the mouth. The articulation of these speech sounds gives the hearing-impaired child the most help in speechreading. The lips, tongue and mouth opening provide the most useful information. Some visual cues are not easy to perceive, however, especially for cognate consonantal groupings, such as /f/ versus /v/, where the distinction is conveyed by slightly different positioning of the upper teeth on the lower lip, and /p/ versus /b/, where the lips are first shut and then separated. The reader is referred to Jeffers and Barley (1971) and Berg (1976b) for a description of the speechreading cues for English phonemes. There is a large literature devoted to the performance of hearing-impaired people on speechreading tests, and on test development, materials, talker characteristics, environmental conditions and non-verbal cues (O'Neill and Oyer, 1961; Berger, 1972; Berg, 1976b; Farwell, 1976; Davis and Hardick, 1981; Sims, 1982; De Filippo and Sims, 1988).

Although we know a great deal about the performance of hearing-impaired people on speechreading tests, and about many factors which affect their speechreading, we are not so well informed about how their linguistic ability affects their ability to speechread, despite the well-established connection between linguistic ability and hearing loss (Berger, 1972; Bench and Bamford, 1979; Conrad, 1979; Quigley and Kretschmer, 1982). It is difficult to know whether the performance of children in tests of speechreading is due to perception of information from the talker's lips and face, or whether it is the child's knowledge of language which is being assessed. Conrad (1979), for example, argued that there were two parts to the question of the proficiency of hearing-impaired children in speechreading. The first was how well the children use speechreading as a perceptual skill involving both vision and residual hearing; the second was how to devise the language material to be speechread.

A recent study by Fletcher (1986) has provided evidence that hearing-impaired children may have a special skill in processing visual information analogous to the lip openings characteristic of English vowels. He set up target dots on a video screen which could be moved vertically through intervals representing the range of lip openings found in the production of vowels. The children's task was to align a feedback dot with the target dot via small light-emitting diodes attached to their lips. Fletcher used children aged 5;7 to 14;1 years for this task. His group of 10 severely to profoundly deaf children showed higher velocities of lip movement, and shorter latencies in reaching goal positions, than a group of 10 hearing children, though both groups were equally accurate. Since the hearing-impaired children performed the task more quickly than the hearing children, it followed that they were more skilled. It was not clear, however, whether the higher skill lay in more rapid perception of the target shift, or in exercising the lips to align the feedback dot with the target, namely whether the skill was enhanced in the perceptual or motor aspects.

Coding for speechreading

Oral education of profoundly deaf children can also affect their speechreading ability, which raises the question of how the speechread information is coded in perception. Dodd (1976) showed that a group of prelingually profoundly deaf children aged 9–12 years consistently employed phonological rules in the use of consonants to name pictures. Their phonological processes were very similar to those of younger hearing children but, although it appeared normal, the phonological development of these profoundly deaf children was delayed. This finding raised the question of whether the phonology was acquired through an acoustic trace reinforced by speech teaching, or through internalising a speechread trace. In a second experiment with 12- to 16-year-old children, Dodd used nonsense words, which the children could not have been taught to speak, and which they could not hear in the experiment. In one condition the children had to speechread the nonsense words and, in a second condition, to read them. The results showed that the phonological rules had in the first, real word-naming experiment predicted the pronunciation of the nonsense words in the second. Further, the children speechreading the nonsense words performed more like the children in the first experiment, than when reading. These results implied that speechreading was the source for the development of the phonology. This outcome was supported by a further study (Dodd and Hermelin, 1977), in which profoundly congenitally deaf children made significantly fewer speechreading errors for homophone pairs predicted as easy to speechread than pairs predicted as hard to speechread.

The overall conclusion to be drawn from Dodd's work is that prelingually profoundly deaf children can acquire a spoken phonology derived from speechreading, similar to that of hearing children, but at a slower rate, possibly because of more slowly developing language ability. Those errors which do not follow the same pattern of errors found in hearing children can be explained on the basis of speech segments which are hard to speechread.

This explanation was supported by Campbell and Wright (1989), who assessed immediate recall for written CV lists in orally educated congenitally deaf teenagers and hearing controls. The deaf teenagers showed a significant consonant 'lipreadability' effect. Thus, the written syllables were harder for them to recall if those syllables contained consonants such as /D, SH and Z/, whose place of articulation is not visually distinctive. By contrast, syllables were easier to recall if they contained visually distinctive consonants, such as /F, TH and B/. Campbell and Wright concluded that phonological representation was poor for written consonants which are hard to speechread. No such effect was found for the hearing controls. Therefore, while the deaf teenagers were using a phonological code, that code produced a different performance in the immediate recall of written CV lists from that of the hearing children.

Conrad (1979) argued that we did not know, in an absolute sense, how well hearing-impaired children could speechread in everyday communication if we did not know about their language ability. In this sense the validity of results obtained on many tests of speechreading is open to question, with the exception of a few studies which have assessed both speechreading and language ability, usually finding a positive correlation (De Filippo, 1982; Meadow, 1968). Conrad's conclusion from his own work was that not only did children show a decline in speech comprehension with hearing loss because they knew less language, but they also speechread less of what they knew. Even when language ability was considered, the hearing-impaired children continued to have greater difficulty in speechreading with increasing hearing loss. A possible explanation is that hearing-impaired children are weak in the information-processing skills associated with speechreading (see below).

The large range of individual differences in the speechreading ability of hearing-impaired individuals has led to investigations of possible covariates, besides linguistic ability. Several reports have presented results for the effects of intelligence on speechreading. The results are generally very variable (Farwell, 1976; Conrad, 1979), with an overall picture of low to moderate positive correlations. Possibly the more intelligent hearing-impaired individuals are better able to use their language ability as a key to the sequencing and meaning of visemes in speechreading. However, the low values of the reported correlation coefficients suggest that speechreading is difficult to learn. Thus the view of speechreading as a learned communication skill is somewhat questionable. Speechreading appears to improve with age (Farwell, 1976) but whether this improvement is due to an increase in visual perception skills or in language ability (De Filippo, 1982) is unclear.

In conclusion, more research is needed on the development of speechreading skills and their coding, with suitable controls for language ability and intelligence.

Neurophysiology and speechreading

To date, neurophysiological covariates have not proved to be particularly illuminating in speechreading, though significant advances have been made in study of the hemispheric lateralisation of differences in visual information processing (Keenan et al., 1989). Earlier suggestions of a link between visual–neural speed and aspects of speechreading skill (Shepherd et al., 1977; Samar and Sims, 1983) were not supported in a more recent study by Ronnberg et al. (1989). The picture is complex, as Ronnberg et al. did find significant correlations for some context–free word discrimination and sign-alphabet conditions for visual–neural peak-to-peak amplitudes.

Further, the neurophysiology involved may be at a lower level of brain organisation. Mead and Lapidus (1989) reported that for 62 hearing and mild to moderately hearing-impaired children, of mean age 10;4 years, the ability to speechread sentences from a silent film was significantly related to psychological differentiation, as expressed in cognitive style, and pre-task skin conductance level, but not to hearing capacity or skin conductance level during the task. Speechreading ability was predicted best by performance on a Rod and Frame test and large increases in skin conductance from pre-task to task, implying that speechreading performance improves with a marked increase in level of arousal. This outcome is congruent with the research of Samar and Sims (1984), who suggested that sensitivity to the timing of a light flash was related to their subjects' expectations in speechreading.

Use of cues in speechreading by hearing-impaired individuals

We saw that only some 40% of phonemes are visible on the lips, and that speechreading is slow to be learned. Also, a relatively high proportion of hearing-impaired individuals have visual defects (Johnson et al., 1981; Gottlieb and Allen, 1985), a large proportion of the profoundly deaf population has poor acoustic short-term memory and coding skills for speech, and profoundly deaf people can have difficulties in dealing with information that is ordered sequentially (Hermelin and O'Connor, 1975; Grove et al., 1979; Grove and Rodda, 1984). We may therefore wonder if speechreading is a realistic option for many prelingually profoundly deaf children, despite some undoubted successes. Speechreading ability, even with the help of residual hearing, develops too slowly for many children to attain sufficient language ability in their early years, creating a linguistic lag which is difficult to overcome (Brasel and Quigley, 1977) and which, in turn, reduces the efficiency of speechreading.

Little is known about how profoundly deaf people who are good speechreaders go about perceiving speech compared with poor speechreaders, although the issue is not new (Kitson, 1915; Markides, 1989b). This means that the processes underlying speechreading are uncertain, although there are many clues – several of which have been described earlier – to go on. Although there is information about the background to speechreading, such as the articulation of the mouth and lips, the visibility of speech segments, styles of speech, types of speech material, lighting effects, paralinguistic cues, etc. (Lott and Levy, 1960; Erber, 1972; Franks, 1979; De Filippo and Sims, 1988; Markides, 1989b; Silverman and Kricos, 1990), little is known of how the expert speechreader uses them, or even if some of them are used to any great extent in any given condition. Research into the skills used by expert as compared with inexpert speechreaders is therefore a matter of pressing need.

A method of investigating some of the processes involved was suggested by the work of Busby et al. (1984), who investigated vowel perception in four profoundly deaf children aged 13–14 years in auditory-alone, vision-alone and audiovisual conditions. They used multidimensional scaling analysis of the confusion matrices to assess the underlying dimensions, and the individual differences found on the dimensions (compare Erber, 1972). Significant individual differences were found in parameter emphases in the auditory and audiovisual conditions. In a further paper, Busby et al. (1988) assessed the identification of consonants in /a/ – C – /a/ nonsense syllables by four profoundly deaf children aged 13–14 years. Performance was better with vision alone than with aided hearing alone. In an audiovisual condition the children predominantly combined the acoustic parameter of voicing with the visual signal. There was considerable consistency for the visual perception of vowels by lip opening, and consonants by place of articulation. These two studies suggest, in the context of identifying what makes expert readers, a method for assessing how vowels and consonants are perceived, which may be used with speechreaders of varying speechreading expertise.

Speechreading of connected speech in some hearing-impaired individuals seems to be influenced by their skills in information processing rather than their hearing loss. Lyxell and Ronnberg (1989), for example, explored verbal inference-making ability by sentence- and word-completion tests in hearing and in mildly to moderately deaf adults, finding that only sentence-completion was correlated with speechreading performance. The contribution from working memory and word-completion was mainly through their contribution to sentence-completion, for both hearing and hearing-impaired speechreaders, whose performances were similar.

Given evidence that hearing-impaired individuals are generally less able or no more skilled at speechreading than hearing people (Conrad, 1977b; De Filippo, 1984), do they use the same psychological processes in speechreading as hearing subjects? According to Dodd et al. (1983), orally educated prelingually profoundly deaf children could not be distinguished from hearing children in serial recall behaviour, including the recency effect, for speechread lists. They also reported that both hearing and profoundly deaf children did not demonstrate the recency advantage when the speechread lists are followed by a speechread suffix. Since it is likely that phonological processing is required for these effects to occur, it appears that both the hearing and hearing-impaired children used a phonological code. This is not so surprising since even congenitally profoundly deaf users of sign language show some evidence of phonemic confusions in recalling words (Hanson, 1982).

At the present state of knowledge, differences between speechreading in hearing and hearing-impaired people seem to be due principally to differences in information processing skills and language ability including inner speech, provided that allowance is made for possible visual defects.

Training in speechreading

We have referred to the study by Raney et al. (1984), who found that, for young hearing adults, the ability to understand CID Everyday Sentences presented in the audio-only mode did not correlate well with the ability to understand these sentences when presented by video-channel. This result suggested that auditory and visual skills can operate separately, as well as in conjunction. High-level visual skills do not necessarily imply high-level auditory skills, and generalisation of skills from one modality to the other need not occur. Although separate training for consonant perception of the visual and auditory systems will improve combined visual and auditory sentence recognition (Walden et al., 1981), unimodal training may be limited to the system used and not generalise well to other systems. However, Crawford et al. (1986) have argued that improvements in speechreading are likely to be affected by methodological and subject differences. It may be, for example, that subjects with low pretraining scores on speechreading tests will improve significantly with extended training, but show little or no change with short-term training.

Generally, it is hard to find evidence for successful training in the visual modality (De Filippo, 1990), which is a worry if we wish to regard speechreading as a skill which can be learned. However, Dodd et al. (1989) have recently described a study in which hearing-impaired students used a 3-hour videocassette containing nine lessons over a period of 5 weeks. The students showed a significant increase in speechreading performance in comparison with a control group which did not study the lessons. This report provided more convincing evidence than some of the earlier work on speechreading training, especially since speechreading generalised to unfamiliar speakers and materials.

Practice alone, rather than specific training, improves speechreading performance in both hearing and hearing-impaired subjects (Bannister and Britten, 1982; Squires and Dancer, 1986; Lesner et al., 1987; Warren et al., 1989). The improvement in performance typically ranges from about 3% to 10%. This percentage is of the same order as effects often ascribed to training, and occurs with both massed and distributed practice. Most subjects tend to show an increase in performance in the early trials, soon reaching a performance plateau, which continues for an extended period of time. Hence controls for practice effects are needed before claims for the efficacy of training in speechreading can be accepted as valid (Warren et al., 1989), particularly in the early phases of training. Few studies have included such controls up to the present time.

Given also that until quite recently there has been surprisingly little research on talker effects, which are known to be significant (Kricos and Lesner, 1985; Lesner, 1988), and that extended training may be confounded with improvements in language ability (Conrad, 1979), much of the research which argues for improvements in speechreading ability with training has to be regarded as suspect. The situation is yet further confounded with performance measures, type of material and task, type and amount of feedback, etc. (Fenn and Smith, 1987; Lesner et al., 1987; Small and Infante, 1988; Markides, 1989a).

In concluding, we note that the area is now the subject of extensive research, and hence useful findings can be confidently expected in the near future. Nevertheless, definitive work on training in speechreading will need to control for practice and language learning effects, which now bedevil the interpretation of most published research.

Chapter 4
The Produced Speech of Hearing-impaired Children

Deaf speech is characterised by features that give it distinctive properties, as described in this chapter. Also outlined are some approaches to speech training and work with speech-training aids. Deaf speech is generally difficult to understand. An account is given of studies that have attempted to explore some of the reasons for the poor intelligibility of deaf speech, with suggestions for further work.

Children who are born severely or profoundly hearing impaired or become deafened soon after birth have great difficulties in acquiring speech. Such children not only hear the speech of others very imperfectly, even if aided, they also have problems in monitoring the sounds of their own voices through auditory feedback. Thus differences in babbling have been found between hearing and hearing-impaired infants as early as the second 6 months of life (Oller et al., 1985). The greater the degree of hearing loss, the more difficult it is to learn speech, whether monitoring and controlling the loudness and the rhythms of the speech, in articulating speech sounds, or in co-articulating combinations of speech sounds (Smith, 1975a; Geffner and Freeman, 1980).

However, this is only part of the problem. Having learned some speech, hearing-impaired children need to maintain it. To do so involves monitoring their speech by hearing, touch and kinaesthesis, but this monitoring is impaired because of the impaired hearing, and so the speech tends to deteriorate. It is therefore not surprising that deaf children differ from hearing children in cerebral control of their speech production. Hearing children's cerebral control for produced speech appears to be left-lateralised, whereas deaf children show more symmetrical patterns of cerebral control (Marcotte and La Barba, 1985).

Older children and adults who become deafened after speech acquisition also experience deterioration in their speech, because they can no longer adequately hear what they are saying, but the order in which aspects of their speech deteriorate with time is controversial. It has been thought, following short-duration auditory feedback studies with hearing people, that the suprasegmental features deteriorate rather than features at the segmental level (Ladefoged, 1967; Ternstrom et al., 1988; Ball, 1991). Investigation of seven long-term postlingually totally deaf subjects by Waldstein (1990), however, indicated that all classes of speech sounds were affected. There is also evidence that the speech of people who become postlingually deaf in their earlier years deteriorates in both segmental and suprasegmental aspects more than for those who become deafened later (Plant and Hammarberg, 1983; Waldstein, 1990).

Since produced speech in hearing children is accompanied by monitoring the voice, speech is not so much a complex motor skill as a complex perceptual–motor skill. In developing speech, hearing children shape their speech sounds to match the phonology of their language by selecting those sounds which reflect the syntax and semantics of the language. For hearing children, learning to speak is a natural part of development. Hearing-impaired children on the other hand have to be taught their speech. Because they cannot, or can only partly, rely on auditory feedback in monitoring their speech, they have to use their visual, tactile or kinaesthetic senses to a greater degree than hearing children, depending on their degree of hearing loss. It proves very difficult to learn fluent speech through these senses, because the feedback they provide is less precise than feedback through hearing. As a result the speech of hearing-impaired children contains interjections (Smith, 1975b), is rarely as intelligible to the listener as that of hearing children (Bernstein et al., 1988) and the central phonetic processing as well as the speech may suffer (Fletcher et al., 1985).

Selected characteristics of the speech of hearing-impaired individuals will now be reviewed. We will also investigate how their speech may be trained. A substantial portion of the chapter will be spent on the intelligibility of deaf speech, as the understanding of speech is of major importance to communication.

Deaf Speech

The speech of hearing-impaired individuals tends to be characterised by features which set it apart from the speech of others, though the speech of a given deaf person does not necessarily show all of them.

Articulation

The classic study in the area of articulation is that of Hudgins and Numbers (1942), who found five types of vowel error and seven types of consonant error in the speech of 192 mildly to profoundly deaf children aged between 8 and 20 years. The vowel errors, in order of preponderance, consisted of substitutions, vowel neutralisations, creation of two syllables from one vowel, simplification of diphthongs by splitting them into two separate vowels or omitting one component, and vowel nasalisations. The consonant errors, also in order of preponderance, consisted of initial consonant deletions, devoicing of stops, insertions and deletions, final consonant deletions, denasalisations, substitutions, and vowel insertions.

Deaf people learning to speak can develop a different kind of articulatory coordination from that of hearing speakers. For example, their jaw and tongue positions in vowel production following consonants may not vary consistently (Tye-Murray, 1987), although deaf speakers tend to move the body of their tongue in a similar way for all vowels (Tye-Murray, 1991). Further, the speech of deaf individuals is characterised by prolongations of vowels, even in multisyllabic words (Tye-Murray and Woodworth, 1989), associated with vowel neutralisation which involves overlapping of F_1 and F_2 formants (Angelocci et al., 1964; Monsen, 1976; Osberger, 1987).

Vowels are particularly difficult for prelingually profoundly deaf children to learn, probably because the articulators rarely come into contact in vowel production, preventing tactile feedback (Povel and Wansink, 1986). Monsen (1976) showed for hearing-impaired adolescents that F_2 remained stable around 800 Hz, irrespective of the vowel the speaker was attempting to produce. The result was reduced phonological space when accompanied by a restricted range for F_1. Similar findings have been reported for languages other than English (Shukla, 1989).

Vowel production is important in most spoken languages, including English, because vowels form the nuclei of words (Osberger, 1987). They often signal the adjacent consonant by formant transitions, so that a poorly produced vowel may result in misperception of not only the intended vowel but the adjacent consonant as well. Accuracy of vowel production is highly correlated with the speech intelligibility of profoundly deaf speakers (Monsen, 1976). Although F_1 is associated with changes in lower jaw movement and thus with vertical tongue movement, F_2 is associated with forward and backward movements of the tongue (Fant, 1962), which are difficult for hearing-impaired speakers to perceive. Monsen ascribed the difficulties in articulation of F_2 by his hearing-impaired adolescents to this reduced perception. Distorted articulation in the speech of hearing-impaired children is also defined by prolonged articulatory contacts (Angelocci, 1962), slow articulatory movements (Monsen, 1978), and slow articulation of syllables (Stevens et al., 1978; Osberger and McGarr, 1982).

Besides distortion, the speech of hearing-impaired children is remarkable for a high incidence of articulatory errors in the form of consonant omissions at the ends of words, phrases and sentences, which are the result of misplacing the tongue and of poor control of the aerodynamic flow (Markides, 1970; Smith, 1975a; Mencke et al., 1985). The reader will recall, however, that Hudgins and Numbers found consonants were omitted more commonly in the initial than the final position. The apparent discrepancy may be due to sampling differences and/or the type of test material (compare Geffner and Freeman, 1980). Markides (1983) reported for profoundly deaf and partially hearing children of primary and secondary school age that omissions were more common for final consonants, and substitutions were more common for initial consonants.

Smith (1975b) additionally noted interposed sounds in the speech of deaf children. She observed recurring patterns of excrescent or interjected sounds associated with movements of the articulators, and attributed them to slowness of movement, overshoot resulting in a greater than normal degree of constriction to yield affricate-like substitutions or glides, mistimed laryngeal action, and mistimed velar action. Tongue action was involved in 43% and lip action in 29% of the occurrences.

The speech of hearing-impaired people is also notable for the insertion of frequent and lengthy inter- and intra-word pauses (Osberger and McGarr, 1982; Stathopoulos et al., 1986). Their speech contains unusual segmentation, reducing its intelligibility, though Abdelhamied et al. (1990) were able to achieve automatic recognition of deaf speech by using these inter- and intra-word pauses to attain recognition rates as high as 93% and 82% for isolated words and connected speech respectively, only about 5% less than for the speech of hearing people. They argued that deaf speech has its own norm, showing typical and systematic patterns.

Suprasegmentals

Many profoundly deaf children produce suprasegmental features which are traditionally associated with 'deaf speech' (Angelocci et al., 1964; Martony, 1968; McGarr and Harris, 1983). Partially hearing children may show difficulties also, but not always if their language development level is considered (Weiss et al., 1985). Such errors or difficulties are described variously as problems with prosody, intonation, nasality, pitch, breath control and voice quality. Also, timing errors, involving prolonged stop closure duration where the time interval between starting the sound and releasing it with a burst of air is prolonged, have been described in semi-intelligible young hearing-impaired adults (Whitehead, 1991).

Typically deaf children speak stressed and unstressed syllables with the same duration or with less of a difference in duration than hearing children. Tye-Murray et al. (1987) suggested that it may be more problematical for deaf speakers to produce long stress patterns than short ones. Thus not only do hearing-impaired children need to be taught correct articulation at the phonetic level, where the sounds have relatively little individual meaning, but they must also be taught to combine these sounds into connected speech, and to appreciate the contribution of the suprasegmental aspects.

It is of interest to consider whether deaf speakers' problems in producing stress patterns are due to impaired motor control of speech or to linguistic factors. To answer this question, Tye-Murray and Folkins (1990) asked deaf and hearing subjects to speak sets of homogeneous syllable strings which they could tap out with a finger, and hence could understand. Strain gauges monitoring lower lip and jaw movements revealed that deaf and hearing subjects produced different durations and displacements for stressed and unstressed syllables. There was no evidence that motor abilities affected the production of stress patterns in the deaf speakers. Thus when the deaf subjects understood a given stress pattern they could speak it, even when they did not articulate the segments correctly. This outcome showed that the deaf subjects were not aware of phonemic distinctiveness via stress.

Voice pitch and quality

Voice pitch, which can be a suprasegmental feature as well as part of voice quality, is directly related to the function of the vocal folds. It is controlled during voicing by the tension of the vocal folds and the subglottal air pressure. In hearing children voice pitch tends to decrease and show lessening variability with age from early infancy (Robb and Saxman, 1985). Measurements of speech fundamental frequency (F_o) in hearing-impaired people, however, have presented mixed and conflicting results. Horii (1982) reported higher than normal F_o values for 12 hearing-impaired girls aged 16–19 years. Leder et al. (1987) found more recently that F_o was significantly higher in profoundly postlingually deaf than in hearing men, but not all studies have found voice pitch to be higher in hearing-impaired people. Whitehead (1987), using the pitch rating procedure of Subtelny et al. (1980), compared experts' perceptual judgements of pitch level with F_o values for 156 young males of mean age 19;6 years and 104 young females of mean age 19;2 years with severe to profound hearing losses, on an oral reading task. The judgements of pitch level and mean F_o values were significantly related for both male and female subjects. The mean F_o values showed a range of vocal frequencies from below to substantially above normal. The results thus showed that most of the young adults had F_o values not greatly different from those of young hearing adults, and they were judged to have a spoken pitch level at, or not too far removed from, the optimal level. Only a minority, of both males and females, produced spoken pitch judged much above optimal, with associated high F_o values.

Hearing-impaired people may also have unusual voice quality, characterised by over-aspiration, spectral noise and so on. A frequent problem in deaf speakers is over-aspiration of initial voiceless stop and fricative consonants (Hutchinson and Smith, 1976; Whitehead and Barefoot, 1980). The over-aspiration, which may increase the tactile feedback for the speaker, gives a breathy quality to the speech and changes the temporal pattern. It is related to misarticulation rather than faulty laryngeal function.

Harshness of voice, related to spectral noise, in hearing-impaired children has been investigated by Thomas-Kersting and Casteel (1989). They compared spectral noise levels and ratings of perceived vocal effort in the voices of severely to profoundly deaf children in relation to hearing children in the age range of 6–11 years. The spectral noise levels were used as an index of the noise components from 100 to 2500 Hz for sustained vowel production. The results showed that the hearing-impaired children attained significantly higher spectral noise levels and were accorded significantly higher estimates of vocal effort. Thus, this group of hearing-impaired children appeared to expend more effort than the hearing children, which generated 'noisy' speech.

Children with severe to profound prelingual hearing loss have a particular problem in learning to coordinate control of their breathing in producing speech. Without experience to guide them they may attempt to speak on inspiration as well as expiration, using ingressive as well as egressive airstreams. They tend to produce short bursts of speech and then run out of breath, because they do not take sufficient breath before beginning to speak. Their spoken sentences are thus broken up by pauses, which interfere with the speech flow. The pauses make their speech stressful to listen to, and understanding of their message difficult (Hudgins and Numbers, 1942; Calvert and Silverman, 1975; Forner and Hixon, 1977; Monsen, 1979). These problems of coordinating breathing and phonation compound their errors in the articulation of vowels and consonants, and difficulties with suprasegmental features.

Speech Training

To learn speech, congenitally profoundly deaf children must expend very considerable effort and concentration on detail. It is therefore to be expected that so many of them produce speech which is difficult for people with good hearing to comprehend. Deaf children need to control breathing, laryngeal functions and movement of the articulators simultaneously to produce speech. They must do so by controlling these aspects within fine tolerances within accepted time intervals if their speech is to be intelligible.

Thus in training hearing-impaired children in the use of speech, the aims include: producing vocalisations, or phonations, as changes in modes of vibration of the vocal folds; control of voice quality; control of pitch, intensity and deviation; developing and practising imitations; developing, controlling and coordinating respiration, phonation and shape of the supraglottal vocal tract; using residual hearing; acquiring a multisensory feedback system by residual hearing, vision, tactile and kinaesthetic senses; articulating phonemes in meaningful contexts; progressing from phonetic skills to connected speech; and developing a recognition that speech is a means to manipulating and controlling the social environment (Siebert, 1980).

The training of hearing-impaired children to express themselves in speech is a complex, time-consuming and demanding procedure. It requires informed, systematic and sustained effort (Ling, 1976). None the less, even given prolonged training of intelligent, motivated hearing-impaired children by conscientious and competent teachers, it is very rare to find a prelingually profoundly deaf child whose speech is not characterised by some of the properties of deaf speech. Partly as a result of this, formal speech-training drills are losing popularity. The more recent emphasis is on integrating the various stages, especially in integrating phonetic level with phonological level skills (Ling, 1991) and in integrating the teaching of speech with the teaching of language (Ling, 1976, 1979, 1989; Subtelny, 1983; Perigoe and Ling, 1986). There is also emphasis on considering the child's environment, particularly the role of parents and family (Lieberth, 1982).

Besides recommending that speech production be taught with the teaching of language, many writers recommend teaching of speech production alongside training in speech perception (Berg, 1976b; Van Riper, 1978; McDonald, 1980; Novelli-Olmstead and Ling, 1984), because a child attempts to speak by using what has been heard or otherwise recognised. Also, hearing or residual hearing is used to monitor and control speech through auditory feedback and through reference to articulation, the so-called motor theory of speech perception (Liberman et al., 1967). Others have recommended the use of music and singing to facilitate speech and language development (Bang, 1980; Tait, 1986; Dawson, 1990; Heffernan, 1990). Moog and Geers (1985) have reported that intensive instruction with increased teaching effort can improve the academic development and speech production of profoundly deaf children.

A programme for speech training which has significantly influenced the approach of others (Martello, 1981), is that of Ling (Ling and Ling, 1978). Before training, the child's produced speech is assessed. Then the child receives speech therapy, ideally on a daily basis, to attain phonetic and phonological targets in a systematic fashion. This approach establishes stages of speech development, and thus provides targets and goals to be achieved for each stage, following the child from preschool to primary school.

Much of the earlier work had an intuitive–empirical base which has only recently become more experimentally based (Silverman, 1983). Most of the earlier reports were descriptive or anecdotal, without enough rationale, subjects or data, or with insufficient attention paid to experimental design, to permit estimation of their reliability and validity, and potential for generalisation to other cases. Nevertheless, some of the earlier texts remain in current use, because they contain a rich fund of insights, illustrations, tips and techniques on which the speech and language teacher can draw. A distinguished example of such writing is the book by Haycock (1933). The many reprintings of this book provide ample testimony to its usefulness over the years. Haycock (1933) is particularly recommended to the reader who wishes to gain an appreciation of the intricacies involved in the teaching of speech, and who may not have a grasp of the phonetic terminology required by the more modern texts. However, it is not concerned with the use of residual hearing in training speech production, having been written before the widespread use of hearing aids.

There is not space here to review the many recent accounts of speech training programmes, but one informative description is that of Osberger (1983), who considered the role of several important variables in training speech, although no controls were used. She employed an adaptation of Ling's system to conduct and evaluate a speech training programme in both segmental and suprasegmental speech for 21 severely to profoundly deaf preschool children. It appeared from her work that the rate of progress in speech production was very variable, requiring individual instruction. Many children could learn speech patterns through hearing alone, though others needed a very systematic and structured programme to develop their auditory–kinaesthetic or tactile–kinaesthetic feedback loops. The ability to produce a given speech pattern preceded and facilitated its perception. Hence training in the production of a particular speech pattern need not wait until there is evidence that it can be discriminated by hearing from other speech sounds – often a difficult task for young children.

Osberger (1987) has also described in some detail the improvement in vowel production by two profoundly deaf adolescents, one boy and one girl, in training again based on Ling's work. This study included controls for test learning effects, and for training, although the controls for training were hearing individuals. There may be some question about how far the findings can be generalised given the small scale of this study, and about the appropriateness of the controls given the highly individualised nature of the vowel changes observed during treatment. On the other hand, these queries illustrate how very difficult it is to design appropriate studies in this field.

Another noteworthy investigation is that of Abraham and Weiner (1985), who compared the use of meaningful and non-meaningful words with ten severely to profoundly deaf children of mean age 9 years. One group of five children was trained in eight daily sessions by direct imitation of words which could be illustrated by pictures. The words were spoken by the experimenter, with oral and aural cues. The other group of five children received nonsense syllables presented in the same way. Two phonemes were selected for each child from those which the child misarticulated with one phoneme, chosen randomly, as a training phoneme and the other as a control phoneme. Training was conducted with the training phoneme in the initial position for both words and syllables, while the control phoneme was not trained. Abraham and Weiner found that both word and syllable training improved the imitation of target phonemes. Word training was more effective than syllable training for improving correct spontaneous production of trained target phonemes in untrained generalisation words. They rightly pointed out that the efficacy of speech training is directly associated with how well it facilitates generalisation, a characteristic of a skill (Bennett, 1978).

A further well-designed study was that of Perigoe and Ling (1986), in which 12 profoundly deaf children aged from 5 to 8 years were arranged in two groups of six, matched as closely as possible for gender, age, hearing loss, phonetic and phonological speech ability and non-verbal intelligence, and who had similar language abilities. The 'context group' was taught speech by focusing on transferring old and new phonetic level skills to nouns and verbs. The 'function group' was taught by concentrating on transferring phonetic level patterns into the structural elements of language. The children's classroom teachers did not know to which group the children were assigned, though they had children from both groups in their classes. All children received phonetic and phonological training for 15 minutes daily for 40 sessions, and were tested over a year at 3-monthly intervals. Regular classroom speech training was given for the first 3 months, followed by 3 months of no intervention and a final 3 months of intensive speech training. The subjects in both groups improved significantly in both measures of speech after intensive training. The function group also improved significantly in language ability as shown by mean length of utterance scores, and scores on a word-morpheme index. Thus phonological training which emphasised the use of function words also enhanced selected language skills.

Descriptions and reviews of other interesting speech training programmes are conveniently offered by Ling (1976), Subtelny (1980), Lieberth (1982) and Blackwell (1983).

To summarise, we can see that there is increasingly good experimental, as opposed to empirical and descriptive, evidence showing that deaf children can be trained to improve their speech, though success is still limited. The evidence accrues from some well-designed and conducted studies which demonstrate significant gains in speech production for selected variables. It is less clear, however, that the gains persist over time or can be generalised to cognate speech skills. There is obviously a need for well-designed, multivariable speech training studies to resolve such issues.

Speech Training Aids

Boothroyd (1972b) identified many of the requirements for valid work in speech training. Until the early 1970s speech training aids mostly offered somewhat unsophisticated visual or tactile analogues of speech sounds. Most of the early devices were not fully evaluated as aids to speech therapy and, individually, they had relatively little impact on speech training (Prinz, 1985). Some of the devices presented oscilloscope traces of visual likenesses of rather gross aspects of speech sounds, such as the overall speech intensity envelope versus time. They were also physically cumbersome, and frequently fell into disuse after a short initial burst of enthusiastic work.

Some modern speech training aids

Recently speech training aids have become more sophisticated, with the possibilities of selection and identification of salient features of speech. They have also become better engineered to meet the needs of the user. Maki (1983) has reported on applications of the speech spectrograph display as an aid to the development of articulatory skills in adults, enabling identification by the user of significant spectral differences. Visual feedback is useful as an aid to speech therapy, since the visual information may be received confidently as a more objective and immediate source of feedback than the advice of a teacher or therapist (Risberg and Spens, 1967; Maki, 1980) and the user can practise alone once the visual display parameters have been set or modelled by the teacher.

In the 1970s work on the development of tactile vocoders accelerated (Oller et al., 1986). At about the same time the advent of the microprocessor offered increasingly sophisticated options at reasonable cost for speech training aids. A number of computer applications became available, with oscilloscope displays of intensity, frequency, voicing, aspiration, tongue position, etc., sometimes with a cartoon face that could be modified to display selected features. Although such instruments may provide the opportunity to work on a number of speech features, it is usual to concentrate on a few at any one time to avoid confusing the child (Martony, 1972). Boothroyd et al. (1975) used this kind of instrumentation on 42 hearing-impaired, mostly profoundly deaf, children, with both meaningful and non-meaningful speech material. The children were able to reduce speech errors in rehearsed, and to a lesser extent in unrehearsed, speech. However, their overall speech intelligibility did not improve, except in a few cases.

Because the use of most speech training aids requires considerable effort and concentration, they are not suitable for hearing-impaired infants and very young children. Hence, by the time they come to be considered for training with speech aids, these children will already have some speech, acquired from non-instrumental approaches. Invariably, this speech will contain errors. So a common way of beginning the use of speech training aids is in speech error analysis. For example, profoundly deaf children often produce stop consonants which are not clearly identifiable. They may, for example, produce a sound which is not clearly either /p/ or /b/, as a result of a voice-onset time (VOT) which is too short to be clearly /p/ but too long to be readily perceived as /b/. A speech spectrograph display can assist the child to produce /p/ or /b/ with less ambiguity by displaying the differences in VOT. Thus the error is first identified for the child, the correct production of the speech sound is illustrated, and the child is then given repeated practice, commonly as a set of drills (Houde, 1980).

Correct vowel production is difficult for hearing-impaired children, as already noted. The production of vowels may be aided by devices such as the laryngograph (Fourcin and Abberton, 1975; Ball et al., 1990; Ball, 1991), which measures the frequency of vocal fold vibrations via electrodes attached to the throat on either side of the larynx, and pitch extraction devices, such as the Visipitch (Key Elemetrics Corporation), which display voice pitch contours against time, with storage to allow for measurement and analysis of vowel formant frequencies. Povel and Wansink (1986) have described a computer-controlled vowel corrector, which provides information about the identity of vowels spoken in isolation or in monosyllables. The vowels appear on a screen in different locations, the coordinates of which are derived from the vowel spectra. Preliminary results showed that the device was useful for exploring vowel space as well as for learning global differentiation for the vowels. However, the discrimination of spectrally similar vowels was limited, as might be expected. Gulian et al. (1986) have also described a computer-based approach to vowel training with profoundly deaf children. Using the Computer Vowel Trainer to provide visual feedback, they found that changes in perception were feedback- and age-dependent. Younger children taught with the trainer showed more mobility in articulation, and they approximated target vowels more closely than control counterparts taught by conventional methods, with evident progress for back and central vowels particularly. There was also a marked reduction in substitutions with central vowels – a characteristic of deaf speech.

New speech training computer-based aids suitable for use with children have been described by Bernstein et al. (1988), Ferguson et al. (1988), and Mashie et al. (1988). They reviewed the characteristics of deaf speech, and proceeded to devise several computer-based aids. Included were two personal computer-based aids, one for use in the clinic, and the other for use in the child's home. The first assessed speech production by microphone, electro-glottograph, and pneumotachograph and was used for diagnosis, speech training and specification of speech exercises. The second assessed speech by microphone alone, and was used for practice at home between therapy sessions. This combination of personal computers was evaluated with five profoundly deaf children over a 1–2-week period, using an activity log and questionnaire completed by the children's parents. The first system, using both acoustic and physiological measures, was evaluated over 15 months with 15 children, when it was easily incorporated into the clinic and found useful for diagnosis and therapy. These preliminary findings appear encouraging, but further reports of more extensive use on larger numbers of hearing-impaired children are awaited.

Rosen et al. (1987) developed a body-worn microprocessor-based aid which presented only the larynx-frequency pattern of speech, as a sinusoid, because they believed it to be of greater value to profoundly deaf people than the complete acoustic signal. Seemingly, the presence of higher harmonics can give poorer labelling of isolated intonation contrasts, and often minimal gain in spectrally based segmental distinctions. Hence simplification of speech can lead to enhanced speech reception in the auditory modality. We might expect similar simplification of speech to be of advantage in speech training aids, because with some apparatus the complexity of the information provided can reduce the motivation of the hearing-impaired child to improve speech because of perceptual overload. This complexity may even embarrass the therapist with the number of available options.

We conclude on the basis of these comments that the human end-user of speech training aids needs to be considered carefully in the engineering of the device. We also conclude that the initial stages of speech training need to be completed thoroughly and to be well internalised before progressing to subsequent stages.

Cochlear implants as speech training aids

Conventional hearing aids and cochlear implants can be considered as speech training aids, because of the role played by the auditory feedback of speech in speech production. We do not discuss here the use of hearing aids as speech training aids, as this topic has been treated comprehensively elsewhere (e.g. Berg, 1976b; Northern and Downs, 1984), but a few words on the use of cochlear implants are in order.

We would expect cochlear implantees to show improved speech production, and this seems to be the case. Svirsky and Tobey (1991) concluded from a small-scale study that cochlear implantation helped in the production of some vowels. Tobey and Hasenstab (1991) found a significant increase in imitation of the non-segmental aspects of speech (loudness, pitch and duration) after the use of implants in a group of 78 profoundly, and mostly prelingually, deaf children. This increase occurred in only the first year after implantation, whereas imitation of segmental aspects, as in syllables, continued to improve with experience over 2 years. The children's speech intelligibility was significantly higher after implantation than before, though their mean length of utterance remained relatively low. Overall, the improvement in speech production was modest, as found also by Busby et al. (1991), who observed some improvements for consonant, but not vowel, production with training following the cochlear implantation of three prelingually profoundly to totally deaf patients with a multi-electrode device. However, the improvement for consonants rather than for vowels, and the lack of a general corresponding improvement in speech perception, suggested that the improvements were due to tactile–kinaesthetic rather than auditory feedback.

Despite the improved design and engineering of cochlear implants and other speech aids, which makes them increasingly more successful and easier to use, and despite some resulting improvements in speech characteristics and intelligibility, the speech of prelingually profoundly deaf children remains problematical. Apparently, to date, the developments in the engineering only partly help to address the formidable demands on the learning abilities of the deaf child.

Intelligibility of the Produced Speech of Hearing-impaired Children

The perceived intelligibility of speech depends on both its suprasegmental and its segmental features. Speech intelligibility is influenced by stress as the loudness/duration aspect which characterises the relative emphasis given to syllables, words and phrases (Levitt, 1971); intonation, or pitch variations across syllables; voicing, with the production of vowels, voiced consonants and diphthongs; the oral/nasal distinction, which governs the distinction between /m/ and /b/, /n/ and /d/, etc. ('met' versus 'bet', or 'not' versus 'dot'); the limitation of airflow through the oral cavity, which may be closed briefly for the stop/plosives (/b/ and /p/), relatively restricted for voiced consonants (/d/), and relatively open for the vowels; and the position taken by the tongue, lips and so on.

Children with mild to moderate prelingual loss of hearing develop normal articulation of vowels and normal or near-normal voice quality. Such children, however, will often have articulation problems with the liquid /r/ in the initial position, fricative consonants (/s/, /sh/, /th/) and the affricates (/dʒ/ and /tʃ/). They will often omit final consonants and voiced fricative consonants, and seldom produce voiced consonants with a back, lingual placement (/g/, /ŋ/, /ʒ/ and /dʒ/), as shown in a study of a 4-year-old hearing-impaired child by West and Weber (1973). Nevertheless, their speech is usually quite intelligible.

The situation is quite different for children with greater hearing losses. Because of problems in producing and harmonising the several facets of speech, their speech is generally hard to understand. Although the speech intelligibility of children with severe to profound losses varies considerably from child to child, the mean intelligibility figure is relatively constant for listeners not used to the speech of hearing-impaired children, at between 18 and 25%. The evidence on this point is very weighty. We now outline several studies to show just how strong this evidence is, though Monsen (1981) has indicated that clinically the speech intelligibility of hearing-impaired children is seldom measured.

A report of the Department of Education and Science in England and Wales (1964) on conversations by a medical practitioner with 359 children revealed that about one-third of the children with hearing losses in excess of 80 dB HL had unintelligible speech. This one-third may have been an optimistic estimate (see below). Brannon (1964) found that the mean intelligibility of 20 day-school students aged 12–15 years, with severe or greater hearing-losses, was 20–25%. He found also that their speech was more intelligible during sentence production than during the utterance of single words. Markides (1967, 1970) studied 85 day and residential school-children in two groups, one of 7- and one of 9-year-olds. For 58 profoundly deaf children, with a mean hearing loss of 95 dB HL, the intelligibility of spoken words was 19% for 'naïve' listeners and 31% for teachers of the deaf. The speech intelligibility for the remaining 27 partially hearing children, with a mean hearing loss of 57 dB HL, was 76% for naïve listeners and 83% for the teachers of the deaf. The product–moment correlation coefficient between hearing loss and speech intelligibility was -0.75 for naïve listeners, and -0.71 for the teachers. Thus teachers tended to score the speech intelligibility of hearing-impaired children higher than listeners who were not used to deaf speech, though Smale (1988) argued that hearing people who are not used to deaf individuals can improve their understanding of the speech of prelingually profoundly deaf adolescents after a short period of familiarisation.

Conrad (1979) also found that teachers tended to uprate very deaf children, but they downrated the partially hearing, while Doyle (1987) reported that audiologists given bogus audiograms rated a given speech sample as of poorer intelligibility if the audiogram showed a high degree of hearing impairment, and gave a high rating if the audiogram showed a low degree of hearing impairment. Such issues of listener experience in evaluating speech are clearly problematical. They have been discussed by Boothroyd (1985), who argued for a forced-choice paradigm to minimise their effects.

Forty-six severely to profoundly hearing-impaired residential school-children aged 3–15 years with hearing losses of 60 dB or more were found by Nober (1967) to have speech articulation age norms of 4 years if their hearing loss was 60–80 dB, and 3 years for hearing losses of 80 dB or more. Heidinger (1972) asked three experienced teachers of the deaf to score the speech of 20 severely to profoundly deaf residential school-children aged 10–14 years. For words in short sentences, only 20% were scored as intelligible.

The Department of Education and Science (1972) issued a further report in which 23% of 167 children with hearing losses of more than 80 dB were assessed, in a similar way to the 1964 investigation, as having unintelligible speech. This result was an apparent improvement on the 1964 report, but could have been due to differences in assessment and/or sampling differences. Also, 54.7% of the children had 'partly intelligible' speech, but it was doubted if the speech of many children in this group could readily be understood by people who were not familiar with the speech of deaf children. Again, 40 residential school-children with hearing losses of 80 dB or greater at 1 kHz and aged 8–10, and 13–15 years, were found by Smith (1975a) to have a mean spoken word intelligibility of 18.7%, and Weiss et al. (1975) obtained a mean speech intelligibility of 37% – a somewhat better result – on 60 preschool children from a number of day and residential programmes. However, the hearing losses extended down to some 75 dB. Levitt et al. (1976) repeatedly assessed the speech intelligibility of more than 100 hearing-impaired children aged 10 years, for whom no hearing loss data were given, but who were probably severely to profoundly hearing-impaired, from 10 schools over 4 successive years, to age 14. Scores of speech intelligibility in tape-recorded picture description tasks made by three listeners, who were familiar with the speech of hearing-impaired children, yielded more than 70% of children rated as impossible or difficult to understand on all test occasions.

On the other hand, 67 severely to profoundly deaf students aged 11 years and older at the Central Institute for the Deaf were assessed as having a mean speech intelligibility of 76%, atypically high, by 50 hearing listeners (Monsen, 1978). This high level was attributed principally to the shortness of the sentences of 4.5 syllables spoken by his subjects. Monsen found that three out of nine measures of consonant production, vowel production and prosody gave a multiple correlation coefficient of 0.85 with intelligibility scores. The mean VOT between /t/ and /d/ and the mean second formant difference between /i/ and /ɔ/ accounted for about 70% of the variance in speech intelligibility. The correlation coefficient between speech intelligibility and hearing loss was −0.60.

A wide-reaching study of speech intelligibility was conducted on 978 hearing-impaired children receiving special education by Jensema, Karchmer, Trybus and colleagues (Jensema et al., 1978; Trybus, 1980). For children whose speech was intelligible, or very intelligible, the percentage of children with hearing losses above 90 dB amounted to 23%. For hearing losses of 71–90 dB, 55% of children had intelligible or very intelligible speech, and for hearing losses up to 70 dB, 86% of children were rated as having intelligible or very intelligible speech. The correlation coefficient between hearing loss and speech intelligibility ratings was −0.68, reasonably close to that of Markides (1967, 1970). Taken together, the work of Jensema and colleagues, and Markides, indicates that up to half the variance for speech intelligibility is associated with degree of hearing loss. The effect of hearing loss is relatively small up to 85 dB, following which there is a marked effect.

In his investigation of 468 prelingually deafened children aged 15–16 years in the UK, Conrad (1979) tape-recorded the speech of each child speaking a set of ten sentences, and had the tapes judged by a panel of 4–6 inexperienced assessors, mainly housewives. He found that the speech of only 26.5% of the children with hearing losses of more than 90 dB had speech which was better than barely intelligible. Similar findings were reported by Geffner and Freeman (1980) who found that the speech intelligibility of 67 children aged 6 years, with a mean hearing loss of 104 dB HL, was only 24%.

Although several of the above reports may be criticised on various grounds, the general outcome shows very clearly indeed that only a minority of profoundly deaf children have reasonably intelligible speech. This depressing finding is universal, and is only moderately offset by differences in approach from one training centre to another. Markides (1983) felt that the only conclusion was that the speech of the large majority of these children was unintelligible to the layman.

Causes of poor speech intelligibility

The next steps in examining the speech intelligibility of hearing-impaired children are to consider, first, what factors are associated with it and, second, what it is about the speech of prelingually profoundly hearing-impaired children that contributes most to its poor intelligibility. Answers to both questions will be of great practical interest to teachers and therapists.

Intelligence, age and orosensory perception

We have seen that the degree of hearing loss is negatively correlated with speech intelligibility, a relationship found consistently by many workers over many years (Hudgins and Numbers, 1942; Markides 1967, 1970; Kyle, 1977; Monsen, 1978; Conrad, 1979; Sims et al., 1980; Whitehead, 1991). As for other factors, intelligence appears to be only moderately highly correlated with speech intelligibility, if at all (Quigley, 1969; Markides, 1970; Ling, 1976; Conrad, 1979). The effectiveness of speech training procedures which seemed to have little more impact on bright than on dull children was therefore queried by Conrad (1979). He wondered, alternatively, whether speech could be taught to deaf children any more than it is 'taught' to hearing children, thus casting doubt on its status as a skill. Correlations between age, beyond the first few years, and speech intelligibility are around zero (Babbini and Quigley, 1970; Jensema et al., 1978). Nor is speech intelligibility correlated with reading ability (Conrad, 1979). It does, however, appear to be correlated significantly with linguistic ability (Markides, 1967; John et al., 1976) perhaps because deaf children will be able to speak more fluently if they appreciate the rules of syntax and have a fair knowledge of vocabulary and semantics (Markides, 1983).

Despite Conrad's pessimistic remarks, there is evidence that deaf children can improve their speech intelligibility, if only moderately, with speech training (Wedenberg, 1954; Markides, 1967; Calvert and Silverman, 1975; Ling, 1976; Siebert, 1980; Subtelny, 1980; Lieberth, 1982; Hochberg et al., 1983; Osberger, 1983, 1987; Abraham and Weiner, 1985; Perigoe and Ling, 1986; Moores, 1987), even though several of these studies have design problems. This evidence is associated with a trend for speech and language specialists to enter the field (Silverman, 1983). Also, Markides (1967) reported that children who were making good use of their hearing aids showed significantly superior speech intelligibility to children who were not using their aids to such advantage. The implication of these studies is that to concentrate on spoken language development, use of hearing aids and aspects of speech training can bring about some improvement in the speech intelligibility of prelingually deaf children.

Since muscle movements are involved in the production of speech, we may suppose that problems of deviant articulation which contribute to poor speech intelligibility are related to a deficit in orosensory (tactile and kinaesthetic) feedback (Ringel et al., 1968; Fucci and Robertson, 1971; Fucci, 1972). Orosensory feedback is important to speech production by hearing-impaired individuals who lack adequate auditory feedback in monitoring articulation (Bishop et al., 1973; Waldstein, 1990).

Lieberth and Whitehead (1987) investigated the use of orosensory perception in hearing-impaired individuals by comparing the articulation errors and speech intelligibility of 75 young adults with a mean hearing loss of 92 dB HL to their errors on an orosensory test, modified from Ringel et al. (1970). They used stem-mounted forms (shapes) from the USA National Institute for Dental Research. Lieberth and Whitehead found no significant correlations for total errors between articulation, speech intelligibility, and orosensory perception. Nor did they find significant relationships between total orosensory perception errors and degree of hearing loss or history of amplification usage. However, between-class orosensory errors, in which the subjects did not perceive the shape of the objects, were correlated with vowel errors, phoneme omissions, and errors where the produced phoneme came from the same place as the intended phoneme. Substitution errors were significantly related to those orosensory test errors in which differences in size were not perceived. The orosensory test errors in which the subjects perceived two identical items to be different were related significantly to total articulation errors, and consonant, vowel and substitution errors. Lieberth and Whitehead concluded that the relationships between the types of errors could be used to develop strategies to remediate articulation disorders through further research.

In summary, apart from hearing loss, factors such as intelligence, age, type of training and orosensory perception seem to be only weakly related to speech intelligibility.

The characteristics of deaf speech and its intelligibility

What are the characteristics of the speech of deaf children which tend to make it unintelligible? We touched on some of these characteristics earlier, and now try to answer this question by considering the segmental and suprasegmental features of deaf speech in a little more detail. However, since the speech of children with the same number of segmental errors can show large differences in intelligibility (Smith, 1975a), it is possible that suprasegmental problems account for the differences. In other words, suprasegmental difficulties may or may not contribute to poor speech intelligibility caused by segmental errors (Markides, 1983).

At the segmental level, negative correlations have been found between vowel and consonant errors and speech intelligibility for the speech of hearing-impaired children (Brannon, 1966; Markides, 1967; Smith, 1975a). Generally the totalled vowel, diphthong and consonant errors contributed most to the problem, namely, up to about 80% of the variance ascribed to speech intelligibility but, within these totalled articulatory errors, difficulties with consonants caused more intelligibility problems than difficulties with vowels. Brown and Goldberg (1990) thought that VOT was a primary factor among consonant features. Initial and final consonants were roughly equally problematical, but consonant omissions caused more difficulties than substitutions or distortions, the latter having only a small effect. This finding is in alignment with that of Warren (1970), whose hearing listeners 'heard' speech sounds that had been removed from recorded speech and replaced by coughs, breaths or other non-speech sounds.

On analysing speech samples from 22 deaf children with an acoustic and a physiological distinctive feature system, Mencke et al. (1984) obtained moderate to high correlations with both systems for speech intelligibility scores. Higher correlations were found for final than for initial position-in-word phonemes, regardless of listener experience or feature system. More recently Porter and Dickerson (1986) investigated the relationship of syllabic complexity to speech intelligibility in 11 students who possessed some intelligible speech. These students were aged 12–18 years old, with hearing losses from 75–103 dB. The results showed that their errors had a marked tendency to reduce syllable complexity, that is, to reduce the number of consonants preceding and following vowels. Also, hearing-impaired speakers with high speech intelligibility tended to make errors on the more complex syllables, thus reducing syllabic difficulty. The results implied that an appropriate approach to therapy for the speech production of hearing-impaired people should introduce phonemes systematically in increasingly complex syllabic structures.

Suprasegmental features were thought to play an important role in speech intelligibility by Hudgins and Numbers (1942), John and Howarth (1965) and Levitt et al. (1974). Hudgins and Numbers (1942) suggested that prosody had as much to contribute to speech intelligibility as articulation of consonants, and more than the articulation of vowels. Such observations led to a study of the importance of syllabic structure in explaining the phenomena associated with deaf speech (John and Howarth, 1965; Calvert and Silverman, 1975). However, correlations between prosody and speech intelligibility have proved to be rather small, perhaps not very surprising in view of the large proportion of variance taken up by articulatory features. Further, if deaf children can appropriately combine syllables into words and manage their phonation, the control of rhythm and intonation does not contribute very much to the intelligibility of their speech (Bernstein, 1977; Osberger and Levitt, 1979; Maassen and Povel, 1984; Maassen, 1986).

Suprasegmental deviations have led to the characterisation of deaf speech as 'staccato', with abnormal grouping of syllables (Gold, 1980), perhaps associated with control of breathing. There is also a relationship between the intelligibility of deaf speech and the number of pauses it contains (Parkhurst and Levitt, 1978). Removing the pauses decreases the intelligibility. Maassen (1986) attempted to compensate for the staccato nature of deaf speech by artificially inserting silent pauses between words, so that the word boundaries were acoustically marked. He therefore marked the word boundaries of 30 sentences spoken by ten prelingually profoundly deaf children aged 12–14 years with 160-ms pauses inserted between words. The insertions significantly increased the speech intelligibility, from 27% to 31%. Lengthening of phonemes to obtain the same sentence duration, as a control measure, showed that this effect was not due to the slowing of the speech. Thus Maassen obtained a small but useful improvement in speech intelligibility at the suprasegmental level.

In a particularly valuable study which produced information about the effects on intelligibility of both segmental and suprasegmental features, Metz et al. (1985) investigated three measures of speech intelligibility: single word identification using isolated words; contextual word identification using key words embedded in sentences; and scaled intelligibility of a paragraph of connected speech using direct magnitude estimation, for 12 segmental, prosodic and hearing parameters in 20 young adult speakers with a mean hearing loss of 91.5 dB. A regression analysis showed that speech intelligibility on isolated and contextual words was strongly associated with differences in VOT for cognate pairs, such as /p/ and /b/, and mean sentence duration.

A principal components analysis produced four factors, of which the first primarily reflected segmental production processes related to the temporal and spatial differentiation of phonemes, whilst the second reflected prosodic features and stability of production. Thus speech intelligibility had high positive loadings on both factor 1, showing differentiation of temporal and spatial events underlying the production of distinct phonemes, and on factor 2 which appeared to be due to prolonged sentence duration, instability in control of sentence duration, and instability in the production of cognate phoneme pairs. Factor 1 was positively, and factor 2 was negatively, correlated with estimates of speech intelligibility. Factor 1 accounted for twice the variance of factor 2 on isolated word intelligibility, for about four times the variance on contextual word intelligibility, and for slightly less of the variance for scaled intelligibility than for isolated words or contextual words.

This work confirmed the indications of previous studies by Monsen (1978) and others that speech intelligibility in severely to profoundly hearing-impaired speakers is determined independently by segmental features and by prosodic characteristics. Segmental features tend to be the more influential, though Metz et al. (1990a) found that the predictive capacity of the factor structure was somewhat reduced. The Metz et al. (1985) study revealed also that subjects with low speech intelligibility showed high variability in some aspects of speech production. This outcome was confirmed and extended by Metz et al. (1990b), who found that hearing-impaired speakers with poor speech intelligibility may fall into two groups: those who consistently produce aberrant speech, and those who have an inconsistent error pattern. Highly intelligible speakers were consistent in their speech patterns.

Given that there is available a corpus of knowledge showing that speech intelligibility in prelingually severely to profoundly hearing-impaired children can be impoverished primarily by segmental, but also by suprasegmental aspects, why do the problems of poor speech intelligibility persist? Ling (1976) suggested forthrightly that teachers did not have, or were not using, approaches which integrated current knowledge with compatible traditional strategies. Subtelny (1982), writing of adolescents, thought that, for segmental aspects, the errors were due to faults in hearing, faults in learning the morphological features of English, or to faults in control of breathing and articulation, especially for word, phrase and sentence endings. It was probable, she also thought, that poor speech intelligibility due to articulation errors was associated with poor linguistic ability (compare Abraham and Weiner, 1987). Thus a child who does not understand the significances of plural -s endings at the linguistic level may not produce them in spontaneous speech production (compare Markides, 1967; John et al., 1976). A similar explanation may account for problems in speech intelligibility at the suprasegmental level, where failure to appreciate the contribution of pausing, stress and intonation to the linguistic domain may go hand in hand with failure at the level of speech production.

Such arguments clearly suggest that training in language could be explored further as one key to improving speech intelligibility. Carney (1986) has recommended that clinical work to assess speech intelligibility should proceed on a basis of maximising contextual and experiential effects, as well as on a basis which minimises them. Meantime, we conclude that for most prelingually profoundly deaf children, and for many children who are prelingually severely deaf, the intelligibility of their speech is so poor as to cause the most serious problems for their communication. Speechreading of the deaf child by hearing listeners (Subtelny et al., 1980) may sometimes assist such communication. However, the situation is not clear, since Kricos et al. (1990) noted that visual information produces considerable variability in judgements of the speech-accuracy of hearing-impaired children.

Conclusion

Calvert (1986) wrote that, over 400 years, there was no clear record of steady improvement in teaching speech production to deaf children, nor had there been significant breakthroughs to reduce the effort required of the deaf child in learning speech. The speech intelligibility of deaf children has not been shown to have improved over the centuries either.

It appears from review of the area that much detail is now known about the characteristics of deaf speech, but less is known about why deaf speech gets to be the way it is and, in general, training for acceptable speech production and intelligibility is not successful. Notably absent in the literature are well-designed studies which compare different speech training procedures with different teaching styles and teacher–child interactions. Although the practical difficulties of conducting such work are very considerable, they are not insuperable. Without the information from such investigations, the present generally unsatisfactory situation seems bound to continue.

Chapter 5
Hearing Impairment and
Manual Communication

Most profoundly deaf individuals prefer to communicate with their deaf peers in sign, though they need to communicate verbally with hearing people. There has been fierce debate about whether deaf sign language is properly a language, rather than a communication system which is less than a full language. Following an account of manual systems other than sign language, this chapter considers the characteristics of sign language as language. It comments also on the neuropsychology of sign and the ways in which sign language is learned or acquired. The chapter concludes with a review of total communication, which is included here as its dominant mode is usually manual.

For mildly to moderately prelingually hearing-impaired children communication is oral and aural. Although such children may show delayed communication skills, and need special help in their linguistic and educational development, they should succeed with oral means of communication. The situation is less certain for the child with a prelingual severe hearing loss, and much less certain for the child with prelingual profound deafness.

Manual Communication

In 1880 an important International Congress on Education of the Deaf was held in Milan. This Congress was driven by a mood of change in European schools in the 1870s, resulting in a strong emphasis on oral communication. Despite this thrust by educators of the deaf, the dominant form of communication in the social inter-actions of one profoundly deaf person with another, especially if prelingually deaf, has been manual communication. We consider later the issue of which mode of communication may be used in the education and rehabilitation of the deaf. For the present we note that, despite the stress laid on oralism, the preferred communication mode of most profoundly deaf people amongst themselves is the manual mode. Manual communication is preferred, despite the availability of hearing aids and experience of aural rehabilitation.

The salient feature is the mode of communication which deaf people use among themselves. Clearly, only oracy will be effective in communicating with hearing people unless they have learned manual communication. Thus most orally educated deaf people communicate orally with hearing individuals and manually with their deaf peers. Profoundly deaf people who have not been educated orally, but by manual or by some mixed form of communication will, of course, have greater problems in communicating with the hearing world, and will be all the more predisposed to manual communication with deaf associates.

The Natural Language of the Deaf

When young profoundly deaf children are left to communicate among themselves, they develop a gestural system of communication. For example, Heider and Heider (1941) studied 14 profoundly deaf children at the Clarke School for the Deaf in the USA, who were observed in communication with other deaf children and with hearing adults. These children communicated by spontaneously acquired signs or symbolic gestures, different from conventional signs, whose meaning was inferred from the social context. The Heiders found that, while several gestures served genuine symbolic functions, considerable use was made of pointing and expressive movement. The communication was bound to the context, especially the social context. Some gestures were global, in that they could not be analysed into single word equivalents. Other gestures were combined in a kind of syntax to provide a 'phrase' or 'sentence', equivalent to the syntax of hearing children up to about 2;6 years of age. Thus gestural communication emerges naturally in groups of young deaf children, together with elementary syntax, without being taught. Such gestural communication is not a developed gestural language, but it shows that every deaf child has some means of communication, and the motivation to develop this means of communication is very strong.

Since most profoundly deaf people universally communicate with one another by some manual form, the suggestion has been made that manual communication is the natural language of the deaf (Charrow, 1975). Standard English is not the native language of deaf people who acquire a manual form of communication. Further spoken language is not perceived and acquired naturally by prelingually profoundly deaf children. If they are to learn it they have to learn it over a long period of instruction. Further, also their learning of standard English is imperfect. They make syntactic errors not made by hearing children; they are generally poorly skilled in reading and in writing; and they produce the unusual expressions commonly referred to as 'deafisms'. The outcome, according to Charrow, is 'Deaf English', a form of English equivalent to pidgin, which serves to cover the gap between manual and oral education for social interaction, and which crystallises in the teen years.

Most profoundly deaf children are born to hearing parents, and their first experience of language will be through oracy. However, it is likely that from an early age they will be brought into contact with other young deaf children, when some gestural communication will ensue. For these children, their first language is thus unlikely to be 'pure'. It will involve at least some gestural forms (Tervoort, 1979), and hence will involve aspects of bilingualism. On the other hand, the minority of profoundly deaf children who are born to profoundly deaf parents will have a monolingual manual form as their first language. Whereas profoundly deaf children born to profoundly deaf parents will have a unitary, gestural native language, the native communication system of profoundly deaf children born to hearing parents is likely to be some unsatisfactory mixture of attenuated standard English and gesture (Mohay, 1982).

The manual form of communication used by profoundly deaf people amongst themselves is deaf sign language. Until quite recently, this gestural form of communication was not seen as a language in its own right. Thus Furth (1966a) tended to argue that prelingually profoundly deaf children functioned as a group without language. He thought that since these children had no language, their performance would be weak in cognitive tasks, such as thinking and problem-solving. However, it became clear that, provided the tasks are not verbal, profoundly deaf children perform at about the same level as hearing children (Furth, 1971; Furth and Youniss, 1975). It also came to be recognised that verbal language is not essential for the performance of non-verbal cognitive tasks. This realisation left the way open for the exploration of deaf sign language as a language in its own right, as a code through which ideas could be communicated, with a vocabulary and semantics of its own, and with a generative capacity in the sense developed by Chomsky (1971).

Manual Systems Other than Sign Language

Before we consider deaf sign language further, it will be informative to cover briefly other forms of gestural communication used by profoundly deaf people.

Fingerspelling

Communication by fingerspelling for hearing-impaired people is one of the oldest known forms, though it has not received much research (Akamatsu and Stewart, 1989). It is sometimes used to connect signs into sentences, or to add stress in sign languages. Fingerspelling is particularly useful for introducing names, neologisms and technical terms, such as 'cruise missile' or 'virtual reality'. The manual alphabet is a one-to-one cipher for the letters of an alphabet on the fingers of the hand. In the UK the manual alphabet is two-handed, but elsewhere it is usually displayed on one hand. For English, there are 26 positions, or combinations of finger placements and handshapes, corresponding to the 26 letters of the English alphabet, which hence are shown without ambiguity and can be used to spell out a word with the fingers, as with conventional spelling of English letters. Clearly, fingerspelling is a slow form of communication. Bornstein (1979) has reported a maximum transmission rate of about 60 words per minute – roughly three times slower than rather fast speech or signed communication.

Fingerspelling is rarely used alone, but its frequent use in combination with signed communication has led to its partial integration into sign languages. American Sign Language (ASL) contains items borrowed from fingerspelling, and hence from standard English (Battison, 1978). Changes in handshape can show the first letter of the corresponding English word, a tactic known as initialisation (Evans, 1981). Thus although fingerspelt material is different from signs it may be 'borrowed' for use in sign language. Thereupon it becomes more sign-like and subject to the constraints of the sign language, such as not more than two parts in each sign. It takes considerable time to learn the rules for fingerspelling and its relationship to signs and to printed and spoken words (Maxwell, 1988).

Fingerspelling can be used in other ways. Evans (1981) suggested that, besides its direct use for names and technical terms, fingerspelling has a role as a lexical tool for the learning of such items, and can reinforce the written form of new words. He also observed that signs tend to communicate content words, whereas fingerspelling is useful for function words, such as articles, prepositions, etc. Thus fingerspelling plays a complementary role to signs, when it may significantly increase understanding of the signed message (Savage et al., 1981). Fingerspelling can be internalised in profoundly deaf subjects with poor speech (Locke and Locke, 1971). Their deaf subjects showed visual and dactylic confusions in their error patterns in recalling lists of consonants.

The Makaton Vocabulary

The Makaton Vocabulary was developed in the UK (Walker, 1976; Walker and Armfield, 1982; Walker and Buckfield, 1983). It was based on basic signs from British Sign Language (BSL) to produce a simple vocabulary of approximately 350 signs, graded to reflect difficulty in acquisition. The Makaton Vocabulary has been widely used in the UK, mainly with intellectually disabled people, for whom it appears to meet a keenly felt need (Kiernan et al., 1979). However, it is not generally suitable for the prelingually profoundly deaf population, as its vocabulary is limited to the 350 signs. Further, because it is essentially a lexicon of signs, its function is that of an elementary system of communication. It is not a language.

Linguistics of Visual English

Linguistics of Visual English (LOVE) was devised by Wampler (1971) for profoundly deaf children attending preschool and kindergarten. The LOVE signs were thought to correspond to the rhythms of speech. They consisted of hand positions as symbols for morphemes, designated in terms of meaning, speech sound similarity or spelling. The syllables of standard English could thus be represented by hand positions, one for each syllable. The LOVE system is of interest in that it represented an attempt to develop a manual system which in several respects was isomorphic with standard English. It is now little used, in part because it represents no natural system.

Mouth–hand systems

Mouth–hand systems use hand signals presented near the lips to supplement speechreading. In particular, they provide information about those speech sounds which are not readily seen on the lips. Hence mouth–hand systems may be described as oral communication with a manual supplement.

Mouth–hand communication systems have a long history. They were used in France in the mid-nineteenth century (Børrild, 1972). Early in the present century, the mouth–hand system was explored by Forchhammer (1903) in Denmark. Forchhammer recognised that speechreading was difficult because the speechreader could not see the position of the invisible speech organs. He set himself to illustrate these positions with one hand. Hand and finger positions were developed to illustrate the movements of the vocal folds, the palate, and the positions of the tongue. It was possible to illustrate all the vowels and consonants in this way. The system could be learned in 15–20 lessons, and could be used without slowing the speech rate. For well-trained users it gave a marked increase in the effectiveness of speechreading (Børrild, 1972). However, subsequent work showed that the users depended more on the hand than on the lip movements for speech perception, and even then only a small minority of users obtained mastery. Forchhammer's system thus proved in practice to be more like manual than oral communication, and for manual communication there were more natural alternatives.

The Rochester Method

The use of fingerspelling with speechreading, which came to be known as the Rochester Method, was developed in the USA in the latter half of the nineteenth century (Scouten, 1964). This method allowed the talker to write in the air, as it were, while speaking. Because fingerspelling is slower than speech, the use of simultaneous fingerspelling can only be used to indicate salient words or emphases, unless the speech is unnaturally slowed. A study of the Rochester Method was described by Moores (1987), who considered a number of programmes to find the preferred educational approach for a given child at a given developmental stage. The programmes investigated were auditory, oral/aural, Rochester Method and total communication (TC), in different settings (day or residential school), orientations (traditional nursery, academic, or cognitive), emphases (parent- or child-centred), and placements (integrated or self-contained). Moores found marked differences amongst the programmes, particularly for receptive communication. The programmes using the Rochester Method, as a combination of sounds, speechreading and fingerspelling obtained results superior to those using printed words, sounds alone, and sounds and speechreading, but not sounds, speechreading and signs.

Cued Speech

Despite some advantages, the Rochester Method is cumbersome. Although fingerspelling is still used to supplement speech (Savage et al., 1981), it is so employed rather informally and, as the Rochester Method, is no longer widely used. To some degree, the Rochester Method was superseded by Cued Speech (Cornett, 1967), which also uses manual gestures to supplement speechreading. Like Wampler

(1971), Cornett recognised that the rhythm, intonation and inflection of speech are intimately associated with the syllable, and hence designed Cued Speech to follow the spoken syllables precisely. Cued Speech allows for complete dependence on the lips for that part of speech information which they can supply, thus differing from Forchhammer's (1903) and the Rochester Method. The hands are used only for speech information which cannot be seen on the lips. The cues of Cued Speech cannot be read alone, which forces the hearing-impaired child to monitor the lips of the talker and to take only supplementary information from the hand. Also, the hearing-impaired child who is the talker must move his or her lips fairly normally to be understood, and cannot rely only on producing the hand cues. Thus (Cornett, 1972, 1985) Cued Speech requires complete use of and dependence on information from the lips. Any information besides that from the lips must be compatible in meaning and rhythm with the spoken form. All the essential detail of speech must be made evident and the method must be suitable for learning by the child in the home, namely, without formal teaching. Hence the method must be suitable for average parents to learn.

There is much to be said for Cued Speech. It does not disrupt the simultaneous talking, as occurs with fingerspelling. Cued Speech can keep up with speech (Nicholls and Ling, 1982) as it emphasises the syllables rather than individual phonemes. Since it signifies the syllables it is also in accord with the rhythms of the speech. It is therefore not necessary when using Cued Speech to single out hearing-impaired students in classes of mainly hearing students (Beaupre, 1985).

Cued Speech was heavily promoted, but there was little systematic study of its effectiveness in the years following its introduction (Quigley and Kretschmer, 1982), despite continuing favourable reports from many countries (e.g. Gregory, 1987). Clarke and Ling (1976) reported on a group of eight profoundly deaf children aged 8–12 years as receivers of 2 years of Cued Speech training. These children showed significantly improved reception of Cued Speech over this training period in their written responses to material presented via Cued Speech. They apparently performed at a level superior to that when using residual hearing and speechreading.

Three children, one severely and two profoundly deaf, aged between 1 and 3 years, were studied in a Cued Speech programme by Mohay (1983), with evaluation of their linguistic abilities before and after training in programmes of between 6 months and 2 years duration. She found a number of problems arising with Cued Speech. For example, the frequency of communicative gestures fell off with the introduction of the programme, but without a corresponding increase in the amount or the diversity of spoken language. As a result, there was an overall reduction in the frequency of communication. There was, however, a change towards the production of longer spoken utterances.

Although its use has been fairly widespread and it is employed in special applications, including the teaching of speech (Quenin and Blood, 1989), Cued Speech has not become highly popular in the USA (Calvert, 1986) or elsewhere. Only a proportion of deaf children manage to acquire full competence in perceiving and producing the cues, since they will have had no experience of the underlying speech sounds, and since they experience difficulties in responding to the complex combined visual inputs of lip and hand movements (compare Jensema and Trybus, 1978).

Seeing Essential English

Seeing Essential English (SEE$_1$) uses ASL signs together with introduced signs to cover the roots of words, and verbal inflections, namely prefixes and suffixes. This system, developed by Anthony (1971) closely followed standard English, with English words translated into the equivalent ASL sign plus a signed affix. The order of English syntax was maintained. Since ASL signs do not correspond exactly to English words the three criteria of meaning, spelling and sound were used to direct the choice of a sign. Compound English words often have a single sign as their ASL equivalent. In such cases, the sign for each component was used, unless the result appeared to be incongruent, when a new sign was introduced. SEE$_1$ has tended to be superseded by Signing Exact English (SEE$_2$), as shown below.

Signing Exact English

Signing Exact English (SEE$_2$) was produced by Gustason et al. (1972, 1983), because SEE$_1$ contained too many signs distanced from ASL (Bornstein, 1973). A distinction, then, between SEE$_1$ and SEE$_2$ is that generally SEE$_2$ uses signs to represent whole words rather than the roots of words. In SEE$_1$ these words would also need an affix if they were complex. SEE$_2$ requires only some 70 affixes, as opposed to the 118 affixes of SEE$_1$, 18% of modified ASL signs and 21% of introduced signs. Gustason (1983) claimed that in five SEE$_2$ school programmes across the USA children younger than 10 years performed better than their age norms on the Test of Syntactic Ability (Quigley, 1978). Writing samples from some of the children also proved to be superior. However, these results were indicative only, as this study was not designed as a controlled experiment (compare Gustason, 1981). SEE$_2$ can be used with young deaf children and has enjoyed widespread use. A difficulty for both SEE$_1$ and SEE$_2$ is that both are compromise systems, because words cannot be converted from the one language to the other with the same form and meaning. Further, the use of inflectional markers in the signed versions is inadequate for transmitting complex English, and they are onerous to learn (Bornstein, 1979). This results in constraints on learning by parents for use in the home, with consequent mismatches between the performance of child and parents (Moeller and Luetke-Stahlman, 1990), though Luetke-Stahlman and Moeller (1990) found that parents can be trained to improve their SEE$_2$ performance.

Pidgin Sign

Pidgin Sign, a variant of which is Siglish (Signed English, or Ameslish in the USA), may be used by deaf signers when they wish to use a manual form which approximates to standard English, rather than their native sign language. Pidgins arise when users of two separate languages meet, usually on a short-term basis, for social exchange. In such situations deaf signers may use signs or fingerspelling in the word order found with standard English, and without the use of English inflections. Such Pidgin Sign English (Bragg, 1973) is not a language, but an elementary communication system. It is far removed from the fluency and generative nature of a recognised language. Despite its limitations, however, Pidgin Sign proves to be remarkably persistent. It is found universally, because it meets a need keenly felt from time to time by deaf signers. Brasel and Quigley (1977) found that Pidgin Sign produced better linguistic and educational progress in early childhood than ASL or oral methods. It should however be noted that what is referred to as Pidgin Sign English, as used in the classroom between deaf children and hearing teachers, is a more developed form than a basic contact pidgin (Lucas and Valli, 1989).

The Paget–Gorman Sign System

The signs of the Paget–Gorman Sign System (PGSS) were developed in the UK (Paget and Gorman, 1968). They provide for a basic idea or concept together with a qualifier to convey specific meaning. Although originally designed for deaf people, the PGSS has more commonly been used for children with severe speech problems, and learning and intellectual disabilities (Fenn and Rowe, 1975; Kiernan et al., 1982; Rowe, 1982). The PGSS is a contrived system of signs devised quite separately from BSL, to which it bears little resemblance, apart from occasional correspondence of icons. Crystal and Craig (1978) thought that PGSS, with its 21 hand positions and 37 basic signs, could well represent standard English, with its logical progression of signs from the general to the particular ('cats' = animal + whiskers + plural marker). The PGSS has gone out of favour for use with deaf individuals probably because it is artificial when compared to deaf sign language, but it enjoys popularity in work with intellectually impaired children because it offers an alternative to standard English for children who have no natural and consistent sign system of their own.

Interim conclusion

Of the forms of manual communication for hearing-impaired people mentioned so far, we can say with some confidence that apart from TC, which is discussed later, and SEE 2 which in some ways resembles TC, only some form of Pidgin Sign is likely to endure in the future as a principal means of communication. Pidgin Sign is a special case. It meets a continuing need for communication when the users of two dominant but different languages, such as standard English and a sign language (see below), meet from time to time and share a need to communicate.

There is serious doubt about the lasting nature of any system which requires great learning effort by hearing parents for use in the home, which will not necessarily be used by the deaf child later in life, and which makes heavy perceptual or cognitive demands on hearing and deaf individuals alike. It is interesting that there are few indications that the systems so far considered have been put to anything like a thoroughgoing test in experimental studies, despite the clear desire of the authors for the utility of their systems to be well researched (e.g. Cornett, 1972). The efforts made to bring sign to conform to standard English, the use of manual supplements to standard English, and the development of contrived sign systems over the past 20 years or so, have generated much empirical work, strong statements of opinion, and a plethora of ideas and hypotheses. There is little consensus about their relative efficacy with deaf children, because the necessary research has yet to be done. For the reasons given, and the increasing recognition given to sign language (see below), we suspect that it may never be done, though others may be more optimistic.

Sign Language

A language is a complex code for conveying information to communicate meaning, and is governed by rules which are accepted by convention among users. These rules set the manner in which the meaning is to be conveyed. The simple sum of the rules does not make the language because, by themselves, the rules only partly direct the meaning. The message to be conveyed also depends on the selection of the words used. In standard English, however, the rules of syntax, governing word order, profoundly affect the meaning. The importance of syntactic rules in English is shown by the newsworthy sentence: 'The man bit the dog', where the rule that the subject normally precedes verbs of active voice makes it clear that the man did the biting, and not the dog. Not all languages ascribe such importance to word order. Some languages use verbal inflections to show subject, verb, object, etc. However, the language provides the meaning or message, not just the rule system. So a consideration of how a language functions must include an explanation not only of the arrangement of the words, but which words may be used, and the role of the words and word groupings in communicating ideas (Kretschmer and Kretschmer, 1990). The explanation must also allow for the generative capacity of languages to permit novel expressions.

The study of signed communication over the last 20 or so years, as used by hearing-impaired people, has shown that it is a complex and sophisticated means of communication. There is a sense in which sign is similar to spoken language if sign is considered as 'articulatory gesture' (Neisser, 1976), or if communication is seen as an articulatory as much as an acoustic phenomenon, where gestures take the place of speech, with their own rhythmic structure (Allen et al., 1991). Communication by signs is thus commonly referred to as communication by sign language (Bellugi, 1980; Bonvillian et al., 1980; Wilcox, 1990). However, not all workers in the field agree that sign language is indeed language. Some argue that sign has no grammar, cultural content or literary tradition, though these arguments have been challenged (Frishberg, 1988; Fromkin, 1988) and sign is gaining academic respectability as language (Wilcox, 1988). Notable amongst the critics of sign language as language is Van Uden (1986). His criticisms will now be considered, as they prove helpful in understanding the nature of sign language.

Van Uden wished to know whether sign language was comparable to pidgin, to a creole, namely, a 'language' developed from pidgin to form an elementary language with some syntax, noun declension and verb conjugation, or to a fully elaborated spoken language. He also wanted to know if sign language was none of these, but was unique. Although this is an argument about sign language as language, it is important to our interests. If sign language is not language, then signed communication is impoverished communication. Its users will not be able to exchange sophisticated messages as do users of verbal language.

Iconic and arbitrary signs

Van Uden began his analysis of sign language at the word level, asking to what extent signs were iconic (resembling reality, especially visual reality), esoteric (known only within a restricted circle of users), or arbitrary (arising adventitiously). For example, iconicity may be shown in sign by indicating whiskers, for a cat. In standard English, analogous instances would come from onomatopoeia such as the 'popping' of a cork. Esoteric signs are those whose meaning is not clear, or not immediately clear, except to a relatively small closed group of habitual users as, for instance, the terminology used in cricket. Many esoteric signs may be indirectly iconic, in that their iconicity becomes apparent when the meaning is explained. Some signs are arbitrary, where there appears to be no observable relationship between the sign and its meaning. However, most standard English words seem arbitrary if we do not delve into their etymology. Even then their origin may be arbitrary.

Sign languages are remarkable for their use of icons. The major proportion of signs is directly or indirectly iconic (esoteric). Only the minor proportion is arbitrary. Thus most signs are relatively transparent as to their meaning and only a minority are semantically opaque, though Miller (1987) found that even transparent signs were opaque to 3-year-old hearing non-signing preschool children. Van Uden argued that the dominance of iconicity in sign language sets it apart from spoken language. Such argument is accepted (Hoemann, 1975; Schlesinger, 1977b; Newport and Supalla, 1980; Sternberg, 1981; Luftig et al., 1983), but it is a relative argument, for both sign and spoken languages contain iconic forms, and esoteric and arbitrary items. It is the proportion that is different. Frishberg (1975) suggested that over the years there has been a trend towards more abstraction and less iconicity in ASL. To what extent this trend will progress, and the precise reasons for it, are difficult to estimate at present.

There is evidence that thinking via icons can retard thinking in the abstract (Furth, 1973; Paivio and Begg, 1981), but sign language does contain signs for abstract ideas (Bellugi and Klima, 1978; Klima and Bellugi, 1979). There seems to be no a priori reason to stop the development of more arbitrary signs to represent abstractions. A further consideration is that the opportunity for iconic, or indirectly iconic, representation is greater for a vocabulary expressed in sign rather than through oracy, which may aid memory in the learning of sign (Beykirch et al., 1990; Lieberth and Gamble, 1991). Intuitively it seems that most spoken vocabulary is simply not suited to iconic representation. Although sign language differs from natural spoken language in the ratio of iconic to arbitrary signs, this difference scarcely prevents sign language from consideration as a language.

Before leaving this aspect, we note that esoteric signs are esoteric only by the definition of the closed circle of users in relation to the culture. If we take the non-signing main culture as the reference, then signs used by deaf people, when the meaning is not apparent, are esoteric. However, if the population of deaf people is taken as the culture the signs clearly are not esoteric. It all depends on where we start from.

Phonology and cherology

We saw in Chapter 2 that a spoken language can be regarded, at one level, as comprising a number of phonemes. Although the acoustic nature of a phoneme may vary depending on the phonemes spoken before and after it, and with voice parameters, such as differences between male and female voices, its function for the listener remains constant.

In a classic paper, Stokoe (1960) proposed an analogous function in ASL. He argued that signs were comprised of a number of essentially meaningless individual features which could be combined in different ways to produce a vocabulary of signs. He named these features cheremes, or manual phonemes. Each sign could be considered as having three simultaneous features, a tabula (TAB) corresponding to the location, a designator (DEZ) corresponding to hand configuration, and a signation (SIG) corresponding to the hand movement. Some signs would need more than a single TAB or DEZ. For a sign to be recognised as a part of ASL, it would have to conform as to TABs, DEZs and SIGs to a set of rules. Stokoe identified 12 TABs, 19 DEZs and 24 SIGs, and gave each one a special symbol. He was thus able to produce a sign language dictionary (Stokoe et al., 1965) which was a marked departure from the 'pictogram' dictionaries in use up to that time. Sign language dictionaries, representing cheremes, have now been prepared for many countries (e.g. Johnston 1987 a, b, for Auslan). Lane et al. (1976) pointed to distinctive features in the geometry of the hand when used to indicate signs, analogous to the distinctive features of spoken language. Cognitive studies with deaf signers have shown that signs serve as perceptual units (Hass and Sams, 1987) and are coded in memory by Stokoe's features (Bellugi and Klima, 1975; Siple et al., 1977; Hanson, 1982; Shand, 1982).

Van Uden (1986) took issue with cherology for signs as analogous to the phonology of natural spoken language. He argued that the features of signs are determined by content, and are essentially iconic. Hence Stokoe's cheremes were integral parts of the icon of the sign, rather than arbitrary functional features, as with the phonemes of spoken language. It has to be admitted that the idea of cheremes seems to fit oddly with iconicity. However that may be, whether arbitrary features are present or absent does not tell us much about whether the system of which they are part is, or is not, a language, as Van Uden himself recognised. What is important is that the phonological, or cherological, rules of a language are the accepted convention, and that problems arise when they are broken.

Inflections

In discussing the morphology of sign language, especially ASL, Van Uden concluded that the morphology was extremely poor, particularly for expressing relationships. The morphological inflections of standard English to signify plural forms, comparatives and superlatives were largely absent in sign. However, as with iconicity, this is a relative argument. In standard English some nouns, for instance, are not inflected to show case. Van Uden quoted Stokoe (1978) to the effect that sign languages do not have the inflectional systems of Indo-European and related languages. However, this quotation missed the point. Sign language can be highly inflected, but it uses inflections in a different way to their use in standard English (Hanson and Feldman, 1989).

Singularity and plurality in English are commonly marked by the absence or presence of the suffix -s for nouns and for third person verbs. Instead of inflecting the sign, sign language uses repetition, or reduplication, of the sign, or precedes the sign by a number, to convey the plural marking. However, signs can be inflected to show classifiers. For example, Kyle and Woll (1985) described the BSL verb stem which means 'to go under a bridge', shown by moving the right hand under the left hand, where the shape (inflection) of the right hand conveys what is going under the bridge.

In an English sentence, such as 'The man bit the dog' the syntax shows that the man did the biting. In BSL (Kyle and Woll, 1985), the role, or who did what, is conveyed by inflecting the verb with conventionalised manual locations. Alternatively, each hand may be used in simultaneous articulation, not possible in a spoken language, by coding separate roles, one on each hand, following which the hands act on each other. Kyle and Woll (1985) illustrated other uses of manual morphology to represent time, aspect and quality, namely, manner or degree. Van Uden argued that purely functional inflexions, rather than the 'semantic' inflections of the type outlined, do not exist in sign language. Whether or not this is the case does not determine whether sign language can be regarded as a true language, however, if the meaning is conveyed in other ways.

Structure

In addition to his arguments that sign language has no 'phonology' and no functional morphology, Van Uden also argued that it has no linguistic syntax. In both ASL and BSL, for example, it is difficult to find a basic order of signs. However, it is arguable that a language must have a basic syntax, like the subject–verb–object (SVO) syntax of English. Rather, ASL and BSL may be topic-comment languages (Friedman, 1976; Deuchar, 1983), where the topic is first introduced and then elaborated. The characteristic structure thus shows semantic or pragmatic linkages rather than syntactic relationships (compare Fontana, 1990). Deuchar gave the example of 'TEN P PUT-IN' = 'I put in ten p', where ten p (pence) was the topic and was made first with the dominant right hand, then the right hand remained in the fingerspelling position for 'p' while PUT-IN was signed with the non-dominant left hand. Deuchar observed that studies of spontaneous signing (Hansen, 1975) accepted topic-comment as the base for signed sentences, whereas formal research using elicited sentences tended to find an SVO structure (Liddell, 1978b). She regarded the situation in which the sign was produced, or the influence of the dominant spoken language, as affecting the data. Hence both Deuchar and Friedman felt that indications of SVO structure in sign were caused by exposure to English, and were not basic characteristics of sign language. We conclude that Van Uden may not have been too far from the truth in stating that sign language does not possess a linguistic syntax, at least in the sense that sign language is not as dominated by word grouping or word order as English, though it does contain its own syntax-like arrangements (Wilbur, 1987; Lillo-Martin, 1990) for wh- questions, for instance. Natural, spontaneous sign language looks to be largely a topic-comment language. As such, there will be some sentence constructions in English which are difficult to convey directly via sign. Crystal and Craig (1978) have given some instances.

In response to Van Uden (1986), Stokoe (1987) observed that opposition to sign as language came from using the wrong kind of linguistics, originating from a particular social orientation. As we ourselves have argued, it depends where we start from. Although there is much to be learned about sign before it can be characterised fully and with confidence, the work reviewed fails to convince that sign language is definitely not language. It does show, however, that sign language has a very different structure from standard English. The real test of whether sign language is truly language depends, nevertheless, not so much on its structure, but on its success in carrying out its function. We need to ask, then, if sign language is as effective as English in coding meaning and information, in getting messages across, in generative capacity, and in facilitating the flow of discourse.

Communication by sign

How effective is sign language as a means of communication? For profoundly deaf individuals with no other form of communication it is 100% effective. Deaf children born to signing deaf parents know no other way of communicating. But we can look at this question in another way, asking how effectively is information transmitted by sign between deaf people in contrast to the transmission of the same information by speech between hearing people?

In one of the earlier referential communication studies, and in one of a number of experiments, Schlesinger (1971) found that deaf subjects had problems in conveying which one out of several pictures had been selected for communication. Each picture contained three characters in three roles – the agent, the object, and the indirect object ('A bear hands over a man to a monkey'). Six pictures, covering all possible permutations, made up a set, with each character appearing once in each role. The sender was required to describe one of the pictures, in Israeli sign language, following which the receiver had to select the correct picture from the set of six. The deaf subjects performed poorly. Schlesinger thought that the reason was because there was seemingly no rule in Israeli sign language which could be used consistently to distinguish between the subject, direct object and indirect object.

Schlesinger's work was criticised by Bode (1974), who thought it unreasonable to conclude that the main form of communication of any group lacked the means of conveying these relationships. Everyday communication required the frequent use of all three roles. Bode's well-founded criticisms included the absence of hearing controls using spoken language, who may also have found the task difficult. Bode also remarked on the lack of testing for competence in Israeli sign language, since some subjects may have been immigrants without developed skills in Israeli sign language. Bode's criticisms seem very pertinent. Schlesinger's (1971) study helps little to answer our question about the effectiveness of sign language in communicating meaning.

In an often-cited report, Hoemann (1972) compared information exchange by 40 mainly profoundly deaf and 40 hearing children in referential communication. The deaf group was acquiring ASL in a school where manual communication was allowed outside the classroom. The age of onset of hearing impairment, where known, was before 3 years of age. Half the hearing-impaired children had a mean age of 8;4 years and half of 11;4 years, while half of the 40 hearing children were of mean age 8;0 years and half 11;5 years. The genders were approximately equally distributed among all four groups. The two groups of hearing children had overall a higher performance IQ than the hearing-impaired groups. The children were studied in pairs of the same age grouping, as 8-year-olds with 8-year-olds, for example, and hearing status, as hearing with hearing and deaf with deaf. The pairs of children took part in three tasks: a description task, involving the description of various picture referents; a perspective task, requiring the construction of referent descriptions from the receiver's perspective; and a game-rules task, explaining the rules of a game.

Results for the description task showed significant differences for age and for hearing status, with no interaction, on sending scores. Older children obtained a higher communication accuracy than the younger children. Higher communication accuracy was also attained by hearing as compared with deaf children. Receiving scores were significantly higher than sending scores. Generally, the deaf children showed a 3-year lag in performance, as the scores of the 11-year-old deaf children were roughly the same as those of the 8-year-old hearing children, on all three measures assessed, namely sending, receiving and communication accuracy.

For the perspective task the hearing did better than the deaf children at both ages, and benefited more from a demonstration of perspective and from a prior experience as receivers. The older children, irrespective of hearing status, did better than the younger subjects, but the older hearing children only were able to establish whose perspective – sender's or receiver's – was to be taken. The younger deaf children produced more ambiguous or egocentric messages both before and after the demonstration, whereas the other groups changed their approach after the demonstration, but not always appropriately in all cases. The performance of the 11-year-old deaf children was again similar to that of the 8-year-old hearing children.

In the game-rules task, few deaf children explained the rules adequately. Both young and older deaf children behaved inappropriately, signing that they could not proceed, simply labelled the materials, or fixated on a single aspect of the game. However, all 40 deaf children were able to teach the game successfully when allowed to show the rules in action. Therefore, they knew the rules, but could not explain them manually. The 11 older deaf children, rated as explaining the rules adequately, used several manual modes of communicating, such as conventional ASL signs, fingerspelling and improvised iconic signs.

Hoemann concluded that peer-to-peer communication by deaf children was handicapped even for manual methods. The only tasks in which all his children succeeded were the descriptions of simple pictures. The 11-year-old deaf children were generally at the same performance level as the hearing 8-year-olds. Even when the hearing and deaf children were equated for IQ, the hearing children still showed significantly better performance on all three tasks. However, it is by no means clear that the differences between the deaf and the hearing children were due to differences in communication channel. As Hoemann himself pointed out, the relatively poor performance of his deaf children may have been due to a general experiential deficit affecting the acquisition of both linguistic skill and the development of formal communication skills. Hoemann's tasks were relatively formal. It is thus interesting to note that, in the game-rules task, the deaf children could convey the rules well by signing when allowed to demonstrate them in action, when they were able to draw on informal ways of communicating. Further, the deaf children would have begun school at 5–6 years of age with a poor knowledge of English, and with limited manual communication skills.

It would be instructive to repeat this study with deaf children of deaf signing parents as the group to be compared with hearing children. Such a comparison would allow a more balanced assessment of the effectiveness of conveying information by manual communication in referential communication tasks. That the performance level of Hoemann's deaf 11-year-olds was better than the deaf 8-year-olds suggested strongly that experience significantly increased formal communication skill, the learning of communication skill, and the learning of communication roles (compare Flavell, 1968). However, this study, though well designed in many aspects, does not allow us to decide whether sign language is sufficiently language-like in conveying meaning, as the deaf children were not necessarily competent users of sign language for their age.

Bode (1974) attempted to improve on the design used by Schlesinger (1971), described above, by trying to obtain comparable linguistic backgrounds for her hearing and deaf subjects. Her 16 English-speaking subjects were all native speakers of English. Her 16 deaf (probably profoundly deaf) subjects were ASL users. All but three had begun to learn ASL by 6 years of age. Those three acquired ASL at approximately 10, 14 and 17 years. All subjects were university undergraduates. All the deaf subjects were judged proficient in ASL by a mature deaf ASL user, who had acquired ASL from his deaf parents and siblings. Bode used one set of black and white picture referents illustrating three characters in which a first character handed a second character to a third, corresponding closely to the descriptions given in Schlesinger (1971). Another set of animals was prepared in which each character was of a different colour and shape and in which the depiction of time sequence was less ambiguous than in the first set ('a throws b overhand to c who stands with arms out' as in: 'The fish throws the cat to the pig'). Eight pairs of subjects were used for the spoken English part, and eight for the ASL part. For pairs of subjects, the two kinds of pictures and two kinds of instructions, brief and detailed, were balanced in two sequences. After a sender had described a picture indicated by the experimenter, and which the receiver could not see, the receiver tried to identify it from the complete set of six pictures.

For hearing pairs of subjects, 95% of the referent pictures were identified correctly. For the deaf subject pairs the proportion was 86%. Correct selection by chance would have been 17%. A comparison of the frequency of errors showed no significant difference between hearing and deaf groups. Nor were there other significant differences in scores. Bode concluded that ASL could communicate information about agent/object/indirect object which was comparable to that in spoken English. Her subjects performed uniformly well with both sets of pictures, when the linguistic abilities of deaf and hearing subjects were relatively comparable. Even so, and although they were judged to be proficient users of ASL, the deaf subjects had begun life with a marked communication disadvantage, as they had not begun to learn ASL till 6 years old. This delay, and the fact that they had not learned ASL naturally from deaf signing parents, may explain why their performance on the referential tasks was a little poorer than that of the hearing subjects, though not significantly so.

Before leaving this account of Bode's study, we comment on the nature of the referential communication task, which, as with Schlesinger (1971), was naturalistically very obscure. After all, man-handling bears and cat-throwing fish are not part of everyday experience. This obscurity was shown by some descriptions quoted by Bode, such as 'Fish hold cat/pig laugh' – a signed description – and 'On the bottom left there's a pink pig holding a yellow cat. On the right bottom there's a green glob' – a spoken description. These examples* show that some of both the deaf and the hearing children did not understand the action the pictures were meant to convey. Similar comments can be offered about the pictures used in other picture-description referential communication tasks. In a study by Oléron (1978), for example, sketches were intended to depict a man showing a boy to a woman, a woman showing a man to a boy, etc. It is not clear from the pictures what the action, namely 'showing', was meant to be. Hence the material was ambiguous. Such ambiguity adds 'noise' to the experimental design.

For all three studies reviewed, we have argued that a fair test of whether or not sign language can be used as effectively to transmit meaning as natural spoken language requires subjects who have been able to use sign as their natural means of communication from very early in life. Hence these subjects can communicate in a way that is comfortable and natural for them, and which they can fully understand (Erting, 1980). The use of signs by deaf children born to deaf parents begins before, or at least as soon as, the use of words by hearing children born to hearing parents, and the acquisition of a vocabulary of signs develops rapidly (Bonvillian et al., 1983). Hence it is particularly important to base studies of the effectiveness of sign by deaf users on those whose signed fluency approaches that of their parents. This emphasis on the use of deaf signers born of deaf signing parents is not trivial. Marmor and Petitto (1979) and Strong and Charlson (1987) have observed

---

* © *Perceptual and Motor Skills*, 1974; reprinted with permission.

that hearing teachers of the deaf may delete important signed information when speaking and signing to deaf children of school age. This observation clearly indicates that deaf children who learn to sign at school in TC may not experience full sign language instruction.

Use of parts of the body other than the hands

Important facets of sign language are produced with parts of the body other than the hands, though it is conventional to refer to sign language as a manual language. Parts of the body to which reference has been made include the face, eyes, head, upper limbs and trunk (Dittman, 1972; Baker and Padden, 1978; Baker 1980; Liddell, 1980; Ruggieri et al., 1982; Kluwin, 1983; Stokoe, 1991), for both hearing and hearing-impaired people. Generally, native speakers of standard English make relatively little use of kinesic communication (Harris, 1989), and as a result there has been a rather late realisation of the potential importance, in the sign language of deaf people, of signs other than the obvious manual gestures.

The signer's eye, face and head movements may help to form signs, serve a function as adverbs and adjectives, and indicate aspects of grammar (Baker-Shenk, 1985). Some signed communication may be conveyed with the face alone. Reduplicated verbs in Swedish Sign Language may be accompanied by different mouth positions. Such verbal modification is adverbial in nature. Another form, referred to as 'initial hold', is a modulation of degree meaning 'very'. Here, the movement begins with a short hold and is then completed quickly while the head is turned away to the side, giving a visual impression of an enlarged sign, since the distance between the hand and head is increased (Bergman, 1983).

Similar combinations, of which at least 20 are known, can occur in ASL (Baker-Schenk, 1985) when movements of the eyes, face and head serve as adjectives and adverbs to modulate the accompanying manual signs. Thus, to make the sign meaning 'write' whilst producing the facial adverb which means 'carelessly' produces the meaning of 'write carelessly'. Grammatical forms showing whether a message is a question, assertion, command, is conditional or negated, or includes a special topic or a relative clause, can also be indicated by movements of the eyes, face, head and trunk. In such instances, the grammatical signals are presented immediately before the relevant part of the message starts, and usually continue until it ends. The signal for the conditional part of a contingent message, for example, consists of raising the eyebrows and leaning the head and/or body to the side, and is offered throughout the presentation of the conditional segment. When this conditional segment has been completed another grammatical signal may be used to signify an ensuing 'main clause' statement, question, etc. Although 'if' may be signed manually in a conditional message, it need not be so signed when the non-manual conditional form is used. Even when it is signed manually, the signer still generally uses the non-manual signal throughout the presentation of the relevant segment. Similarly, a message which offers a negative statement can be presented with a manual sign for 'not' or with a non-manual negation signal which includes shaking of the head and a negative expression on the face with the corners of the mouth turned down. Baker-Schenk (1985) has presented pictorial representations of the above.

A combination of facial expression and head position marks topics in ASL where the eyebrows are raised with the head tilted slightly backwards (Bellugi and Fischer, 1972; Liddell, 1980). This combination is presented at the same time as the topic sign and then ceases. Liddell also described other non-manual signals giving grammatical information. Thus, head tilt is used to indicate relative clauses (Liddell, 1978a). Yes–no questions may be cued by raising the eyebrows, and leaning the head and body forward.

Research in facial expressions has developed to the degree to which a coding system is needed to record and analyse signed discourse, especially when overlaid with facial expressions of emotion. Baker-Shenk (1985) described a coding system based on the Facial Action Coding System of Ekman and Friesen (1978). This system uses 44 Action Units to describe the range of possible movements of the face which are closely related to movement of the facial musculature. It allows for separate coding of all positions and movements of gaze, face, head and trunk. Together with coding of manual signs, including onset and offset, via their English counterparts or glosses, the whole communication signal can be recorded against a timeline, giving a record of what was produced and when.

Baker-Shenk found that the affect of the signer could change the nature of the grammatical signal, so that it continued to be recognizable but changed its characteristics. Thus, the raised eyebrows in yes–no questions are usually at a mid-intensity level, with the upper eyelids slightly raised. But when the signer asks a question in surprise, the raising of eyebrows and eyelids increases in intensity and the jaw drops to leave the mouth open. Changes of facial expression in sign language are thus analogous to the role played by intonation in spoken English. Baker-Shenk remarked that facial movements could function as signs, components of signs, modifiers (adverbs), and as grammatical signals. Further, the movements and positions of the head of the signer had a function in the syntax of sign language. She felt that, as a result, sign languages should be referred to as visual–gestural, rather than manual, languages.

Mimicry and role-taking

Users of sign language may take the role of a person or animal to which allusion is being made, when the signer represents the person or animal with his or her own body, to show what that person or animal is doing. Such role-taking, mime, mimicry, or even dramatisation is very useful for representing indirect discourse (Hoemann, 1976, 1978a; Suty, 1986; Mindess, 1990). Hoemann (1976) reported the cumbersome indirect message: 'The doctor said that I should stay home. She said I could come to her office, but she told me not to go out for any other reason' as the signed 'STAY HOME. COME SEE ME, OK. OTHER OUT NO', with the signer acting in the role of the doctor. Signals that the signer has changed roles are given by facial expression, body posture and position, and manner of expression, in this case to simulate the authority figure of the doctor. Role-taking results in a considerable saving of effort. It may also produce a gain in clarity of who is saying what to whom, especially when the message involves a number of agents interacting with one another, when the role of each agent may be taken in turn.

ychology of communication by sign

erstand communication by sign, we need to appreciate the ways in which sign and other gestural forms, are organised in the brain. It is generally accepted that the left cerebral hemisphere plays the major part in monitoring and controlling speech functions in hearing people (but see Efron, 1990). It is also generally accepted that, for almost all right-handed people, speech functions are left-lateralised. The situation is less clear for left-handers. Their speech functions may be left-lateralised in about two-thirds or more of cases (Kimura, 1983). It is further well accepted that right-handed hearing people predominantly make right-handed gestures while talking. This effect is less marked for left-handers. Left-handers do not make left-handed gestures to the same extent as right-handers make right-handed gestures (Kimura, 1973a, b; Dalby et al., 1980; Kimura and Humphrys, 1981). The left cerebral hemisphere controls both the speech functions and the predominantly right-handed gestures which accompany speech in right-handed talkers (Kimura, 1973a).

Feyereisen (1983) concluded from work on non-fluent speech that gestures were related to speech function. Feyereisen reviewed evidence showing that, when hearing talkers are stuck for the correct words to communicate what they want to say, they may shift to use of gesture; gestures are more often used by bilingual people when using the less familiar of their two languages; and people with impaired speech, or expressive aphasia, use gestures more frequently than non-impaired people when communicating, but not in other activities. Were such gestures to occur more frequently on the right than the left side, when assessed against the proportions of right- versus left-hand gestures which occur during normal fluent speech, this finding would strongly support left cerebral lateralisation as mediating both speech functions and gestures in hearing people.

In his review of the rather slim evidence available, Harris (1989) observed that the increase in gesture was disproportionately greater on the right-hand side. He also took Kimura's (1973a) argument a stage further in concluding that the right hand is generally more expressive in serving communication among hearing people. In considering handedness and use of gestures by deaf people, the evidence suggests that right-handed deaf signers make gestures more with the right than the left hand (Harris, 1989). The inference is that signing is left-lateralised for right-handed deaf signers, but more work is needed before firm conclusions can be drawn. There is some suggestion that use of the dominant hand is less marked in deaf signers than is the use of the dominant hand for gestures during speech by hearing people, indicating that sign may not be as strongly lateralised as speech functions.

Further evidence of cerebral lateralisation in sign language comes from the area of the neuropsychology of visual perception – the so-called visual hemifield studies. Such studies are of practical interest because deaf children can identify signs presented well into their visual periphery (Swisher et al., 1989; Swisher, 1990), although studies investigating peripheral vision for signs and cerebral lateralisation have yet to be done.

Visual stimuli which impinge on one side of the retina are transmitted directly to one of the two cerebral hemispheres. Thus visual stimuli presented from the right side, that is, from the right visual field, go directly to the left cerebral hemisphere. If the stimuli move across the visual field from right to left, they will first directly stimulate the left side of the retinae and the resulting nerve impulses will travel from both eyes to the left hemisphere. They will then stimulate the right side of the retinae, with resulting nerve impulses travelling to the right hemisphere. Studies which demonstrate this effect require fixation on a central point, while stimulus material is introduced into the visual periphery. There is a right visual field (left hemisphere) advantage for verbal stimuli and a left visual field (right hemisphere) advantage for visual spatial stimuli (Mishkin and Forgays, 1952; Cohen, 1977; Hellige, 1980), though Moscovitch (1979) has argued that this kind of laterality effect occurs in relatively late stages of processing, and that analyses of the physical features of stimuli occur in both cerebral hemispheres. The right visual field advantage for verbal material seems to occur because the left cerebral hemisphere has an advantage in processing serial information, whereas visuospatial information is processed favourably by the right hemisphere (Cohen, 1977). Alternatively, the left hemisphere may be specialised for processing codes, while the right hemisphere may be superior in processing novel stimuli.

Neuropsychological processing has been studied in both deaf and hearing people. Phippard (1977), Ross et al. (1979) and Scholes and Fischler (1979) among others found that deaf signers showed a small left visual field (right hemisphere) advantage for words as compared with hearing individuals. Other workers (Poizner et al., 1979) have found a right visual field advantage in deaf subjects for English words, which was, however, less marked than the right visual field advantage for hearing subjects. Manning et al. (1977) observed that hearing subjects, as expected, showed a significant left hemisphere advantage for English words while deaf subjects showed only a tendency in the same direction. The results for the deaf subjects may have been due to variable familiarity of this group with ASL (Wilbur, 1979). Phippard (1977) studied a group of orally educated deaf and another group educated orally and manually, together with hearing subjects. The latter showed left hemisphere advantage for English letters and right hemisphere advantage for lines and faces. The orally educated deaf group showed right hemisphere advantage for English letters and lines (they were not presented with faces). The group educated both orally and manually showed no marked hemispheric advantage for different types of stimuli. Again, the extent of familiarity with the stimulus modality for the last group was not recorded, and may have been a confounding factor. The visual field effects found in these studies of verbal stimuli with deaf subjects were small and conflicting. This conflict may have been due to differences in method between the studies, or because of a lesser experience with written English amongst the deaf subjects (Zaidel, 1980).

For signs, both hearing and deaf people show a left visual field (right hemisphere) advantage when the signs are stationary (Manning et al., 1977; Poizner et al., 1979). Moving signs may show a small left visual field (right hemisphere) advantage (Poizner et al., 1979), but not when they are temporally redundant, such that parts of the signs are similar at the beginning and the end (Kyle and Woll, 1985).

These studies taken together do not present a convincing case that signs are processed in a neuropsychologically different way to standard English. More recent investigations tend to confirm that sign language, like English, is processed in the left cerebral hemisphere. Thus, while Boshoven et al. (1982) observed a left visual field advantage in deaf subjects for drawings, they did not find an advantage for words, dots or ASL, in comparisons with hearing subjects and interpreters for the deaf. Panou and Sewell (1984) also obtained a right visual field advantage in deaf subjects for English words and BSL signs. Poizner et al. (1984) found that four unilaterally brain-damaged deaf signers, fluent in ASL, processed linguistic and non-linguistic visual stimuli in essentially the same way as would have brain-damaged hearing people. Their three patients with left hemisphere damage were poor at processing linguistic signs, but processed non-linguistic visuospatial stimuli appropriately. The single patient with right hemisphere damage performed poorly with the non-linguistic visuospatial stimuli, but performance for the linguistic stimuli was adequate.

In a later significant review of neuropsychological work with deaf signers, Bellugi et al. (1988) concluded that hearing and speech were not necessary for hemispheric specialisation to develop. Hence hearing for speech was not crucial for hemispheric specialisation. This conclusion casts further doubt on aspects of the critical period hypothesis of the importance of early hearing ability for language development (Chapter 2), although auditory and sign languages may differ in other neuropsychological aspects. Bellugi et al. further concluded that patients with left hemisphere damage show marked deficits in the syntax of sign language, for example, but adequate facility for non-language visuospatial material such as spatial relations. Patients with right hemisphere damage showed the reverse. In sign language, although grammatical information is conveyed by the visuospatial modality, this did not appear to affect complementary hemispheric specialisation, which was similar to that by which hearing people process standard English and non-linguistic material. Bellugi et al. also found that aspects of sign language, such as lexicon and grammar, could be impaired selectively, suggesting that the brain's functional organisation for sign language may be modular. They concluded that the left cerebral hemisphere had an innate predisposition for language irrespective of language modality, and that views of hemispheric specialisation which based a distinction of function on a difference between language and visuospatial function were oversimple (compare Kimura, 1990). Sign language, in the visual modality and involving an interplay between visuospatial and linguistic relations, was processed neuropsychologically in the same way as standard English.

Similar conclusions were drawn by Bellugi et al. (1989) and Sanders et al. (1989). However, the situation is less clear for facial expressions. Corina (1989) found that deaf signers' visual field asymmetries for affective and linguistic expressions were affected by the order of presentation, whereas hearing subjects showed left visual field advantages for both kinds of signals. Thus for deaf signers, hemispheric specialisation for processing facial signals, which are of particular salience to them, may be affected by the differences which those signals serve. Sanders et al. (1989) have also presented results suggesting a left visual field advantage for semantic categorisation of words and static BSL signs, but their adolescent subjects were not all profoundly deaf and all had been instructed in sign-support-ed speech. The issue of lateralisation was therefore confounded with subject and experiential variables.

Although it may be relatively difficult to find them, work in this area will con-tinue to be hard to interpret unless the deaf signers employed are congenitally profoundly deaf signers born to deaf signing parents, with no use of speechread-ing or residual hearing, and with no other interfering handicaps.

Acquisition and learning of sign language

Sign language is far from an elementary system of communication requiring only basic skills for its acquisition. It appears as a language in its own right, containing complex structures and its own intonation, semantics and pragmatics. Although its lexicon and sublexical material is relatively iconic, there is often an iconic corre-spondence between form and meaning in syntax and morphology (Fischer, 1978; Klima and Bellugi, 1979). Sign languages convey the meaning in communication pervasively by transparency and translucency of form.

Profoundly deaf children come from varying social and economic backgrounds. Their backgrounds also differ in whether their parents and siblings are hearing, or prelingually or postlingually deaf. Further, different members of their family may be deaf or hearing. What profoundly deaf children do have in common is a reliance on vision as their main means of acquiring language and communication skills (Russell et al., 1976). Where neither parents nor siblings are deaf, the deaf child will use speechreading supplemented by residual hearing and improvised gestures, or perhaps by manual communication if the parents have learned manu-al skills. On the other hand, deaf children will communicate most readily with deaf relatives by manual communication. There are thus different familial situa-tions which direct a young hearing-impaired child's modality of communication. That modality seems likely to be purely manual only when both parents and any siblings are themselves deaf, and habitually use sign language in their everyday communication, including communication with visitors (Siple, 1978a). On attain-ing school age, deaf children born to hearing parents may communicate with each other in several ways, both in and out of the classroom. Much or all of this com-munication will be non-linguistic, a poor relation of sign language, especially if it is 'prohibited' by teachers (Lewis, 1968). It is likely to be an imperfect kind of communication (Tervoort, 1961). The reader is referred to Quigley and Kretschmer (1982) and Volterra and Erting (1990) for reviews of this area.

We now consider what is known of the early acquisition of sign language by deaf children born to deaf signing parents, where such children are congenitally deaf, or deafened before the acquisition of spoken language.

Schlesinger and Meadow (1972) reported a small study of two hearing children and one deaf child born to deaf parents. All three children learned to sign before they learned to speak, with the first sign for the deaf child produced at 10 months of age. Williams (1976) found that the first sign of a deaf child born to deaf par-ents was produced at 9 months. McIntire (1977), in a study of an infant with a borderline hearing loss, born to hearing-impaired parents, found 85 signs at 13 months of age and more than 200 signs at 21 months, with 2-sign productions at 10 months. Bonvillian et al. (1983) investigated 11 children from nine families with deaf parents. Both father and mother were deaf in seven families, one family was a single-parent family and one family had a deaf mother and a hearing father. Nine of the children were firstborn, with the remaining two second-born. Ten children were normally hearing, while the remaining one had a severe bilateral hearing loss. The children and parents were visited once every 5–6 weeks over a 16-month period. Seven children were studied from before their first birthday, from 4–10 months, together with a 12-month-old and an 18-month-old. Two older children, aged 2 and 3 years, for whom their parents had kept detailed developmental diaries, were also included. The infants' acquisition of the various motor milestones was in accord with accepted norms. While infants produce their first words between 11 and 14 months of age, the first sign was produced at an average age of 8.5 months. Ten signs were produced by 13.2 months as compared with norms of 10 words at 15.1 months, and the first combination of signs appeared on the average at 17 months as compared with norms for first word combinations at 18 to 21 months. Of the first ten signs produced, 30% were considered to be iconic, 37% were metonymic, being based on a relatively small or unimportant feature, and 33% were arbitrary. This distribution differs considerably from that discussed by Van Uden (1986), who reported relatively few arbitrary signs. The use of signs, then, was in advance of the norms for the use of words for these infants, who were all but one hearing, but all of whom had deaf parents who habitually used ASL in the home. Caselli (1983) reported on four deaf children without recording details of hearing loss or the hearing status of the parents. She concluded that the first gestures of both deaf and hearing children were deictic, such as pointing, and that these deictic gestures were then followed by signs, or words.

The parallel between the early acquisition of sign by deaf children of deaf parents and the acquisition of verbal language by hearing children of hearing parents continues into the later years. Thus Prinz and Prinz (1985) observed that 24 profoundly deaf children, mostly born to deaf parents and aged from 3 to 11 years, showed signed discourse strategies in peer interactions comparable to those used by hearing children in spoken conversations. They adhered to discourse rules, including soliciting attention, obtaining and holding eye contact, handling conversational topics, turn-taking, and remedial interruptions.

Deaf infants, then, acquire sign language at the same age as hearing infants acquire verbal language, or earlier, perhaps because the body-motor system develops earlier than the control of speech musculature (Sperling, 1978). The rate of increase in mean length of utterance with age, for example, is strikingly similar for deaf manually communicating and hearing verbally communicating infants around the age of 30–36 months. There are similarities, too, in infantile expressions or 'baby talk' (Siple, 1978a), and overgeneralisation of rules, similar to 'camed' and 'wented' in young hearing children acquiring standard English (Wilbur, 1979). It may therefore be argued that language acquisition develops in stages (Brown, 1973), which are not modality-specific (Schlesinger and Meadow, 1972; Collins-Ahlgren, 1975; McIntire, 1977). However, specific language structures, such as syntax, depend on particular mechanisms which may be modality-specific (Klima and Bellugi, 1979).

Although published research relates to studies of only small groups of children, it seems likely that deaf children acquire sign language structures developmentally in a similar way to that in which young hearing children acquire verbal language. Further, since languages need to be learned or acquired, this fact sets constraints on their structures (see below). Sign languages have the same type of analytic structure as spoken languages, in so far as both have a limited number of variables, each of which may contain a limited number of discrete values which shape language acquisition, together with a set of rules which control the ways in which the discrete values may be used. Further, the process of language acquisition sets limits on the structures languages may adopt, because languages are constrained by the processes of language acquisition (Newport and Supalla, 1980).

In learning any language, people like to establish one-to-one relationships between its basic semantic aspects and its surface forms. They also like to see clear relationships between meaning and form (Slobin, 1980). In the jargon used by linguists, people like the semantic aspects of a language to be transparent. Slobin argued that, in acquiring their first language, children strive for transparency and regularity, even beyond the natural regularity of the language, and only gradually adjust to the more opaque aspects of the language. He also argued that when the opacity is too great there is a shift to new and more transparent forms. These arguments suggest that the transparency of sign languages, and their noted iconicity, confers on sign a learnability beyond a characterisation of mere modality difference from spoken languages, and beyond the possible benefits of a clearly perceived association between signs and their referents. Under some circumstances, there is a tendency to regress towards transparency which seems to put sign languages at an advantage in their learning. It would also help to explain why the iconicity of sign is so pervasive and persistent.

Hearing children develop their expertise in spoken language subconsciously, without apparent effort. The same might be said of deaf children born to deaf signing parents and who have deaf signing siblings, in their progress with sign language. Older hearing children and adults are able both to acquire by unconscious assimilation and to learn by conscious effort in expanding their first language. They become aware, through learning, of its rule structure and lexicon, while retaining some continuing facility for acquiring it. The use of both acquisition and learning holds true for second-language learning by hearing older children and adults (Krashen, 1982), and for verbal language development by native deaf signers, for whom verbal language is a second language. For the orally communicating young congenitally deaf child, born to hearing parents and with hearing siblings, spoken language is the first language. But the difficulties imposed by poor auditory inputs are so great that a first spoken language for deaf children develops more like a second than a first language. The learning effort required is very considerable, and the part played by acquisition is small.

For most young deaf children who are born to hearing parents, sign language is a kind of second, second language, because the first oral language, with which they communicate with their parents, is nearly always imperfectly developed for their age. Thus most deaf children, who are those born to hearing parents, have to learn sign language. However, their motivation to communicate with other deaf individuals is likely to be so strong, especially if their oral communication is limited, that they usually become far more fluent in sign language, if permitted to do so, than hearing people who set out to learn it.

It is generally reported that deaf children born to deaf parents, or who otherwise begin their experiences with manual communication early in life, learn sign language more effectively and attain other advantages in cognitive skills and academic attainments. Nevertheless, there may be exceptions. Parasnis (1983) compared congenitally deaf college students, with deaf parents and who were native ASL users, with congenitally deaf college students who had hearing parents and learned ASL between 6 and 12 years of age. Comparisons were made of cognitive ability, the cognitive style of field dependence/independence and English language presented and produced in the spoken, written and signed modes. As expected, the subjects who had learned sign language performed significantly better than the native ASL group in speech perception and production. However, the latter group did not show differential effects which might be ascribed to early signed communication with their deaf parents. The lack of difference between the native ASL users and the group who learned to sign between 6 and 12 years may have occurred, however, because the relevant test involved English language presented via sign. Such a test would probably have been in a manual form more familiar to those who learned ASL rather than those who acquired it as their native language. Thus there was possible confounding with the type of test used, so Parasnis' work cannot be seen as clearly negating the general reports.

We saw earlier that young deaf children will develop a gestural form of communication for interaction with deaf peers, in the absence of any specific direction or modelling. Goldin-Meadow and Mylander (1984) have reported analogous findings for young deaf children of hearing parents, who developed a system of gestures for communicating with hearing individuals. Such gesture creation was observed in four deaf children aged 1;4 to 3;1 years, when each child, without usable conventional linguistic inputs, either oral or manual, developed a system of gestures comparable in semantic content and structure to the early spoken and signed systems of children acquiring conventional languages. As with Heider and Heider (1940) and Mohay (1982) the results suggested that signed communication can develop in markedly atypical language-learning environments, without a tutor's modelling or otherwise shaping the structure of the communication. It is not clear whether the development of such kinds of communication is acquired or learned. Certainly it will be far from the apparently effortless acquisition of the usual first steps in normal language development. Nevertheless, it is clear that the children themselves played the major role in developing these communication systems, as with the private verbal languages developed between hearing twins, implying that the gestural systems were not learned in the sense that they were not explicitly taught.

Research in volume into sign language learning has appeared only in recent years, and probably as much or more with hearing people and the intellectually disabled or communication-disordered as with the deaf child. This research followed earlier investigations of the nature of sign language, which emphasised the linguistic and psychological factors involved (Hoemann, 1975; Bellugi and Klima,

1976; Klima and Bellugi, 1979). The translucency of the sign and the correctness of its gloss were seen as important in sign language learning by Luftig and Lloyd (1981). Lloyd and Doherty (1983) considered production strategies that may be helpful for the learner of signing. Recent developments have been reviewed by Volterra and Erting (1990).

Much of this work has been conducted with the learning of sign language semantics and vocabulary – the relationship between the referent and its symbolic, manual representation (Robinson and Griffith, 1979; Orlansky and Bonvillian, 1984) in terms of iconicity, transparency and translucency. Page (1985a) also studied the perceived translucency between ASL signs and their glosses in hearing preschool and school-age children and adults. She found that her 4- and 7-year-old children and adults perceived signs that convey action, excluding stative verbs like 'feel' and 'is', to be more translucent or more iconic than signs representing nomination, which in turn were more translucent than signs conveying attribution. Page ascribed these results to Newport and Bellugi's (1979) categorisation of objects into the three levels of basic, superordinate and subordinate, as *chair* is basic to the superordinate *furniture* and the subordinate *recliner*, for which ASL has rather different forms in sign. Thus signs for basic terms are usually of single-unit form, signs for superordinates are compounds of basic level signs, and signs for subordinates consist of basic elements together with visual descriptive gestures. Page argued that translucency is that aspect of iconicity which is closest to usual sign learning, and that translucent signs are to be preferred to non-translucent signs in preparing materials for instruction in sign language.

Exploration of the relationship between signs and their verbal glosses should be a powerful tool for developing academic achievement. For example, Akamatsu and Armour (1987) drew the attention of six severely to profoundly prelingually deaf residential high-school students to signing, making explicit some of the ways in which signing differs from writing. Their results indicated that translating between sign and writing made the students more aware of the rule differences between sign and written English. In analysing the construction of ASL and Pidgin Sign English, the students began to perceive a common base to signed and written English modes of communication, signing in English and signing in ASL. A further useful outcome was that the students improved in the grammar of their written English more than a matched control group of deaf students who did not receive the analytical instruction.

This report by Akamatsu and Armour, showing a positive attitude to the use of sign in formal training of deaf children, also draws attention to the large proportion of teachers who now agree that sign input is very important to the development of communication skills in the profoundly deaf child, and to the level of skills needed for general conversation. This attitude now is regularly found in Australia (Ballge-Kimber and Giorcelli, 1989) though the development is recent (Treloar, 1985), Canada (Wickham and Kyle, 1987), the UK (Child, 1991) and the USA (Crittenden, 1986; Stewart, 1983). However, it is the majority view that signed English should be used in the classroom rather than sign language.

As regards the use of technology in the learning of sign language, Seal (1987) has discussed the preparation of instructional videotapes for signing deaf preschoolers. Slike et al. (1989) used an interactive video system to teach an introductory course of sign language vocabulary to 20 hearing students, while a control group, also of 20 students, learned the same signs by a traditional classroom method. Comparison of the groups after training showed no difference in the ability to recognise signs. However, the group that learned signed vocabulary via the interactive video system took only two-thirds of the time taken by the group learning the signs by the conventional approach. If these findings can be generalised to deaf students, then such students may be able to learn signed vocabulary more efficiently if use is made of interactive video technology.

Sign language learning clearly involves motor learning. It strikes the observer as involving perceptual motor skills rather more obviously than spoken language. There have been several studies concerned particularly with the motor aspects of sign learning to a greater or lesser degree. Dennis et al. (1982) proposed that motor factors played a part in facilitating the learning of sign vocabulary, since signs with high motor complexity will tend to dissuade the child from using them frequently. Hanson and Feldman (1989) devised a sign decision task in which deaf signers made a decision about the number of hands needed to produce particular ASL signs. They found significant facilitation of such decision-making by repetition among signs that shared a base morpheme, thus illustrating a practice effect in a motor aspect of sign learning. Also, a lexical decision task with English words showed facilitation by repetition of words that shared a base morpheme in both English and ASL, but not among words that shared a base morpheme in ASL alone.

Polar coordinates were used by Montgomery et al. (1983) to demonstrate patterns in signing, but the way in which students learn to express sign language movement patterns has only very recently been investigated by spatial analysis of motion. Thus Lupton and Zelaznick (1990) examined the changes in movement trajectories of two right-handed young female adult hearing students, from shortly after the beginning until the end of an introductory ASL course. These students had no knowledge of sign language to begin with. Lupton and Zelaznik, using infrared apparatus, found that the movement patterns increased in speed, symmetry and replicability, and became more limited in amplitude of movement as instruction progressed over a semester's course. Although users may show some preference for one-handed signs, interlimb coordination is important for many recognisable ASL signs. Thus (Battison, 1978; Hamilton and Lillo-Martin, 1986) there are constraints of symmetry in ASL such that when both hands are moving they display the same movement and shape, whether moving in- or out-of-phase. Because Lupton and Zelaznick's subjects developed such skill easily, their ease of learning supported the notion of such symmetry constraints.

From observations of an infant over age 13–21 months acquiring ASL in a family of deaf signers, McIntire (1977) suggested four stages, concerned with positions of fingers and thumb, in acquiring ASL handshapes, which are based on a child's developing cognitive and physical control of the weaker fingers. Thus the child became increasingly able to produce the more difficult features. McIntire's findings were similar to those observed in infants acquiring phonemic competence in spoken languages, where there are different stages for the acquisition of segments of speech sounds (Schick, 1990). In a study of the acquisition of classifiers, Schick explored whether handshapes were accurately produced in both structurally simple and complex predicates, and whether errors in production of handshapes occurred only because of anatomical factors. She found, in severely to profoundly deaf children aged between 4;5 and 9 years, that morphological complexity affected the accuracy of handshapes. But whereas earlier studies (Kantor, 1980) had suggested that the earliest handshapes used by children to form classifiers depended on both anatomical and cognitive complexity, Schick found that the children's production of handshapes was affected by complexity of morphology and by morphosyntactic aspects. There was no evidence, from analysis of handshape errors, to suggest that stages in the acquisition of handshapes depended only on anatomical complexity. Hence, in developing ability in ASL, the deaf child's performance depends on linguistic organisation rather than on motor learning or acquisition.

To summarise this section on the acquisition and learning of sign language, there is good evidence to show that deaf children born to deaf signing parents acquire sign readily, at a rate comparable to or faster than the acquisition of spoken language by hearing children. Deaf children born to hearing parents, however, have a harder time of it in learning sign, if such is available to them. A very recent area of research is the use of sophisticated techniques to investigate the geometry of sign, including the ways in which sign develops spatially. These techniques have revealed that sign develops as a coordination of speed and symmetry, with increasing replicability, in adult learners, and as a staged process increasing in complexity in infancy.

Total Communication

Despite the emphasis on oralism following the Milan Congress in 1880, a proportion of hearing-impaired children, especially those born to deaf parents, continued to acquire sign language as their first language, and used sign in communicating with other deaf individuals. To this day, both deaf children and adults who are competent in sign tend to seek out the deaf individuals in mixed groups of hearing and deaf people, and carry on communication in sign.

Sign language began to aquire official and linguistic respectability in the 1960s, notably boosted by the work of Stokoe (Stokoe et al., 1965), which initiated a status for sign as a language in its own right. This seminal work was followed by a burst of research into sign language, still continuing, from which it seems that the more that is known of sign language, the more accepted is its status as language. Further recognition of the potential of sign language came from the 'oral failures', an unfortunately large proportion of deaf children who had been educated orally but who did not perform well in academic achievement tests and whose speech was unintelligible. Those mentors who based educational attainment on the development of good communication skills argued that deaf child signers, who were expert in their native sign language, could benefit educationally from good signed communication with their teachers (Schlesinger, 1986). However, this attitude quickly ran into problems, because few of the teachers, who were mainly hearing, were fluent in sign language. Rather they used some form of signed English. The educational attainments of deaf children as a whole continued to be unacceptably low (see Chapter 6), whether the children were educated orally or manually.

The advent of TC

In the mid to late 1960s in the USA, soon followed in the UK (Montgomery, 1966), and Australia (Burch and Hyde, 1984) proposals were made to combine oral and signing approaches (Schlesinger, 1986) in what became known as Total Communication (TC), very similar to what is known as simultaneous communication (Newell et al., 1990). In theory, TC goes beyond oral plus manual approaches to permit other forms of communication. TC thus allows aural, manual and oral modes of communication (Gannon, 1981; Ling, 1984a; Johnson, 1988). In practice it may amount to not much more than a manual approach, occasionally augmented by other methods, such is the attraction of manual communication to the profoundly deaf. Hence TC is included in this chapter.

In retrospect, it is odd that it took so long to consider what seems to be an obvious alternative to oral-only or manual-only forms of communication. One reason was a fear that successful use of one alternative could be hindered by introduction of the other. The main reason, however, was probably that the positions of the oralists on the one hand, and the manualists on the other, were so entrenched, and defended with so much vigour and emotion, that for a long time consideration of a compromise was out of the question. However, in fairness, it should be pointed out that when a parent, therapist or teacher has expended great effort in learning an approach, the chosen approach will be defended stoutly and is unlikely to be altered except on the basis of very clear and overwhelming contraindications.

It was recognised at an early stage that TC should help to reduce the dominant position taken in class by teachers of the deaf, because TC would help to induce rapport between teacher and child, besides assisting a deaf child to communicate with hearing children and adults. TC also offered a prospect of the deaf child participating in an educational curriculum more like that of hearing children, and promised insights into spoken language learning by providing continuing opportunities for the deaf child to analyse and compare spoken and manual languages (compare Akamatsu and Armour, 1987). By 1975, White and Stevenson could report that in the USA the current trend was towards classroom use of TC.

TC and other communication methods

Since TC was introduced when oral and manual communication both had a long history, it is understandable that adherents of TC wished to 'prove' its usefulness against the established methods. White and Stevenson (1975) conducted an interesting study of the effects of learning-equated factual information by TC, manual communication, oral communication and reading by children in residential schools for the deaf. They were at pains to point out that most of the TC research conducted previous to their work was *ex-post-facto*, with recognised difficulties of interpretation, rather than experimentally based. Their subjects were all, or almost all, prelingually deaf with hearing losses of more than 65 dB, IQs in the range 60–140, and aged between 11 and 18 years, selected as a stratified random sample into nine subgroups, each of five children. An interpreter presented factual information from books at second- to fourth-grade level, following which the subjects were asked a standard set of questions about the information. All subgroups were found to have assimilated more information through reading, and more through total and through manual communication than through oral communication. No significant difference was found between total and manual communication, nor were there significant differences between high-, middle- and low-IQ children in assimilating information presented orally. However, the middle- and high-IQ children learned significantly more information than the children of low IQ when the information was presented by TC, manual communication or reading. There was thus an interaction between method of instruction and IQ, implying that conveying information orally to the brighter of these children resulted in them learning below their ability level. The addition of speech to manual communication (TC) did not increase these students' ability to learn the information but depressed it slightly, perhaps because the children lost information in shifting attention between speech and the manual signals, or because they experienced perceptual overload. This possibility is a continuing worry for adherents of TC (Nix, 1983). Further research is needed to establish to what extent it is a major issue.

The use of TC and oral communication in the UK were compared by Grove et al. (1979) with 26 adolescents, aged 16–21 years, all or most of whom were prelingually severely deaf. In this study each subject was presented with messages in their chosen mode of communication and instructed to tick a picture which meant the same as the message. Ten subjects relied on oral communication, and 16 on TC. The TC system was found to be the more effective method of communication for a number of different message structures. Grove et al. concluded that their results, and also the results of Montgomery (1968), and of White and Stevenson (1975), showed that TC and manual methods were no less effective in representing conventional language structures than oral communication, and were superior when used by those for whom they were the natural mode.

Grove and Rodda (1984) continued to obtain similar findings and to draw similar conclusions in a study of reading, TC, manual communication and oral communication with 118 severely and profoundly prelingually deaf subjects aged 9–20 years in Canada and New York. In checking pictures against a message, reading was the most effective method of communication, followed by TC and then manual communication. Oral methods were the least effective. From analyses of communication time, Grove and Rodda suggested that the relative weakness of the oral method was due to its low signal-to-noise ratio, and to short-term memory overload from ambiguous information caused by the hearing loss. Combining the oral and manual approaches, however, seemed to produce a stronger trace in short-term memory.

Using a video-taped test, five different communication modes – TC with audio, TC without audio, manual communication with no mouth movement, oral communication with audio, and oral communication without audio – were compared by Crittenden et al. (1986). The comparisons were made with 52 profoundly deaf children aged 6–12 years, all of whom used TC for their instruction over at least the previous 2 years and communicated outside the classroom in sign. The children were assessed on vocabulary, with a test standardised for deaf and hearing-impaired populations. The results showed that modes involving manual communication gave significantly better scores than all other modes. Oral communication added little to the manual mode for these children, confirming a view that deaf children communicating by TC communicate predominantly in manual language.

Despite such promising findings, TC has not been without its critics. Champie (1984) was concerned that although signs were used, preferably in combination with speech for TC, sign language was not being studied linguistically by deaf children. Their educational curriculum, she felt, should include the study of ASL as a language and as the communication system of deaf people. ASL was important for its effects on students' self-concepts, and because comparisons of ASL and English could improve their understanding of the rules of English, and hence their academic success. Nix (1983), mentioned earlier, took a more directly critical approach. He pointed out that the manual component of TC was typically either Manually Coded English (MCE), which required every word and morpheme present in the spoken version to be presented manually, or Pidgin Sign English (PSE), which was a conceptual approach that did not require a one-to-one relationship between the spoken and signed modes. On the one hand, the use of MCE cannot keep up in time with fluent speech, so that its users omitted up to 80% of it; on the other hand, users of PSE tended to decrease their speaking rate, but still spoke faster than they signed. They also omitted some of the signed material (compare; Marmor and Petitto, 1979; Strong and Charlson, 1987; Cokely, 1990). Nix's principal criticisms were that the overall transmission rate was decreased, the normal rate and rhythm of speech were changed, and the omission of MCE and parts of the spoken message produced ungrammatical and inconsistent models of English. Further, children using TC tended to show poor performance in specific areas related to spoken English, such as vocabulary and reading comprehension. However, Kluwin (1981) noted that more experienced teachers used more sign language, and less MCE, suggesting that as they became experienced they became more concerned with the function than the form of communication. It is hence interesting to note that Maxwell and Bernstein (1985) found MCE/sign mismatches in morphemes to be structural rather than semantic, and that the great majority of expressions conveyed the information appropriately, despite morphological differences. Certainly, the reader should not think that the problem is caused by the use of signs per se, as Emmorey and Corina (1990) have shown that fluent users of ASL can identify signs faster than has been found for spoken language. Much 'phonology' in sign is available simultaneously, in contrast to speech, resulting in faster lexical identification.

Knell and Klonoff (1983) obtained few differences between TC and orally educated severely to profoundly deaf children aged 7–11 years in verbal language output, but their orally educated children were significantly better in syntactic measures. Geers et al. (1984) also found that profoundly deaf children educated by TC experienced problems in the production of selected English language structures.

They assessed 327 children from oral/aural and TC programmes across the USA with the Grammatical Analysis of Elicited Language–Simple Sentence Level (GAEL-S) test, analysing the results separately for the oral productions of oral/aural children; the oral productions of TC children; the manual productions of TC children; and the combined productions of TC children. They found that the TC children gave oral productions substantially below the same children's manual scores, and below the scores of the oral/aural children for all sampled GAEL-S grammatical categories. The manual and combined scores of the TC children were significantly lower than those of the oral/aural children in over 50% of the grammatical categories, though the manual scores of the TC children significantly exceeded the oral/aural children's scores in up to 20% of these categories. This outcome suggested that spoken English did not develop along with MCE. Geers et al. also remarked that children in TC programmes, using MCE, did not show an advantage in the learning of English syntax over the orally/aurally educated children.

Much of the work described was conducted with single-item and/or short duration material, such as sentences. However, Gallagher and Meador (1989) found that in conversations between two adolescent hearing-impaired twin boys who had been TC-trained, there was use of an integrated bimodal form of English. Analysis of proportional frequencies of modes and the structural elements of spoken utterances showed that the bimodal English form used did not alter with the presence or absence of simultaneous signs in either the individual's or the partner's speech. Markides (1988) has found that in another specific area of spoken English, the speech intelligibility of a group of severely deaf children in a TC programme deteriorated over time. On the other hand, the intelligibility of the speech of a matched group in an aural/oral programme improved significantly over the same time interval.

A large number of studies which investigated the use of TC in educational programmes has been summarised by Schlesinger (1986), to which the reader's attention is drawn for a broader overview of the area. Her review concluded that, apart perhaps from deaf children whose background suggested that they would have success with oral methods and who could meet the demands a successful oral approach implied, such as well-educated and motivated parents of above average intelligence, TC could produce quite positive results. TC was valuable because it provided both a means of communicating and a way of assisting oral communication. TC could also help by stimulating the child's attention span, motivation, social interaction etc. As a recent report comparing oral, TC and cued speech approaches with hearing-impaired children in Hong Kong suggests (Lai and Lynas, 1990) TC could be also decrease behaviour problems. Schlesinger concluded her overview with a plea urging a truly bilingual approach, since for the great majority of deaf children, the situations with which they are faced require bilingual solutions involving both sign and speech.

In a considered and penetrating review, Maxwell (1990) has pointed out that TC or simultaneous communication mean different things to different people, and what is seen as a deficiency in a bimodal approach depends on the perceived purpose of the approach. Thus although a complete and exact translation of every spoken English morpheme into signed form is rarely achieved, except perhaps for the more simple or more easily translated constructions, such exactitude may not be the purpose of the teacher. It is therefore interesting to note (Mayer and Lowenbraun, 1990) that educators in kindergarten to fourth-grade educational programmes could produce a full manual representation (MCE) of their speech in TC. Proficiency in MCE may be affected by the teacher's attitude to the need to sign a complete message, the school's educational policy, and the degree to which teacher implementation of MCE policies is monitored. MCE was used in this study with a much higher accuracy rate (up to 90%) than that found by Marmor and Petitto (1979) at 10%.

Thompson and Swisher (1985) argued sensibly that TC was suitable for providing immediate and consistent language inputs for very young deaf children before eventual auditory perceptual skills could be determined. Such early inputs were important, they felt, because most hearing-impaired children have auditory discrimination or auditory perceptual problems which are difficult to assess thoroughly in early life. It also seems possible that TC is better suited to instruction for younger deaf children, who do not need such lengthy and complex linguistic inputs as the older deaf child. It may be particularly suited to deaf infants, who are too young for valid assessment of their hearing loss.

Conclusion

The adherents of TC argue that TC promotes communication, and a resulting increase in facility with language will assist academic learning and improve the production of speech. However, the academic abilities of hearing-impaired children who communicate in TC do not show conclusively that TC has major advantages over other methods. TC has not adequately met the high expectations of it (Eagney, 1987) for reasons such as those described above, although it is generally agreed to be valuable. The current trend is to proceed with TC, while contrary arguments continue.

Chapter 6
Hearing Impairment and Literacy Skills

There is an extensive literature on the reading achievement of hearing-impaired children, which shows a plateau in attainment at around 8–10 years of age beyond which it is difficult for the child to progress. This chapter outlines some of the studies documenting this effect. It then considers work which seeks to explain the processes underlying the reading performance of hearing-impaired children, and which promote intervention for the teaching of reading. An account is also given of the writing abilities of hearing-impaired children, and the reciprocal relationship between their reading and writing is discussed.

Besides the major handicaps imposed on oracy by severe and especially profound hearing loss, similar handicaps are encountered by the severely and profoundly hearing-impaired child in the skills involved in literacy. Such skills are learned by hearing children following the acquisition of oracy, most probably by building on inner speech. This inner speech mediates reading by the silent understanding and rehearsal of symbols or words, and recognition of sequential and contextual cues (Conrad, 1979; Wood, 1980; Nolen and Wilbur, 1984; Bamford and Saunders, 1985; Wood et al., 1986; Hanson et al., 1991). It also assists in the production of symbols or words in writing. Therefore, if children have problems with oracy they are also likely to experience problems with literacy (Vellum, 1979; Hanson, 1986), resulting in overall weak communicative fluency. This is generally also the case for deaf children.

Reading

We read to comprehend, and reading permits us to inform ourselves at our own rate of learning. Reading is particularly useful in allowing us to assimilate detail and considered ideas. Hence reading provides a deep basis of knowledge about events and concepts which add to the depth and flexibility of our communication. The increasing use of microcomputers, either as standalone devices, or more especially as aids to telecommunication, has produced a particular emphasis on skills in reading and writing (typing), not only for hearing people but also for the hearing-impaired, including deaf children.

Problems with reading can be experienced by hearing as well as by deaf children. Hearing children who are prone to hearing impairment as a result of chronic middle-ear infections may have difficulties in beginning reading (Webster et al., 1984; Webster et al., 1989). Also, young children with only a mild sensorineural hearing loss (20–45 dB) may show reduced performance in vocabulary acquisition and reading comprehension (Blair et al., 1985).

Hearing children of school age use complex grammatical structures and enjoy a large vocabulary. Their early reading primers, which contain grammatical constructs and vocabularies which are well within their grasp, are attuned to these linguistic skills. Hearing children can therefore concentrate on learning the skills involved in reading itself, on understanding printed material as a cipher that projects the linguistic code they already know (Smith, 1973).

The situation is quite different for the severely to profoundly deaf child who, in learning to read, is confronted with two main problems (Clarke et al., 1982). The first, and underlying, problem is that most such children are severely deficient in their knowledge of verbal language. The second problem lies in perceiving the written words as reflecting the language code. It is small wonder that, as a result, deaf children of school-leaving age commonly have a reading age of only about 9–10 years (Gentile and Di Francesca, 1969; Trybus and Karchmer, 1977; Conrad, 1979; King and Quigley, 1985). For most deaf children, learning to read means having to learn language as well (Webster and Ellwood, 1985). Of course, there are some deaf children, with well-developed linguistic attainments, whose reading ability is within normal limits, but unfortunately such children are in the minority. Even if a deaf child can recognise individual words, understanding of the written material will not happen without a sure base of language (Quigley and Kretschmer, 1982).

Reading achievement

Early work on reading achievement by deaf children has been reviewed by Quigley (1982), Quigley and Kretschmer (1982), Bamford and Saunders (1985), and King and Quigley (1985). Most of this work, in the USA, was based on tests of reading achievement standardised for hearing children, and was directed towards the demographic assessment of reading age or reading grade level (Pinter and Paterson, 1917; Pugh, 1946; Fusfeld, 1955; Wrightstone et al., 1963; Myklebust, 1964; Furth, 1966b; Balow et al., 1971; Hammermeister, 1971; Di Francesca, 1972; Trybus and Karchmer, 1977).

Quigley and Kretschmer (1982) pointed out that large-scale demographic studies may obscure the somewhat better results attained by some individual programmes, using the study of Lane and Baker (1974) to illustrate this point. Lane and Baker noted from Furth (1966b) and Wrightstone et al. (1963) that only 12% of more than 5000 hearing-impaired adolescents aged 10–16 years had a reading age of 11 years or more. On comparing the performance of this large group of adolescents with the scores of 132 hearing-impaired students of the Central

Institute of the Deaf aged between 10 and 16 years, Lane and Baker found that the CID group's grade level reading equivalent was much higher, though the reading attainment was still below that of hearing children. It was not clear, however, whether this difference was due to the educational approach, namely maximum use of residual hearing in continuous education at school and oral communication at home, as argued by Lane and Baker, or to the socioeconomic advantages of the CID group.

The depressing run of research which found low levels of reading achievement in the USA was supported by work in the UK. Hamp (1972) used a Picture Assisted Reading Test for words with children aged 9–15 years in eight schools for the deaf or partially hearing, to obtain a mean reading age of approximately 9 years for 15-year-old children. In associated assessments of reading comprehension, he found a mean reading age of around 8;10 years. Also in the UK, and using the Southgate Reading Test, Redgate (1972) measured the reading age of 698 hearing-impaired children aged 9–18 years attending 23 schools. At 15 years old the children had attained a reading age of 7;8 years. With the same test, Morris (1978) obtained a very similar reading age of 7;6 years for severely and profoundly deaf school leavers. Wood et al. (1981) found a mean reading age of 7;9 years for 60 children with a mean age of 11 years and a mean hearing loss of 87 dB, also with the Southgate Reading Test.

Conrad (1977a, 1979) used the Brimer Wide-Span Reading Test of sentence completion (Brimer, 1972) to measure the reading skills of 355 mostly orally educated deaf school leavers in England and Wales, all of whom were prelingually hearing-impaired, and aged 15–16 years. Conrad obtained a median reading age of 9 years for this group. He found no significant differences between groups of children with hearing losses in the ranges 86–95, 96–105, and above 105 dB HL. However, he did find that children with losses in the ranges of less than 66, and 66–85 dB HL attained higher reading ages than the children with severe and profound losses. Thus reading comprehension was greatly retarded with hearing impairment greater than 85 dB HL. Conrad also found a highly significant correlation between intelligence and reading age, with coefficients of between 0.30 and 0.53 for his five ranges of hearing loss, where the higher coefficients were associated with the lower levels of hearing loss. He concluded that there is a stage or plateau in the reading attainment of many deaf children which they cannot escape. Quigley and Kretschmer (1982) came to the same conclusion, finding that deaf children tended to progress to about the third- or fourth-grade level at 13–14 years of age, but progressed very little thereafter. This limiting stage or plateau may, however, be more apparent than real, because the reading achievements of hearing-impaired children tend to slow down as they reach the teen years. Also, the difference in reading attainment between hearing and hearing-impaired children increases with age, giving an impression of levelling-off of progress in reading by the hearing-impaired children (Myklebust, 1964; Serwatka et al., 1984).

Very different results, providing some grounds for optimism, were recently reported by Geers and Moog (1989) in a study of factors associated with literacy in profoundly deaf adolescents in the USA. Their aims were to record the literacy levels of a large sample of orally educated hearing-impaired school leavers, and to describe the factors which would predict competence in reading and writing. Their work is commended to the reader for its thoroughness of reportage, besides the significance of its outcome.

Geers and Moog's sample of 100 prelingually profoundly deaf adolescents, 49 boys and 51 girls, was aged from 15–18 years. Non-verbal IQ levels were not less than 85. All subjects had been enrolled in oral education programmes throughout preschool and elementary schooling. Their socioeconomic backgrounds were above average, being middle to upper middle class. Most families had at least one parent educated to tertiary level. Some 90% of parents reported that they had helped their children with speech production, language development and academic studies. Also, they had read to their children and had regularly discussed television programmes with them while they grew up. Only 15% of the subjects were enrolled in classes for the hearing impaired at the time of the research. The remainder were mainstreamed for all or most of the day, the average age at mainstreaming being 11;1 years (s.d. 4;6 years). Hearing aids had been fitted to 54% of the sample by 1 year of age, and to 90% by age 2 years. Seventy-five per cent of the subjects had enrolled in a parent–infant programme by 2 years of age, and 63% had attended a special education preschool by age 3 years. Forty-six per cent of subjects could identify some spoken words with their hearing aids; 36% could make speech pattern distinctions, such as one versus two syllable words, while only three subjects showed no speech perception skills. Fifteen per cent could correctly identify 90% of words in a closed-set word test. On the Minimal Auditory Capabilities visual enhancement subtest (Owens et al., 1985) the sample averaged 57% correct for lipreading alone, and 74% with lipreading and hearing. The mean performance IQ was 111, distinctly superior, probably partly a result of not including individuals with performance IQs of less than 85. The average verbal IQ score was 89, on the low side, as expected. On speech production tests (Monsen, 1981), 65% of the subjects obtained good to excellent results (above 80% intelligible). Sixty-two per cent of subjects knew no sign language, 9% could communicate in signed English, and 13% could converse in ASL. However, spoken English was the primary means of communicating for all.

The characteristics of this particularly well documented sample appears atypical of deaf adolescents. However, Geers and Moog estimated that it contained about 50% of the total American population of profoundly deaf 16 and 17 year olds who were educated orally. Although it comprised only about 5% of the population of all profoundly deaf children in this age range, the sample was thought to be representative of profoundly deaf children who continued in oral education.

In reading tests at the word level, the Woodcock Reading Mastery Test (Woodcock, 1973) was used to assess phonics skills independently of word knowledge, by using nonsense words. All subjects could perform this task. Half scored above, and half below the seventh-grade (13 year) level. Thirty-four per cent scored in the average range for hearing subjects of the same age. Word knowledge was measured with the vocabulary subtest of the California Achievement Test (1977), for knowledge of antonyms, synonyms and multiple definitions of words. Ninety per cent of subjects scored above the third-grade (9 year) level, and 54% above the seventh-grade level. Thirty per cent attained the levels for hearing children of equivalent age.

At the sentence level, recognition of syntactic structures was measured with the Test of Syntactic Abilities Screening Form (Quigley et al., 1978). Two-thirds of the subjects scored 90% or more. Ninety-two per cent scored above 75%, showing substantial mastery of the test's nine syntactic structures. Semantic skills at the sentence level were measured by the Peabody Individual Achievement Test – reading comprehension subtest (Dunn and Markwardt, 1970). Fifty-four per cent of the sample obtained scores below the seventh-grade level, but a quarter attained scores typical of hearing subjects.

At the text level, reading skills were assessed with the reading comprehension subtest of the Stanford Achievement Test (SAT: Gardner et al., 1982). Thirty per cent of the sample scored at their hearing grade-level equivalent, and 57% at the seventh-grade level. Special purpose tests were also devised to test top-down reading skills but as they were non-normed, these are not considered here. Skill at text-level reading was measured with the Gates McGinitie Reading Test (Gates and McGinitie, 1965). Sixty-three per cent of subjects scored at or above tenth-grade (16 year) level in reading speech, but only 44% scored at the same level for reading accuracy. Geers and Moog also included tests for writing and spoken language skills, and conducted a factor analysis for variables predictive of literacy, to be considered later.

For reading ability, it is apparent that Geers and Moog's sample had skills above the average for profoundly deaf adolescents, and above what may be expected on the basis of the studies reviewed earlier. For instance, their mean grade level on the SAT for reading comprehension was the eighth-grade level. Only 15% showed reading skills below the third-grade level, the mean level found for 16- and 17-year-old subjects by Schildroth and Karchmer (1986), while 30% performed at the same level as hearing subjects of the same age. Although this level of reading skill was encouraging, on the whole the sample did not attain the levels achieved by hearing 16- and 17-year-olds. Geers and Moog attributed this lower level of attainment to deficiency in vocabulary development, since the subjects' oral vocabulary was assessed at sixth-grade, and reading vocabulary at seventh-grade level.

Geers and Moog concluded, among other things, that by 16 years of age, profoundly deaf children could achieve, by reading, skills similar to those of hearing individuals, since between 24% and 34% of their subjects attained such skills. They also concluded that profoundly deaf children who had at least average non-verbal intelligence, early oral education, early auditory stimulation, and a middle-class family environment with strong family support, had the potential to attain much higher reading and other skills than generally reported for profoundly deaf people. They found the primary factors associated with the development of literacy in their orally educated sample were good use of residual hearing, early amplification, early educational management, and especially oral English language ability.

We have considered this work of Geers and Moog at length for good reasons. First, it is exemplary in its characterisation of the study sample. Few reports have taken the care to describe their subjects in such detail. Secondly, it is notable for reporting the good level of reading and other skills that can be attained by some profoundly deaf adolescents. The reported levels of reading suggest strongly that it is erroneous to generalise from the demographic studies of reading achievement to subgroups and individual cases. It is also notable that this study goes some way towards substantiating the claims for oral education put forward by its adherents.

However, although Geers and Moog may properly claim that a proportion of orally educated prelingually profoundly deaf children can achieve reading abilities approaching or equal to those of hearing children, the mean grade level, for reading comprehension on the SAT, was the eighth grade. Most members of their sample were retarded in reading ability with regard to norms for hearing children of the same age. Further, the sample was at a distinct advantage in terms of socioeconomic and environmental background. For this sample, the effects of oral education were confounded with environmental variables.

Two methodological aspects need special attention in interpreting the results of this study. The first is the high level of non-verbal intelligence (mean performance IQ of 111), which probably occurred in part because subjects whose IQ was less than 85 points were excluded. The findings were thus about *bright* orally educated prelingually profoundly deaf children. It is not clear how far the results were affected by such preselection. The second aspect concerns possible self-selection bias. The study was conducted at camps lasting 5 days. Although transport costs and other expenses were paid by the research grant, and not by the subjects, other self-selection criteria, such as willingness to leave home, could have played a significant part. Geers and Moog estimated their 100-subject sample as being about 50% of the prelingually profoundly deaf population aged 16–17 years, who had received an oral education. Thus there were approximately 100 other potential subjects, only a small proportion of whom would have included those subjects rejected because of IQ less than 85 points. In fairness, perhaps not all of these further 100 adolescents would have experienced an exclusively oral education throughout their preschool and elementary school years. But this still leaves us with a suspicion that self-selection may have biased the results. There is therefore scope for further investigation to discount these queries.

The results of Geers and Moog's USA study are at considerable variance with those given by Conrad (1979) in the UK (actually England and Wales). The reasons may include differences in national styles of provision for deaf education (USA versus UK), time of study (1974–1976 versus 1986), ages and age ranges of subjects (15–18 years versus 15–16 years), ranges of hearing loss (the UK study included subjects with moderate to profound losses), and possibly a less complete, less intensive or less demanding oral education in the UK. Also, the UK study reviewed the whole population of deaf school leavers and without selecting for intelligence. On the average the UK study subjects would have been less bright, and had no chance to self-select. There were thus considerable differences between the two studies in the characteristics of their subjects, which reflect a notable diversity among hearing-impaired individuals.

Processes associated with reading

Although recent studies of reading by deaf children have continued to confirm the thrust of earlier findings (Bennett et al., 1984; Allen, 1986), attention has turned from reading achievement to possible factors underlying the low levels of reading achievement generally observed.

Method of communication

It has been generally believed that prelingually deaf children of deaf signing parents are favoured in their cognitive and academic achievements. When the literature on the effects of parental method of communication on the reading attainments of prelingually deaf students was reviewed by Kampfe and Turecheck (1987), they confirmed this belief for reading. They concluded that deaf children of signing parents typically have more advanced reading skills than deaf children whose parents do not sign. This conclusion did not necessarily mean that there is a positive general relationship between the use of sign and reading ability. However, the evidence suggested some relationship between specific kinds of manual communication, level of parental skill in signing, and reading ability. Later, Kampfe (1989) reported results for the reading comprehension of 201 deaf adolescents, who used some manual form as their primary means of communication, in relation to the communication strategies and skills of their mothers. The method of communication used by the mothers, which included signing, speech and speechreading, gestures, made-up signs and pantomime, was not significantly related to their deaf children's reading comprehension scores on the SAT. For mothers who used manual communication, no significant relationship was found between reading comprehension and the age of the student when the mother began to sign. There was evidence that the students' reading comprehension was related to the level of skill used by mothers in signing. However, this relationship was not necessarily straightforward because mothers with higher manual communication abilities tend to have higher educational levels and children with higher IQs.

This interesting study thus had limitations. Kampfe also noted that the findings applied to students in residential schools, and the relation between mothers' signing skills and reading comprehension might have been greater had the children remained at home. Further, the measurements for mothers' skills and for students' reading comprehension, which were obtained by questionnaires, may have been applied differently in different schools.

A further complex mix of results was obtained by Moores and Sweet (1990), who assessed literacy skills in two groups of congenitally deaf children. One group had deaf, and the other hearing parents. The latter group was educated in TC from 4 years old. The data suggested similar factors associated with literacy for both groups. Measures of structure in English and vocabulary were important, whereas speech measures and hearing level were of less importance. Fluency in ASL was not correlated with reading or writing for either group.

To summarise, although there is evidence suggesting that native signing deaf children are better readers than deaf children who have learned to sign in later years, the situation is by no means completely clear. Reading competence may be more closely related to text-based competencies than to the type of face-to-face language which the reader brings to the reading task (Livingston, 1991).

Basic processes

Given that hearing-impaired children have problems in reading, we should ask in which aspects of reading are the problems found. In particular, do the problems occur at the more basic levels of letter and word recognition, or at higher levels, as with understanding meaning? Kyle (1980b) provided an answer to this question. He assessed the skills of profoundly deaf, partially to severely deaf, and hearing children of equivalent non-verbal IQ in discriminating letters, associating words with pictures, and reading comprehension. He found that the deaf children had similar vocabulary skills to the hearing children at 7 years of age. By age 9 years, their letter skills had caught up, although their vocabulary was then about 1 year behind. In contrast, at age 9 years, the deaf children had only just begun to read for meaning. The implication is that, since the hearing and deaf children performed at a roughly similar level in the basic skills of letter discrimination and vocabulary recognition, the difficulties experienced by deaf children in reading mostly occur at a higher level of processing, associated with reading for meaning.

The basic skills involved in letter and word matching and identification described by Kyle begin at the prereading level (Clay, 1979; Mason, 1980). Prereading skills need to be acquired or learned, as concepts about letters, words and stories, before children can learn to read successfully (Mason, 1980; Stanovich, 1980; Maxwell, 1986; Andrews, 1988). Normally, children acquire such concepts by identifying printed material in their everyday experiences, by printing letters and a few words, including their names, on their drawings and by listening to stories read from books by their parents. Andrews (1988) found for 23 prelingually deaf kindergarten and first-grade children with severe to profound hearing losses, who used speech, fingerspelling or signs, that all could identify a few written letters, while ten could read and understand simple sentences. The lesser-skilled children lacked practice in labelling pictures with signs, a variant of word recognition.

Tests of reading ability which estimate lower-level skills, up to the level of word recognition, tend to show relatively similar reading achievement in deaf and hearing children. According to Webster (1986), only with more demanding tests of reading ability, involving complex language skills and comprehension above a reading level of 8;6–9 years, will the performance of deaf children fall off sharply. He suggested that the plateau effect observed in tests of reading achievement with deaf children occurred at just this point, when the reading task passed from letters and words to a level of linguistic complexity beyond their abilities.

It seems necessary to qualify the implications of Kyle's (1980b) findings and Webster's (1986) arguments. Deaf children have more than their share of visual and visual perceptual deficits (Cooper and Arnold, 1981). Also, the eye movements of deaf children during reading may be different from those of hearing children of matched reading age and non-verbal IQ (Beggs et al., 1982). Thus deaf children, on average, are at a disadvantage in learning to read because of visual and visual perceptual impairment. However, the situation is not clear-cut. Spencer and Delk (1989) tested visual perceptual processing in 77 hearing-impaired children aged 7–8 years, finding that only those tests which had a memory component, or prevented an approach to a memory task through a non-sequential strategy, produced lower levels of performance than test norms for hearing children. Spencer and Delk's sample, however, contained a substantial proportion of children with moderate to severe hearing losses, who would have been less likely to experience visual perceptual processing problems than profoundly deaf children.

Reading tasks more complex than letter- and word-matching and discrimination are required in order to answer written questions about reading assignments. This point was illustrated by Scouten (1980), who observed that deaf students often tried to match specific words or phrases in a written question with the same word or phrase in the assigned text. This superficial visual matching resulted in the student's copying whole sentences, irrespective of the sense made in answering the question. Similar strategies have been observed by Webster et al. (1981), Wood et al. (1981), and Beggs and Breslaw (1983), where deaf children, unable to comprehend the text, based their responses to written questions on visual similarities of words and phrases, or picked the most interesting picture in a picture-assisted reading test.

This area was investigated further by LaSasso (1985), who compared the visual matching test-taking strategies of hearing and deaf student readers. She found extensive use of visual matching by deaf, but not hearing, students across several kinds of visual matching strategy. Her findings were supported by LaSasso (1986), in comparing the visual matching test-taking strategies on the SAT of 50 hearing children aged 14–17 years with those of a group of prelingually, profoundly deaf children of similar chronological and reading age. Although some visual matching was used by the hearing children, it was used far more by the deaf children. The implications are that care is needed in taking the results of some reading comprehension tests scores of deaf children at face value when the children have been able to look back at, or re-inspect, the text.

There are problems in assessing reading comprehension when the questions used to measure understanding of text are themselves liable to misinterpretation or confusion. Thus mistakes may be due to a failure to understand the question rather than the text. To overcome such problems, LaSasso (1980) and Reynolds (1986) used modified cloze procedures, where each reading passage might include a number of sentences with a single word omitted, with several alternative single word options provided for each omission. Cloze tests obviate errors attributable to the misunderstanding of questions in a comprehension test, and are more direct tests of reading comprehension. However, they have been criticised (Kretschmer and Kretschmer, 1986) because they stress syntactic knowledge in the sentence under consideration, and do not show a reader's competence in understanding the content of a passage of text, nor various literacy devices.

Cumulative cloze, a technique devised to overcome this problem, was proposed by Knight (1989). In cumulative cloze, the same noun, say, is deleted whenever it occurs in a paragraph of about 5 or 6 sentences. As the child reads the text, an increasing number of contextual cues to the missing noun is given by the text. If the missing noun is varied in its syntactic position, the effect of a given syntactic structure on solving for the missing noun is much reduced. Further, if readers are observed as they encounter each noun-gap, their predictions can be recorded. These predictions should be increasingly accurate as the readers receive an increasing number of contextual cues. Using cumulative cloze with ten prelingually deaf and ten hearing readers from each of the grades 4, 6, 8, 10 and 12, with six sentences in short paragraphs, Knight found significant differences between deaf and hearing children up to the sixth exposure point, that is up to the sixth sentence, for grades 4–6. However, there were no significant differences for grades 8–12. Both groups predicted meaning more accurately and their predictions were more semantically and grammatically acceptable as the contextual information increased. Hence, with a reduced load on their knowledge of syntax, the deaf children could improve their scores in reading for meaning. Knight also found that his deaf readers tended to abandon correct choices more often than his hearing readers, possibly because they focused more on the immediate context rather than on the progressive use of context.

Another extension of the cloze procedure was used by Andrews and Mason (1991) to explore decision making by prelingually profoundly deaf high-school youths, aged 17–20 years, in filling deleted words and phrases. Although born of hearing parents, these youths were all skilled signers in ASL. Besides predicting the missing word or phrase, the youths were asked to explain the reasons for their prediction. Andrews and Mason discovered that their deaf youths often relied on re-reading and background knowledge, whereas comparison groups of hearing readers relied more on cues from context. However, the use of re-reading and background knowledge were not as effective as were cues from context. The deaf readers' performance was poorer than that of the hearing readers because their background knowledge was poor in some instances, they experienced linguistic difficulties at the word, sentence and intra-sentence level, had problems with metaphor or recoding from print into sign or inner speech, or used inappropriate graphic similarities.

Cloze tests, free-response question tasks, and question tasks without permitting lookback were found by LaSasso and Davey (1987) to be very sensitive to vocabulary knowledge in 10–18-year-old prelingually profoundly deaf children, possibly because such tasks need more memory or more verbal ability than multiple-choice or lookback tasks. However, LaSasso and Davey observed that vocabulary knowledge, assessed by the Vocabulary Comprehension Subtest of the Gates–McGinitie Reading Tests, was a stronger predictor of reading comprehension, measured by the Reading Comprehension Subtest of the SAT, than cloze tasks, free-response questions, and no-lookback question tasks. Possibly, vocabulary knowledge was more strongly correlated with reading comprehension than the SAT.

Higher-level processes

Higher-level processes involved in reading include the understanding of ideas and meanings, which is associated with the structure of syntax. Here too, hearing-impaired children have difficulties. They develop linguistic skills later and in a different way from hearing individuals. A useful example of this situation was presented by Sarachan-Deily (1982), who examined both the syntactic and semantic relationships used by hearing-impaired readers. She asked 30 congenitally profoundly deaf and 30 hearing children aged 10–18 years to read a set of 12 sentences, one at a time. After reading a sentence once, the child was given a number-counting task for a period, to prevent rehearsal, and then had to recall the sentence in writing. The sentences varied in length from 5–9 words, and in syntax from active to passive. The deaf children, all orally educated, produced more syntactic errors in their recalled sentences than the hearing children, whose errors were relatively minor. Although nearly half their sentences contained syntactic errors, the deaf children produced sentences which preserved the meaning. Sarachan-Deily concluded that although their syntactic skills were frequently in error, the semantic patterns and processing abilities of the hearing-impaired children were similar to those of the hearing children. The syntactic errors, such as derivational or inflectional word endings, were not generally such as to destroy the semantic content.

However, things may not be so straightforward. Strassman et al. (1987) showed that profoundly prelingually deaf adolescents, aged 13–20 years and educated by TC, experienced problems with instantiation in a cued recall task, implying that they had some difficulties with semantics. In a typical instantiation task, the subject has to substitute a specific term, such as a specific noun, for a general term in a sentence to fit the meaning of the sentence ('The fruit was yellow' becomes 'The lemon was yellow'). The task thus requires familiarity with categorisation. Strassman et al. reported that their deaf subjects could instantiate when asked, but did not do so spontaneously. Their subjects' poor overall reading level possibly encouraged the use of verbatim, rather than inferential, recall. Alternatively, while their subjects may have been able to represent the semantics of individual words, the strength of the associations among and between the semantic representations could have been weak, limiting the use of context in comprehension. This study appeared to require a higher order of semantic representation than that of Sarachan-Deily (1982), which may account for the relatively greater difficulty in semantic processing observed in comprehending sentences. However, the studies used subjects of different ages and methods of communication. The large differences between the subjects make it impossible to compare the studies directly.

Conclusion

It appears that hearing-impaired children experience reading problems at both basic and higher levels of processing. The main reasons seem to be difficulties with syntax and the more complex aspects of semantics, and poor reading strategies. These problems become more obvious with age, as the differences between the reading performances of hearing and hearing-impaired children increase over time.

Neuropsychological aspects of reading

As noted earlier, neuropsychological studies of cerebral dominance have typically relied on the split-half visual field technique, in which the individual fixates on a central point while material is introduced into the left or right visual half-fields. Cerebral dominance is assessed by noting for which half-field the individual reports the greater amount of material correctly. This technique is useful in exploring the neuropsychology of reading.

In a test of 18 congenitally deaf undergraduate students, compared with 18 hearing control subjects, McKeever et al. (1976) found only minimal cerebral asymmetry for printed words among their deaf subjects, while their hearing subjects demonstrated left cerebral dominance, as anticipated. McKeever et al. concluded that deprivation of hearing resulted in very reduced asymmetry in cerebral processing. Similar results for word perception were obtained with congenitally deaf students by Manning et al. (1977). Letters were used by Phippard (1977) in work described earlier to compare visual hemifield perception in congenitally deaf students educated by TC or by oral methods, together with a group of hearing students. The hearing students showed dominance in the left cerebral hemisphere, as expected. The deaf students educated by TC showed no cerebral asymmetry, but those educated orally rather surprisingly showed a significant dominance of the right hemisphere. Phippard concluded that the orally educated group were coding the material visually rather than phonetically.

In reviewing these and related studies, Conrad (1979) commented that the differences between deaf and hearing subjects in tasks involving linguistic material was striking in all cases. He cautioned, however, that care should be taken, as the results were presented as group averages. Since a few profoundly deaf children had been shown to develop internal speech, it was not necessarily correct to assume that no deaf child would show left cerebral hemisphere dominance. Nevertheless, the clear implication was that most seriously hearing-impaired children have unusual neuropsychological function. Conrad also remarked that cases of left-hemisphere stroke in deaf patients resulted in disturbance to sign language performance, suggesting a common left cerebral hemisphere locus for all language processing (Chapter 5).

The work outlined above and a review and study with similar findings by Boshoven et al. (1982) were concerned with lower-level abilities associated with reading. As tests of reading ability, they were clearly incomplete. In other areas of reading in hearing children, and in hearing children with reading disabilities, the association of neuropsychological findings with reading is more comprehensive (Marcel et al., 1974; Kelly et al., 1989). In particular, processes associated with cortical function have been demonstrated for naming deficits (Vellutino, 1983), problems with serial order (Denckla et al., 1981), verbal dysfluency (Wolf, 1984), insensitivity to syntax (Rudel, 1985), selective attention (Rudel, 1985), and learning to read (Denckla, 1983). Investigation of neuropsychological processes associated with reading problems in deaf children in these latter areas remains to be carried out.

Bottom-up aspects of reading

Although tests of reading achievement are valuable in outlining the extent to which hearing-impaired children can read, they provide insufficient information about their reading skills. Similarly, the neuropsychological work related to reading suggests that reduced asymmetry in cerebral processing results in linguistic problems with reading, but does not show the nature of such linguistic skills that the hearing-impaired child may bring to reading. We now consider the cognitive processes involved in the bottom-up approaches to the study of reading, the approaches through which the reading difficulties experienced by deaf children were explored in detail by workers in the 1960s and 1970s.

Phonological coding

There is good evidence to show that poor readers do not make efficient use of phonemic information (Shankweiler and Liberman, 1976; Mann et al., 1980; Siegel and Linder, 1984; Hurford, 1988). Good readers bring to reading an ability to identify and discriminate among phonemes (Treiman and Barron, 1981) and hence can learn grapheme to phoneme correspondences (Gibson, 1972; Savin, 1972), where the written material is segmented and decoded into a phonological representation. This view is supported by electromyographic work showing that reading is accompanied by electrical impulses in the speech musculature, particularly when the reader is having difficulty with the material (McGuigan, 1970; Sokolov, 1972). Such phonological coding is thought to allow the reader to make use of inner speech, so that the reader covertly hears, as it were, the material which is being read. When phonemically confusible material, such as rhyming material which can interfere with phonemic coding, is included in sets of consonants (Conrad, 1970, 1972b, c; Liberman et al., 1977), words (Byrne and Shea, 1979; Conrad, 1979) or sentences (Mann et al., 1980), the recall of material is affected more for good than for poor readers. This outcome suggests strongly that poor readers do not rely, or rely less, on phonemic coding. Evidence for the use of weak phonemic coding in profoundly deaf children is found in work by Chen (1976) who reported that, when asked to put a stroke through all instances of the letter 'e' in a piece of prose, profoundly deaf students showed no difference in cancelling silent and pronounceable 'e's, as in 'name' vs 'net'. However, hearing students missed nearly twice as many silent 'e's as the deaf students. Locke (1978) obtained similar results. These studies suggest that hearing children decode written letters through a speech-like code, but that profoundly deaf children do not, or do not do so to the same extent.

Conrad (1979) found that hearing-impaired children who possessed inner speech were likely to be less severely hearing-impaired, better at reading, better at speechreading (compare Williams, 1982), more competent in language use, and to have more intelligible speech. He thus placed heavy emphasis on the possession of inner speech, particularly for phonology. His findings have since been supported by Quigley and Paul (1984) and Meadow (1980).

Visual coding

Conrad's emphasis on phonological coding may have been overdone. Bamford and Saunders (1985) pointed out that Conrad's conclusions were qualified by those of Hung et al. (1981), whose profoundly deaf 14–18-year-old students had to judge whether or not a pair of letters was identical. The deaf students' results were similar to those of hearing subjects in showing lower reaction times for name-identity conditions (*Aa*) as compared with physical-identity conditions (*AA*). However, the reaction times of the deaf students were considerably longer than those of the hearing subjects, showing that the processes associated with the coding of letters operated more slowly in deaf than hearing subjects. Slower encoding is to be expected because deaf children have less experience in reading letters but, as Hung et al. stated, slower decoding is also to be expected, for the same reason. Thus the reading deficiency of deaf subjects may be the result of a failure to develop fast automatic processing for low-level skills such as letter coding. If attention is then directed at letter coding, it is difficult to direct it to higher-level processing. Deaf child readers do limit their visual attention, at least to a word-by-word strategy, as shown in studies of reading and eye movements (Beggs et al., 1982).

Hung et al. also found that in a sentence/picture verification task, the deaf subjects seemed to use a visual imagery code rather than a linguistic code to verify printed sentences. However, this did not necessarily mean that the deaf students were unable to use a linguistic code. When they were given sentences with ASL signs in English frames, their verification reaction times showed a pattern consistent with a general linguistic model.

These observations provide an answer to the question of how those deaf children who do not possess inner speech, manage to code written material. If they do not use a phonological code, they may use a code based on visual imagery (Hirsh-Pasek and Treiman, 1982). Use of such a visual code can still result in reading problems as compared with readers who use inner speech, because if speech is 'special' (Chapter 1), then presumably inner speech is special too.

Use of a visual code is likely to persist into adulthood. Treiman and Hirsh-Pasek (1983) explored recoding strategies, as translation from printed text to some other form, in the silent reading of second-generation deaf readers, namely, congenitally deaf subjects born to deaf parents. Their 14 subjects, aged 28–63, all profoundly deaf and native ASL signers, who had never been fitted with hearing aids, took part in four experiments which recoded sentence material into articulation. The recoding involved phonological recoding, fingerspelling, ASL, or no recoding observed. Fourteen hearing young adult subjects, aged 18–25 years, none familiar with ASL, were used as controls. The deaf subjects did not appear to recode into articulation nor, as a group, did they recode into fingerspelling, even though most deaf individuals have a considerable fingerspelling vocabulary. However, they did recode into sign, as shown by the difficulty they experienced in reading and judging sentences whose sign versions contained similar signs. Thus these second-generation profoundly deaf subjects recoded written English into ASL, their native language, even though there are few direct spelling-to-sign correspondences. Treiman and Hirsh-Pasek concluded that the advantages to be obtained in memory and comprehension by using one's native language weigh heavily in choosing a system for recoding.

Studies of the type described by Hung et al. and Treiman and Hirsh-Pasek are not many, although few doubt that deaf children use some kind of visual code (Webster, 1986). Obviously, more work is required to identify how deaf individuals recode written material into sign and possibly fingerspelling, and the circumstances under which they do so.

Top-down aspects of reading

Conrad's (1979) approach to reading via phonological coding has been subject to a fair degree of criticism. To be fair to Conrad, his deaf poor readers almost all had problems with phonological coding and, besides, this criticism has been levelled at other proponents of bottom-up approaches (e.g. Locke, 1978; Hirsh-Pasek and Treiman, 1982). Bamford and Saunders (1985) remarked that arguments have been levied against non-lexical grapheme-to-phoneme conversion (GPC) processes from a psychological viewpoint (Henderson, 1982) in preference to explanations that unfamiliar words are spoken by analogy with familiar words. Also, fluent readers can use phonetic imagery to trace prosodic features from text. Such a suprasegmental level of operation argues for a higher arrangement of operation beyond GPC, and the emphasis on low-level phonological coding in GPC should be reduced in favour of higher-order factors This top-down thrust is reminiscent of the direction taken by such authors as Stanovich and West (1979), who argued that readers who otherwise performed poorly because of inadequate GPC rules could improve their performance by using top-down information to a greater extent than good readers.

Proponents of this top-down thrust would argue that use of a phonological code in short-term memory tasks does not necessarily imply the use of such a code in other tasks, including reading. Children can change tactics from one task to another, as shown by the different results obtained on reading tasks which force the adoption of different tactics. Since deaf individuals who use signing as their first language can be reasonably fluent readers, they probably use visual coding in reading, either alone or in combination with phonological coding. Further, reading involves more complex operations than phonemics alone. Higher-order linguistic processes have a most important part to play. Hence inner speech as speech may not always be involved in reading, and to rely principally on inner speech as phonological coding is too limiting (Webster, 1986, 1988).

Linguistic and cognitive considerations

Turning to linguistic considerations, Webster (1986) pointed out that deaf children can learn the simple declarative subject–verb–object (SVO) construction, although they have problems up to school-leaving age and beyond with more complex structures such as embedded clauses (Quigley et al., 1976b). Like younger hearing children, they may attempt to apply the SVO sequence not only to written SVO sentences, but to sentences which have other kinds of grammatical structure, using a simple tactic of visual order, in which the first occurring noun is taken to be the subject, followed by the verb, and then the object. Thus a sentence of the type 'The cat was bitten by the dog' may be reproduced as 'The cat bit the dog'. Another tactic that seems to be used frequently by deaf children is the 'Minimum Distance Principle' (MDP) of Chomsky (1965). This tactic makes use of visual contiguity in written text, so that a deleted subject is not inferred, but is taken to be the noun closest to the verb. Thus 'The dog bit the man and ran away' is interpreted as 'The man ran away'.

Both SVO and MDP tactics are used by young hearing children, though there is little agreement on how and why they are used (Romaine, 1984). The lack of agreement does not make it easy for us to explain their use by deaf children (Wood et al., 1986). However, we may explain why their use persists in older deaf children if we regard that persistence as a mismatch between the child's available grammatical skills and the more complex grammar of the printed text. In this case, the SVO and MDP tactics are simple devices to make sense of grammar beyond the childs' linguistic ability.

The issue of how deaf children read can be approached with tests of reading comprehension which permit study of the skills of deaf child readers at various levels. Webster (1986) presented a battery of graded reading material to 80 severely to profoundly deaf children aged 8–11 years. The test battery used familiar vocabulary in sentences with graded amounts of information and with increasingly complex grammar. The reading task was to look at a picture and to choose one sentence, out of 3 or 4, which matched the picture. Two scores were obtained for each child. The first approach scored the number of items passed when the child read sentences with complex grammar for meaning. The second approach scored the number of items where the child had to be shown the right vocabulary to pass the item. If a child failed on the first, but passed on the second, approach, it was assumed that the child was confused by the grammar.

Webster found that hearing loss was not of major importance in determining success in reading, but age was. The older the child, the better were the overall test scores, with little evidence of the plateau found in earlier studies of reading achievement. The plateau may thus be due to insensitive test instruments. The younger children were easily confused by the grammar, but usually succeeded when the vocabulary was highlighted (compare Sarachan-Deily, 1982). The older children made fewer overall errors, and approached 100% success. Many children found that the sentences with higher information (meaning) content were easier to get right, yet these sentences were more complex in their grammar. Webster suggested that deaf children can be helped if they are given more, rather than less, information in making selections from sentences. It is possible that Webster's results could be due in part to guessing. If the children were making guesses, then the greater the amount of information, the more directed would be the guesses. Hence the provision of more information with complex sentences would yield more accurate guessing.

We may envisage that the reading tactics of deaf children can easily be disrupted by imposing a load on their short-term memory. In an extension of his work, Webster (1986) made use of just this technique. For 20 severely to profoundly deaf children aged 11 years, 20 hearing children aged 8–9 years, and a group of 11-year-old hearing children, he set a further task of matching a picture with one of a set of sentences. First, both picture and sentences were presented. Then the sentences were offered without the picture, so that cross-referencing could not occur. After a 10-second delay, the picture was presented, but the sentences were removed. The children were asked to recall which of the sentences fitted the picture. Under the first condition, the deaf children scored beyond 90%, but under the memory test, scores dropped to around 45%. The younger hearing children attained 70% correct scores under the first condition, falling to 52% under the memory test. The older hearing children obtained scores of more than 90% and more than 80% in the first and memory tasks, respectively. Webster concluded that the top-down reading strategies of deaf children are easily disrupted. He explained this outcome by suggesting that deaf children lacked inner speech in which to conduct articulatory rehearsal in short-term memory. He therefore accepted the importance of inner speech in reading, but ascribed its importance not to phonological coding, but to a top-down use in memory rehearsal via an articulatory loop. Deaf children are limited in rehearsing verbal material via inner speech in short-term memory, which explains their problems in tasks related to verbal language.

Others have also been critical of Conrad's (1979) bottom-up approach to the study of reading ability in deaf children. Thus Wood et al. (1986) also argued for a top-down orientation, drawing on a model of poor reading skills developed by Stanovitch and West (1979). This model views poor readers as weak in using automated GPC rules. Poor readers try to make more use of top-down information than good readers by using their general world knowledge and language knowledge to cover the gaps in their poor reading. Such a reading strategy requires considerable conscious effort, is time-consuming, error-prone, and requires a copious store of valid general knowledge if it is to succeed (compare Stanovich, 1986; Andrews and Mason, 1991). Wood et al. believed that deaf children were in exactly this situation.

However, deaf children generally have poorer linguistic and general knowledge than poor hearing readers, giving them an additional handicap. They are likely to use various tactics, some of which may be non-linguistic. They will stretch their intelligence in using general knowledge, and such elementary devices as word associations, to make the most of cues from the reading task and its context to augment their limited linguistic ability. This error-prone approach results in frequent failures, which is hardly encouraging for the deaf child reader. Making a somewhat similar observation, Hanson (1986) suggested that deaf readers with poor speech, likely to be poorer readers, may compensate for their low level of ability in spelling to process nonsense words, consisting of legal consonant and vowel strings, by relying on the statistical redundancies of the orthography.

Storytelling

Several workers have begun to recommend that more attention be paid to conversation and storytelling as foundations for literacy in teaching reading to deaf children (e.g. Gaines et al., 1981; Wood et al., 1986). Their case is supported by the role found for linguistic prediction in reading for hearing individuals (Goodman and Burke, 1980). Studies of the cloze procedure with deaf children (Marshall,

1970; Odom et al., 1967; LaSasso, 1985, 1986) show that they have severe problems in using grammar or vocabulary to complement written material with missing words. The findings of these studies also relate to problems of linguistic prediction, supporting the view that failure to predict grammatical sequences markedly slows the attainment of literacy (Kretschmer and Kretschmer, 1986).

However, conversation and storytelling are more promising as foundations for the discourse and content levels of reading. There are two main types of discourse: narration and exposition (Hidi and Hildyard, 1983; Kretschmer and Kretschmer, 1986). Narration is relatively tightly organised, around a situation of conflict, for instance, and is more easily recalled, whereas exposition is less tightly organised and less easily recalled. Both types of stories have been used in relation to reading by hearing-impaired children.

Tales with a narrative structure can be employed to assess how well hearing-impaired children identify significant intelligence in the story. Thus stories with a narrative structure were presented together with scrambled stories to groups of hearing-impaired and hearing children by Gaines et al. (1981). For scrambled or distorted stories, the children had to rearrange the material to create the story. Both groups of children recalled significant information better than significant detail. The hearing-impaired children recalled more total information from the scrambled stories, but this information was not always about the more important parts of the story. Generally, the hearing children made better use of the narrative stories than the children with impaired hearing.

Expository stories have been used to explore the ways in which hearing-impaired children respond to organisational styles of text. Gormley (1981) found that familiarity with content facilitated the ability of third-grade hearing-impaired children in reading comprehension. Familiar paragraphs were better understood than unfamiliar paragraphs, even though they were structurally equivalent. Gormley (1982) extended this study by comparing the reading comprehension skills of hearing-impaired children at the ages of 8 and 15 years. Seven children formed the younger group, while eight children were the subjects in the older group. All children had hearing losses of 80 dB ISO, or more, and came from a TC day programme. The children read silently short (100-word) expository paragraphs about sports and insects. Two paragraphs were about familiar material (baseball and mosquitoes), and two were of unfamiliar content (curling and aphids). The paragraphs were equivalent in sentence structure, word frequency, readability level (third-grade), argument repetition and idea units. Apart from the reading of the text, communication between child and interpreter was by TC. Having been checked for prior knowledge, the child read the paragraph and then retold it. Additional information could be probed by text-based questions.

Gormley found that children from different age groups did not differ in prior knowledge or understanding of the text. However, familiarity with the material was a significantly differentiating factor for both age groups. Even though the third-grade level text was too difficult for the 8-year-old children at a technical level, they recalled paragraphs with familiar content better than those where the content was unfamiliar. This finding was important, because it showed that hearing-impaired children can obtain a fair reading comprehension of prose, which is too difficult for them at a technical level, if they are able to use their intelligence and general knowledge to assist their knowledge of grammar (compare Wood et al., 1986). Similar comments have been made by Banks et al. (1991a) and Gray et al. (1991) in discussing the use of story schemata in deaf children asked to reproduce a written story by arranging a set of pictures in sequence, a technique aimed to encourage the children to read for meaning and reducing the effect of syntax.

Figurative material

It has been generally thought that deaf children are not able to cope with figurative material in their reading or otherwise, and findings to this effect continue (Payne and Quigley, 1987). However, Fruchter et al. (1984) noted a surprisingly high level of non-literal understanding of idioms, where 13–15-year-old severely to profoundly deaf children read a sentence and then chose one of four pictures to explain the meaning.

In a later study of figurative language, Rittenhouse and Stearns (1990) also observed good figurative understanding in deaf children. Their moderately to profoundly congenitally deaf children aged 8–18 years were given a short original expository story to read. After reading the story, the children answered ten written yes/no questions, with lookback permitted. Vocabulary help was offered as needed. The 14 children were randomly assigned to two groups. One group read a literal version of the story; the other group read a figurative version, in which all textual answers to the questions were marked in figurative phrasing. Results showed that both groups answered the questions, which were all presented in literal form, above chance level. The figurative version of the story was no more difficult to comprehend than the literal version. Therefore figurative language need not always cause problems in reading comprehension for severely deaf children. Rittenhouse and Stearns observed that teachers were often reluctant to expose hearing-impaired children to figurative language, because the children did not use it spontaneously. However, hearing-impaired children can come to understand figurative language, even though they do not use it spontaneously, as also found (Iran-Nejad et al., 1981; Rittenhouse et al., 1981) in studies of hearing-impaired children's experiences with metaphor. It may be that failure to use higher-level skills, such as semantic representation, instantiation and metaphor, spontaneously is the result of over-exposure to low-level reading materials and markedly verbatim recall tasks (Davey and King, 1990).

Intervention in reading

There is a very large number of approaches to the teaching of reading. For example, reading in volume (Eller et al., 1988) and varied reading contexts (Nagy et al., 1987; Sternberg, 1987) have been promoted for vocabulary learning. Regression or lookback has been recommended as a reading strategy (Daneman, 1988; Davey and King, 1990). We cannot hope to conduct a detailed exploration of such methods here. Instead, we offer a few words about selected studies with hearing-impaired children.

Deaf children in UK classes have been been found to stop reading of their own accord more often than hearing children (Wood et al., 1986). They were also stopped in their reading more often than hearing children by their teachers, because they did not pronounce words correctly, and to teach the meanings of words. Generally teachers stopped deaf children in reading both more often, and for more varied reasons than they stopped hearing children. Teachers of the deaf thus viewed deaf children as having a wider range of reading difficulties than did teachers of hearing children. Teachers of hearing children viewed breaks in the reading of their hearing children as signalling breakdowns in grapheme/phoneme relationships, assuming that the children knew the vocabulary and syntax. Furthermore, hearing children tended to be praised more often in relation to the number of breaks than did deaf children.

A spoken reading rate of less than 40 words per minute suggests that the child does not comprehend what is being read, and many deaf children read below that rate (Wood et al., 1986). They thus have difficulty in understanding what they are reading. What is nominally a reading lesson becomes a lesson in the expression of speech and in language learning. Since they read slowly, deaf children have reduced opportunity to use intonation or stress patterns appropriately in their reading. Because of their reduced hearing, they have a more difficult task in dividing their attention between reading materials and the teacher. Together with a less than fully developed vocabulary for their age, and with problems in understanding syntax, it is not surprising that their reading achievements are weak. A possible solution would be to delay the teaching of reading until the child has acquired greater mastery over vocabulary, grammar and speech. Wood et al. also remarked that when the number of breaks for the teaching of language and speech expression are greater than those for teaching reading itself, then clearly the reading text is too difficult. More emphasis might be given to silent reading, as speech articulation is problematical for so many deaf children. Also, more attention could be given to story-telling and to conversations to provide a basis for the development of literacy.

A quite different approach was suggested by Serwatka et al. (1984). Instead of working directly on the children, they chose to promote the educational role of classroom teachers, dormitory teachers who were teachers acting as surrogate parents in after-school hours, and parents. Classroom teachers were treated to workshops by external consultants and project staff, instructional videotapes, and newsletters containing reviews of recent research in language and reading. The dormitory teachers, who had received little instruction as language and reading teachers, were also given workshops by external consultants and project staff, and newsletters on techniques for encouraging reading. The parents of the hearing-impaired children, too, were given workshops by project staff, and newsletters. The 43 students in this study were aged 11–16 years, and had taken the same level of the SAT over at least 2 years. They were thus in a group which appeared least likely to improve in reading without special intervention. Significant gains were found on the SAT for students who were in the project for at least 1 year, albeit less than those gains that would have been attained by hearing children. The results were not fully conclusive, however, as no controls were included. Also, it was not clear as to which of the classroom teachers, dormitory teachers or parents were most responsible for the improvements in reading skills, and/or whether the apparent improvements were due to improvements in language, or reading itself.

The reading material may be based on the ideas and experiences of hearing-impaired children themselves, to improve the meaningfulness or relevance of texts for reading purposes. This approach will help the children to learn that meaning is conveyed by print, as well as other forms of communication. This experiential method for language learning and reading is the Language-Experience Approach (LEA). The emphasis is on the use of whole language, as the text for subsequent reading is based on the child's use of lexicon, grammar and semantics in dictating the original material. LEA thus makes use of oracy and literacy in the preparation and reading of text, into which a child's drawings or pictures may be incorporated (Ewoldt and Hammermeister, 1986). LEA is derived from a sociolinguistic base, emphasising the interactive nature of language, and is aimed to promote the child's interest and motivation, so that success in language-related tasks is more assured. Further, since the original material is generated by the child in dictation to the teacher on an individual basis, there is no need for external controls for familiarity with vocabulary, grammar or semantics. The child's signed or spoken dictation offers its own constraints.

Other advantages for the LEA technique in reading are that a child who uses signs can see how the signed experience is translated into text. The translation does not require matching on a word-by-word basis, but does require the introduction of punctuation. Children who have individually dictated a common experience to the teacher will be keen to see how their peers have reported the same experience, and how it appears in the LEA texts of other children. This interest, so the argument goes, will help the child to learn that a given experience can be reported and written down in a variety of linguistic styles and conventions.

Despite these seeming advantages, LaSasso (1987) found in the USA that basal reader approaches, such as that devised for hearing-impaired children by Quigley and King (1984), were used more often than LEAs as the primary approach to instruction at all teaching levels. This finding was robust, as LaSasso surveyed 478 educational programmes for hearing-impaired children. The 'Reading Milestones' approach of Quigley and King was regarded favourably because it contained appropriate vocabulary, grammar, figurative expression and phonics emphasis.

LaSasso questioned the appropriateness of the continued use of basal readers. However, she remarked that although the LEA method was used quite extensively, it could lack uniform effectiveness, since comprehensiveness and continuity require careful coordination. More than two-thirds of programmes using LEA reported that teachers made independent decisions about which specific vocabulary and reading skills to introduce. This finding highlights criticisms of the LEA technique. First, in its purer form, where the teacher keeps closely to the dictated material of the child, the scope for introducing new vocabulary, grammar and semantics is reduced. However, if the teacher is too adventurous, familiarity with the reading material, one of the main advantages of LEA, is likely to be lost. Secondly, LEA does not prescribe how the teacher should go about the teaching of reading skills. It is only to be expected that teachers of hearing-impaired children more often preferred the basal reader approach. A further possible reason why the LEA method was not as favoured as it might have been, is that teachers of hearing-impaired students may be only moderately accurate in judging the reading interests of their students. When Stoefen-Fisher (1990) asked 20 teachers of the hearing-impaired to judge the top two areas of reading interest for each of 82 severely to profoundly deaf students in residential programmes, their judgements were only partly accurate.

Computer-assisted instruction in reading

Several authors have remarked on the advantages of using computer-assisted instruction with hearing-impaired students, the first really influential computer system for such purposes being Plato (Watson, 1979; Richardson, 1981). Most of the emphasis has been on the use of computer-aided instruction for language learning and problem solving, but some studies have also been concerned with reading (Geoffrion and Goldenberg, 1981; Richardson, 1981; Geoffrion and Geoffrion, 1983; Prinz et al., 1985). MacGregor and Thomas (1988) commented that much of the earlier instructional software for the deaf student required only a simple response to questions or statements. This was a serious disadvantage because it relied on drills and practice exercises. More recent developments include the introduction of computer-mediated text (CMT), in which the computer program changes the text to allow for interactions not possible on the printed page. CMT can also be used in conjunction with such tools as computer dictionaries, text paraphrasing and reciprocal questioning. Thus CMT reduces some of the student's processing load and encourages more interaction between the student and the program (Reinking and Schreiner, 1985). The following two examples show the type of use to which CMT is being put.

MacGregor and Thomas (1988) used five versions of a CMT system plus an electronic dictionary with 45 hearing-impaired children in grade levels 4–6, who had reading abilities between first- and third-grade levels. The children, aged between 7 and 13 years, were severely to profoundly deaf. The five CMT versions included activities with intrinsic motivation in a vocabulary game, extrinsic motivation in a post-reading passage test in the form of a vocabulary and comprehension check, or no given motivation. The information supplied by the electronic dictionary was also varied. Some versions showed a standalone definition, while others gave the definition together with a sentence showing the use of the word in context. The results indicated that the extrinsic motivation activity, assessed with a post-reading vocabulary and comprehension test, was the best motivating condition for developing vocabulary, comprehension and expository writing. The evaluation concentrated the children's attention on the need to know the meaning of words and to understand the text passages. Use of the expanded electronic dictionary, giving a definition of a word and an exemplar of the word in a sentence context, did not however result in improved reading or writing, for reasons which were not clear.

Braden et al. (1989) studied the effects of microcomputer-assisted telecommunication, analogous to reading and writing text, on the language and literacy of 48 hearing-impaired children between sixth- and eighth-grade levels, with a mean reading grade equivalent of 2.76 years. One group of children used microcomputers to telecommunicate with hearing children, another group telecommunicated with hearing-impaired peers, and a control group was given computer-aided instruction without telecommunication. Results showed that the two telecommunication groups improved their syntax skills in comparison to the control group, but not on other measures. However, there was a general tendency for the hearing-impaired to hearing-impaired telecommunication group to outperform the hearing-impaired to hearing group on all measures of improvement, namely in unstructured telecommunicated conversations, written language and scholastic achievement test scores, with both of these groups doing better than the control group. This finding is perhaps of greater importance than the microcomputer-assisted telecommunication. It suggests that it is not so much the language expertise or language model that promotes an increase in language and literacy skills as the need to match like with like, namely to present hearing-impaired children with text at a level familiar to them, though Braden et al. argued that it was the disequilibrium of experiencing conversations frustrated by other weak users of language which prompted the gains in language and literacy skills.

Much work remains to be done in this rapidly developing area, since computers are now favoured as a teaching tool in schools for the deaf. Although they are used commonly to present academic work, and to provide for practice in question-and-answer program, this is a traditional and rather limited expression of their potential. As computers become more sophisticated and user-friendly, we expect to see them being used in an increasing variety of educational applications, including CMT, for instruction in reading.

Writing

Since what is read has been written, and because both reading and writing skills depend on a common knowledge of vocabulary, syntax and semantics, it is to be expected that achievements in reading are related to achievements in writing (Graves, 1983; Walmsley, 1983). Further, most material is written in order to be read but, because reading is the skill learned first, writing is learned after the attainment of some skill in reading. Thereafter achievements in reading and writing tend to progress in tandem.

Useful discussions of the purposes of writing, and of the processes involved for hearing individuals are presented in several papers in volume 87 (1985) of the *Volta Review*. A recent summary of disorders of written expression is available in Gregg (1991). A full review of writing ability would involve consideration of spelling. However, spelling does not play as primary a role in written communication as other factors, and it is not considered here.

The principal purposes of writing for hearing individuals are to communicate information and ideas in a lasting form. Deaf people, however, also write to communicate everyday ideas to persons beyond their nuclear family and their circle of friends. If they do not receive sufficient help from amplification and/or speechreading, they need to rely heavily on written communication. They also need to rely on writing if they communicate manually or if they cannot articulate reasonably clear speech (White and Stevenson, 1975). Remarkably, there is very little published research in this important area. Most reports of writing by hearing-impaired individuals have been concerned with written exercises of hearing-impaired children at school, or similar activities. Necessarily, this is the material which we review.

Written grammar

Writing by hearing-impaired children has been the subject of considerable study and research, conveniently summarised by Quigley and Paul (1984) and Yoshinaga-Itano and Snyder (1985). Although there are large differences between good and poor deaf writers in both content and linguistic style (Gormley and Sarachan-Deily, 1987), the weight of research shows clearly that severely and profoundly deaf children produce grammatical errors in their writing. Even partially hearing children have problems in writing grammatically correct sentences which they can say (Arnold et al., 1982). Children with greater hearing losses tend to omit function words, such as articles, auxiliary verbs and prepositions – a characteristic which continues into post-secondary years (McAfee et al., 1990). In addition to these omissions, their sentences tend to be short, because of problems with some conjunctions, leading to 'jumps' from one sentence to another. Many of their sentences are of the SVO type. Some have no apparent grammar at all (Webster and Ellwood, 1985), or may be grammatically deviant. Overall, the impression for the reader is one of a rigid style of writing, with omissions, sequencing problems and occasional grammatical infelicities ('deafisms') which make it difficult to follow the train of thought (Ivimey, 1977c; Harrison et al., 1991). The semantics of the written message are hence thrown off track for the reader, who may have to study the writing with repeated regression and progression to understand the meaning of such instances as: 'The girl take pencil and drop. Pick-up. Drawing in book. Rub-out'. Inevitably problems of interpretation arise, which cast some question on the validity of syntactic and semantic analysis of the writing (Rodda and Grove, 1987).

Earlier studies approached the analysis of writing from the viewpoint of traditional grammar, with tallies of words, sometimes classified as traditional 'parts of speech' (nouns, verbs, adjectives, adverbs, etc.), and sentences. Studies of type–token ratios were popular, where types referred to the number of different words and tokens to the total number of words (Heider and Heider, 1940; Simmons, 1962; Myklebust, 1964; Schulze, 1965). Some of these earlier authors suggested that the writing of hearing-impaired children resembled that of normally developing children of a younger age. Others (Fusfeld, 1955) saw the writing as a tangled collation of words in a disorderly array, without sequencing or inflections reflecting accepted grammar.

Following Chomsky's (1957, 1965) transformational generative grammar, the analysis of writing by hearing-impaired children was approached in another way (Ivimey, 1976; Quigley et al., 1976a). Instead of traditional approaches, the writing was analysed for syntactic structures which, while not usual, none the less appeared consistently. Hearing-impaired children were seen to have problems with the inflection of nouns and verbs, and with articles and auxiliary verbs into the teen years, although they had mastered straightforward active declarative sentences, such as SVO forms.

Particular problems were experienced with the less concrete verbs, such as 'to be' and 'to have'. Control of verb tenses was weak, and in some cases non-existent (Ivimey, 1981), so that the one verb tense could be used to indicate past, present and future, but modified by an external marker ('He came now'). Similarly, noun modifiers were used to show plurality ('The two cup'). Articles were often appropriately used with the subject but were often omitted for the object ('The family go on picnic'), though the use of determiner and noun as subject was often overused. Relative and other embedded clauses were used rarely. Indeed, Wilbur (1977) argued that hearing-impaired children tended to approach writing as a clause by clause, or sentence by sentence, task rather than as a task in whole composition. There were also difficulties in using the passive voice (Power and Quigley, 1973). However, because these results were found consistently between and within deaf children, it was argued that the writing was not lacking in grammatical rules but had a rule system of its own, or that hearing-impaired children used the standard English rules of grammar together with their own constructions (Quigley et al., 1976b).

It is now generally accepted that the writing of hearing-impaired children is both linguistically delayed and different, or deviant (Webster, 1986). The use of unusual or deviant written grammar is a real problem, because society cannot be expected to cope with idiosyncratic use of grammar. Even if there are consistent patterns of deviancies across groups of hearing-impaired children, there will still be a major problem for them in communicating their ideas to hearing individuals. Thus from the communication viewpoint, it is a pressing issue to discover the extent of the use of deviant grammar in the writing of hearing-impaired children. Papers by Bamford and Bench (1979), Williams and Dennis (1979) and Williams (1986) using the Language Assessment, Remediation and Screening Procedure of Crystal et al. (1976) illustrate methods of how this issue might be explored further.

To explain the findings, it has been suggested that function words are short in duration and often unstressed, so that they are difficult to hear or speechread and hence are poorly learned. The over-use of the definite article with subject nouns and other features has been ascribed to rigid teaching, though Bunch (1979) found no difference in the use of rules of grammar with natural versus formal methods of teaching for hearing-impaired children aged 9–16 years. Problems with writing standard English have also been ascribed to interfering effects from the learning of sign language (Dawson, 1981).

More recent work (Geers and Moog, 1989), discussed earlier in the section on reading skills, has shown that some orally educated profoundly deaf adolescents aged from 15 to 18 years can write at levels much better than the main thrust of the literature would indicate. Geers and Moog reported that the majority of their children could write acceptable essays and business letters, with only some mechanical and grammatical errors. Such reports show that caution is needed in generalising about the abilities of deaf individuals. However, Geers and Moog's subjects were atypical of deaf adolescents as a whole. McAfee et al. (1990), mentioned earlier, reported findings for severely deaf post-secondary students which showed that the written English skills of these students were consistent with the earlier reports, with a high occurrence of errors in function words. Klecan-Aker and Blondeau (1990) have also presented results which confirm the earlier work for use of clauses, and coordinating versus subordinating conjunctions.

Some of the unusual aspects of the writing of hearing-impaired children are similar to the early efforts at writing of young hearing children, an observation which lends weight to the idea that the writing skills of hearing-impaired children are delayed, at least in part. Although the writing of hearing-impaired children improves with age (Myklebust, 1964; Power and Wilgus, 1983), this improvement is relatively slow, as with improvement in their reading skills. It seems that the older children attempt to express more complex thoughts in writing as they develop, but their grammatical ability holds them back. One result is 'deafisms' or deviant grammar. Although the vocabulary may be adequate, the way in which words are put together reflects a less sophisticated style of writing because of imperfectly learned grammatical structures. It seems, then, that difficulties of a linguistic kind, and especially with grammar, retard the ability of hearing-impaired children in both reading and writing. Since reading is problematic for hearing-impaired children, it is scarcely surprising that they also have problems with writing. Difficulties in both reading and writing can be explained by failure to develop an internal language (Quigley and Kretschmer, 1982).

It will be recalled that manipulation of memory rehearsal can shed light on the reading strategies of hearing-impaired children (Webster, 1986). Given a reciprocal relationship between reading and writing, it would seem that manipulation of rehearsal could also be a useful tool in the investigation of writing. In a novel experiment, Webster (1986) has indeed studied the effects of rehearsal on the writing skills of hearing-impaired children, particularly for the writing of longer items. Such longer items need to be held in memory, and hence a child who has poor inner language will be unable to rehearse the material, just before it is written down, through 'articulatory feedback loops' or some similar strategem (Baddeley, 1979). The child will therefore have problems in the fluent writing of sequential connected prose. Webster studied 20 severely to profoundly deaf children aged 11–12 years, and 20 hearing children of the same age. The children wrote about a picture under two conditions. For the first condition, the children were given a sheet of paper and asked to write for 30 minutes about what they saw. In the second condition, the children performed the same task, but wrote with an expired pen on a sheet of paper, under which was a sheet of carbon paper overlaying a second sheet. Thus the children could see what they had written in the first condition, but not in the second.

Webster found, first, that hearing children used fewer sentences and made fewer grammatical errors than the hearing-impaired children. The latter used simple sentence structures, more content words such as nouns and verbs, fewer function words, and many non-standard grammatical forms, confirming earlier work. Secondly, in comparing the two conditions, he found that writing without visual feedback in the second condition did not affect the performance of the hearing-impaired children. The possibility, in normal circumstances, of looking back at what they had written did not affect their subsequent writing, because their use of feedback mechanisms was already disrupted or weak. The hearing children, however, performed badly in the second condition, increasing their errors and reducing their production of complex sentences. Some hearing children produced deviant structures similar to deafisms, such as omission of determiners and auxiliaries. They also used inappropriate word endings. Thus feedback from material already written and rehearsal of material play an important role in writing skills, especially for prose containing more complex structures.

The poor achievement of hearing-impaired child writers can be attributed, in part, to failure to rehearse the material because of difficulties with inner language which prevents rehearsal from taking place. This conclusion is supported by Wood et al. (1986) who found that hearing-impaired children who wrote relatively well also produced relatively accurate spoken messages, suggesting that inner language assisted both writing and speaking. Interestingly, Webster's study suggests that the primary failure, namely failure to rehearse the material, is a cognitive rather than a linguistic problem.

Learning to write

The literature is weak on how hearing-impaired children begin to learn writing skills. In a free-choice exercise, Conway (1985) found that hearing-impaired children of kindergarten age were interested to express meaning and content in their writing rather than form. He argued for an educational focus on the child's capacity to learn rather than on the writing deficits. Ewoldt (1985) used a natural composition approach to teach fluent writing over a period of 3 years to ten hearing-impaired children, born to hearing-impaired parents. The programme began with children at ages 4–5, concluding at ages 6–7 years. Her results, however, did not indicate clear advantages for a natural language approach to writing as a means of overcoming the rigid productions of hearing-impaired children. In any case, and as we saw above, Bunch (1979) found no difference between natural and formal approaches in teaching written grammar.

More informative results were obtained by Truax (1985), who described a 3-week programme of near-daily meetings for 6- and 7-year-old hearing-impaired children. The teacher modelled stories, after which each of six children told short stories, in turns, with the teacher asking questions for clarification. Then the children drew pictures to show the main characters, settings and events in their stories, and retold the stories, which were written up in front of the group. This programme continued, with the children writing words to add to the pictures and progressing to more sophisticated forms of writing. The interaction of the children in telling and writing stories was highly motivating. Presenting their ideas in writing to others, with verbal storytelling and group discussion, spurred them on. Truax's programme appears to be worth pursuing further, particularly as it attempted to integrate reading and writing with group communication. However, her work lacked controls, such as a matched group of children learning to write through traditional methods, which makes the significance of the report difficult to estimate.

The approaches of Conway (1985), Ewoldt (1985), and Truax (1985) look promising as teaching vehicles because they were motivating. The focus was on content, narrative or semantic aspects rather than grammar. Yoshinaga-Itano (1986) continued with this theme. She reported an attempt to expand the semantic properties of the written compositions of hearing-impaired children using a propositional analysis. She also studied the semantic–syntactic links between sentences (Yoshinaga-Itano and Snyder, 1985). She compared the writing of 49 prelingually deaf children aged 10–14 years, who had moderate or greater hearing losses, with the writing of 49 hearing children. A quadratic trend was found for semantic written language variables, peaking at age 12 years for hearing-impaired children and at age 13 years for hearing children. Both groups, however, showed a linear developmental trend for syntactic variables. This linear trend increased with age, with the hearing children outperforming the deaf group. Hence the difference between the two groups was greater in syntactic than semantic performance.

Increasing numbers of researchers have begun to study the written narratives of hearing-impaired children as narrative discourse in the last few years. We have already referred to work in this area by Webster (1986). Sarachan-Deily (1985) gave an account of the ability of hearing-impaired high-school students to recall explicit propositions and inferences, going beyond the literal meaning, by reading and then writing a given story. Although the hearing-impaired students recalled significantly fewer propositions than hearing subjects, they included a similar number of inferences in their written narratives. Further, the better readers among the hearing-impaired students recalled propositions more accurately, but did not differ in recalling implicit content.

Somewhat dissimilar findings were presented for stories written and signed for severely to profoundly deaf children, or written and told for hearing children, aged 8–15 years by Everhart and Marschark (1988). Their hearing children produced comparable numbers of non-literal constructions in spoken and written stories, whereas the deaf children produced significantly more non-literal constructions in sign than in writing, where the non-literal constructions were very few. The deaf children were linguistically much more creative in sign than in writing. However, the children studied by Sarachan-Deily on the one hand, and by Everhart and Marschark on the other, differed in age and otherwise. As Everhart and Marschark remarked, different children may have different preferred ways of creative expression. To separate the different effects and causes would require comparisons of individuals who are matched carefully for their abilities in sign, speech and other relevant variables.

Intervention programmes

Given the emphasis on writing in education, it is not surprising to find many reports of educational programmes to improve the written communication skills of hearing-impaired children. Besides the more conventional approaches, we note the advent of computer-assisted training using word-processing programs (Schilp,

1989), and the use of a journal or notebook to prompt interactive dialogue (Staton, 1985; Teller and Lindsey, 1987). Journal-writing is helpful since it is much more like face-to-face interaction than formal writing assignments, especially where dialogue journals are exchanged between deaf and hearing children (Kluwin and Kelly, 1991). Research on dialogue journal exchange approaches the need we mentioned at the start of this section for studies of the use of writing in everyday communication by hearing-impaired children. Unfortunately to date, reports of dialogue–journal exchange are as far as the literature goes.

We next consider the effects of combining communication modes on the development of writing skills. In one of the better designed studies, Akamatsu and Armour (1987) assessed the effects of complementary teaching in sign language, transliteration as writing in letters of another alphabet, and translation and editing skills on the writing skills of six severely to profoundly deaf students in a residential high school for the deaf. The students had auditory discrimination scores of less than or equal to 15%, and reading comprehension grades between 3.5 and 6.0 on the SAT (hearing-impaired version). Following a pre-test with a spontaneous writing sample and a receptive signing transfer test, the students were instructed twice a week for 45 minutes over a 10-week period. The instruction included information on communication, the way in which sign systems convey information, transliteration and translation skills, and editing/grammar skills for English, to make the students more aware of these features and their interrelationships. Both literal and figurative aspects were taught. In comparison with seven matched controls, no significant differences were found between the groups on pre-test measures, but the post-test scores for the experimental (instructed) group were significantly higher than those of the control (no instruction) group for spontaneous writing and sign-receptive transfer for grammar and accuracy of information. These results showed that drawing the experimental group's attention to signing, and ways in which signing differed from writing, improved aspects of their writing ability. Akamatsu and Armour went on to argue for an increased role for bilingual education in the classroom, with a broad range of teachers. Their results are stimulating. However, as they were aware, their design confounded instructor effects for the experimental group. Also the use of editing skills in writing was confounded with the instruction. Clearly, further clarificatory work needs to be done.

The work we have considered so far has been concerned with identifying the reasons for poor writing performance in hearing-impaired children, and remediating it. There has been little reference to writing as communication. There is, nevertheless, one approach which has taken written communication as its focus. In a particularly interesting paper, Harrison et al. (1991) reported a bold approach where there was no intervention to teach vocabulary or syntax for writing, and written syntax was never corrected. The aim was to allow the child's writing to be judged on its ability to communicate ideas. Samples of the writing, from usual school routines, of 86 moderately to profoundly deaf children aged 5–17 years, who were integrated in ordinary schools in Leicestershire, UK, were grouped into categories according to their syntactic maturity or completeness. Harrison et al. found that 85% of the writing contained fluent and expressive use of complex language allowing easy extraction of meaning, though with immature syntax, up to normal use of syntax. Seventy-seven per cent of the profoundly deaf children also produced writing in this range. The authors believed that the achievement of sentences with the completeness of adult usage was an inappropriate and unnecessary goal for many hearing-impaired children. They concluded that a non-corrective approach to writing enabled the children to develop a confidence and fluency of expression which allowed them to express their ideas using their available linguistic knowledge, and to use writing as a means of communication. This study offers much food for thought. Confirmatory reports of its findings and reports of the degree of community acceptance of its goals are keenly anticipated.

Concluding Remarks: Reading and Writing

This chapter concludes with some comments on the relation between reading and writing as it affects hearing-impaired children.

A first point to note is that although reading and writing depend on both syntax and semantics, the semantic aspects of writing are more closely related to reading comprehension than are the syntactic aspects (Yoshinaga-Itano and Snyder, 1985). The reason is that, within limits, syntax indicates how verbal material is to be processed rather than what it means. This point is particularly relevant to communication, because communication is concerned with the transfer of meaning. In everyday communication, errors of syntax can be accommodated, provided that they are not too glaring. Semantic errors are likely to be much more troublesome.

The relationship between reading comprehension and writing skills may be observed by asking children to read a passage of prose, and then to provide a written summary of it. One such study is that of Peterson and French (1988) with 30 hearing and 30 hearing-impaired college students. Each group read and summarised two expository scientific passages which were controlled for the number of topic or main idea sentences, and which had been judged earlier for the importance of the 'idea units' they contained. The two groups' performances were similar in their use of summarisation strategies, except for the inclusion of comments or opinions in the summaries. The hearing-impaired group was less sensitive to the importance of ideas. They made less frequent use of important ideas, choice of topic sentences, creation of topic statements, and integration of ideas within and among paragraphs. The hearing-impaired college students thus had basic skills in writing summaries, but used summarisation strategies less effectively than the hearing students. However, this study may have underestimated the abilities of the hearing-impaired group. Given a chance to read and revise their own narrative drafts, hearing-impaired high-school students can produce revised drafts which are better than the first (Livingston, 1989).

Arnold (1981) and Exley and Arnold (1987) drew attention to the propensity of deaf children to make fewer written spelling errors because of phonemic confusions than hearing children, since deaf individuals code and store words as visual sequences of letters. The analogy with processes involved in the reading abilities of deaf children, outlined above, is clear. Although deaf children may have this advantage in avoiding written errors caused by phonemic confusions, it is far out-weighed by their lack of inner speech, which causes major difficulties with both reading and writing.

We recall that assessments of deaf children's ability in reading were criticised when based on reading tests for hearing children. The criticism was that such tests are based on expressive language skills which deaf children may not have (Davey et al., 1983). It is tempting to promote a similar criticism of the assessment of deaf children's writing skills. The problem is, however, that there is no general alternative mode such as sign in which to write, for written sign systems are little used. Although Quigley and Kretschmer (1982) suggested that video-recording of signed communication be used in lieu of writing, this novel suggestion is seldom pursued. It proves cumbersome in practice.

The reciprocal relationship between reading and writing is known to hearing-impaired children themselves (Hollingshead, 1982). Practice in the one should therefore promote attainment in the other. Both depend on well developed internal language, which itself depends on a communication system which can convey a wide and complex range of meaningful experiences to the child (Quigley and Kretschmer, 1982). However that may be, it is unfortunately the case, as we have seen, that most severely to profoundly prelingually deaf children presently do not learn to read and write adequately. They are accordingly denied communication via literacy with wider society.

Chapter 7
Hearing Impairment and Cognition

This chapter is divided into three sections dealing with cognition, metaprocesses and central auditory dysfunction in communication. The first section considers cognitive skills in relation to the hearing-impaired child's understanding of speech. There follows a discussion of cognitive processes including memory, temporal processing, semantics and higher-level aspects, and then some comments on the cognitive processes of deaf signers. The section on metaprocesses, where the literature is very slim, reviews virtually all the published research on metaprocesses in hearing-impaired children. The final section on central auditory dysfunction outlines the nature of the phenomenon, making a distinction between central auditory disorders and language learning problems.

Because of the pervasive influence of language in everyday communication, language supports not only oracy and literacy, but thinking, understanding, memorising and so on (Hayes, 1990). The closeness of cognition and language can be seen in questions, for example, where deaf children may experience problems with both the linguistic form of a question and in comprehending its meaning (LaSasso, 1990). In earlier work, language was seen as primary to cognition (Sapir, 1949; Whorf, 1956). Although it was accepted that the very young infant develops some cognitive abilities before language begins to appear, as soon as language emerges it was thought to dominate cognitive development. The work of Chomsky (1957, 1968), which emphasised a unique role for language, added impetus to this direction.

With Piaget's influential work on concept development (Chapter 1), the so-called Whorfian view that language dominates cognition fell out of favour. In its place emerged the idea that language builds on pre-existing cognitive activity. According to this view, cognition is primary to language (Bever, 1970; Slobin, 1979). Language is built on concepts and ideas which have already developed without a linguistic basis. Apparent evidence to support this view comes from research into deafness (Furth, 1964a, 1970; Bond, 1987; Christensen, 1990), since cognitive activity in the signing deaf occurs in the absence of verbal language.

However, since we cannot be sure that such activity occurs without mediation by sign language, the evidence is questionable. More convincing are the studies of object permanence by Corrigan (1978), who found in hearing infants that the beginning of search for objects removed from view occurred at the same time as production of the first words. The early deprivation reports (Chapter 2) also offer support, since several of these reports showed that cognitive activity can develop with little language.

At present, the cognitive-dominant view is the accepted one (King and Quigley, 1985; Christensen, 1990), but the issue is by no means settled. It may be that phonology and syntax are acquired satisfactorily even with severe cognitive impairment, but that semantics and comprehension cannot be (Cossu and Marshall, 1990). Much remains to be discovered about the nature of cognitive and communicative development early in life, before the first words are spoken. We have already seen that active communication takes place between mother and infant in this period, setting the stage for further cognitive and linguistic development, when the need to communicate thoughts and intentions drives the development of language. For the time being, we will settle for a parallel interaction between cognition and language, after early infancy (Schlesinger, 1977a; Wells, 1979). According to this position, thinking, intention and meaning can be developed through experience of language, as much as language may be expanded through cognition. In taking this position we recognise, of course, a distinction between language associated with cognition, and language as a basis for communication (Wood, 1991).

Cognitive Skills

In discussing cognition, it is common to refer to studies by Piaget, reflecting his concern with cognitive development (Duckworth, 1979; Rittenhouse et al., 1981; Peterson and Peterson, 1989; Christensen, 1990). These references relate to Piaget's focus on developmental stages and the interaction of the child with the environment in acquiring knowledge, though Affolter (1985) has argued that developmental patterns follow a continuous developmental progression rather than stages.

It is also common to give an account of cognitive subskills, ranging from such 'lower-order' skills as attention, psychophysical discrimination, and short-term memory, through such 'middle-order' skills as temporal sequencing and rehearsal, to higher-order skills, such as thinking, concept formation, problem-solving and reasoning (Sloan, 1980; Davis and Rampp, 1983; Rodda and Grove, 1987; Gruneberg et al., 1988). There is a logical sense to this kind of treatment, following, as it does, the sequence from sensation and perception to the mental activity which ensues. Also, it allows us to think about cognitive ability in an orderly way. However, the lower-order skills tend to be directly involved in the acquisition of the higher-order skills. In hearing children, for example, an articulatory loop, the phonological memory component of working memory, is directly involved in language acquisition and development, and in the development of oral comprehension (Hulme, 1987; Gathercole, 1990). Further, although it is feasible to analyse cognitive activity into a range of subskills at a conceptual level, it is very doubtful if hearing individuals, in their ordinary conversations, process speech inputs by analysing the speech sounds in detail, and then bring some such sequence as that outlined above to bear on the interpretation of the results. The sheer rate of speech production in even a simple conversation can scarcely allow it (Chapter 1).

We will consider the way in which the information contained in speech becomes accessible to cognition by viewing the task as an exercise in information processing constrained by the phonetic and linguistic properties of running speech.

Information processing

A useful place from which to start is the situation as described by Ivimey (1977a, b, c). He pointed out that the acoustic properties of conversational speech are quite different from what might be supposed from analysis of the 40 or so phonemes identified by classical phonetics. It is false to view the phonemes as making a set of relatively free-standing sounds, some representing vowels and some representing consonants, with each taking between 10 and 100 ms to produce and which, in combination, produce the sounds of speech. The true situation is much more complex. Speech sounds occur concurrently as much as sequentially. There is a relatively slow sequence of vowels which are modified at their beginnings and endings by formant transitions in the production of adjacent consonants. The acoustic cues for consonants are usually different when the same consonant is paired with different vowels, when the consonants are in different positions (initial, medial or final) and for the kinds of cues (manner, place and voicing) that are used (Liberman et al., 1967).

Instead of discriminating among some 40 stable phonemes, the listener has to choose from about 300–400 possibilities. The complexity does not stop there, because different speakers produce distinctly different speech sounds. Male, female and child's speech sounds are quite different. Also, in running speech, the 'target' sounds that the speaker intends to produce are not fully realised because, as one sound is pronounced, the vocal organs are already being positioned to produce the next one. The anatomical speech structures do not have time to attain the ideal configuration for the production of a given speech sound before they start to alter to produce the next. Thus, instead of bringing perceptual and cognitive processes to bear on a relatively small range of speech sounds, presented in a clearly sequential fashion, the listener has to contend with up to perhaps 1000 possible different sounds, many of which are coarticulated, and many of which only approximate what the speaker intended to produce. The task for the listener primarily involves identifying the main bursts of energy, the vowels, which may not be on target, and the initial and final modifications to those bursts of vowel energy, representing the consonants. These identifications must be made so that relative differences between speakers do not disrupt the process. The listener does not so much analyse speech in minute acoustic detail, as analyse for the overall pattern of the speech. Clearly, much more is at issue than the acoustic properties of the speech signal. The listener has to decode an apparently confusing and rapidly changing complex of sounds.

Phonological, prosodic, grammatical and semantic constraints

The interpretation of speech sounds in conversations is greatly facilitated by the characteristics of the language in which the speech is produced and received, because languages are subject to phonological, syntactic and semantic constraints. Under these constraints, only a limited number of sequences is allowed. The result is a marked reduction in the cognitive load on the listener in understanding what is being said. For example, when listening and then repeating a new word, or when reading aloud a new word for the first time, people articulate the word on the basis of the accepted phonology. It is thus easy to articulate a nonsense word such as 'poad' to rhyme with 'road' or 'goad'.

Several authors have attempted to describe how segmental information is processed in spoken words. Salasoo and Pisoni (1985) examined the sources of knowledge from which spoken words can be identified; Grosjean and Gee (1987) reported on the effects of prosodic structure on the perception of spoken words; and Slowiaczek et al. (1987) explored the effects of phonological priming, a form of prompting to manipulate phonological salience, on word recognition. Slowiaczek (1990) manipulated lexical stress by varying the stressed syllable in sets of words. Some stresses were correct and some incorrect ('YELlow' versus 'yelLOW'). She reported that correctly stressed words were produced faster than incorrectly stressed words in shadowing experiments which involved speaking a word immediately following its presentation. Correctly stressed words were also classified faster than incorrectly stressed words in a lexical decision task between words and non-words ('YELlow' vs. 'GHELlow'). Her work further suggested that sequential information was relied on more heavily when the correct lexical stress was absent. Thus prosodic information, and in particular lexical stress, is subject to constraints which must be observed to make sense of a message.

Speech sounds are subject to grammatical constraints of syntax and morphology. For instance, besides using syntax to put words into permissible sequences, we use syntax to organise morphemes. The morphemes can exist alone as free morphemes ('boy', 'girl') or bound morphemes, which have meaning only when joined with other morphemes (-s in 'boys', or -ed in 'played'). Syntax organises morphemes as part of grammar. A sentence such as 'The boys shout and run away' is allowable, whereas 'The boy shout and run away' is beyond the rules.

At the semantic level, the overall context is of particular importance in understanding connected speech. Whereas semantic information is conveyed by the meaningfulness of the words in an isolated sentence, under natural conversational conditions the context of the conversation sets the scene for the whole utterance. In such conditions whole words may be replaced experimentally by noise bursts, analogous to the replacement of phonemes discussed above, and yet the listener may insist that the original word was present (Warren, 1970). At this level of semantic processing expert knowledge of language and everyday affairs is central to skill in communication.

Occasional problems with speech production or perception, such as occasional mispronunciations or mishearings, are no problem because the context and the speaker's and listener's knowledge of the world allows such lacunae to be bypassed. Hearing people who have well developed central cognitive processes and who are well versed in the world of affairs have considerable leeway in overcoming such errors, gaps and breaks. Even when words that make up a sequence of connected speech cannot be perceived, the listener may still be able to make sense of the message if isolated speech fragments can be fitted together in the listener's internal schema (Bever, 1970, 1973). What is said has to be heard as making sense. The constraint is derived from meaning.

The constraints on the semantics produced by the speaker are less particular than constraints at the phonological, morphological and syntactic levels (Garrett, 1980; Meyer, 1990). This relaxation of constraint at the semantic level for the speaker can be matched by the listener's concentration on the meaning of what is being said, as shown by supplying words or phrases for which the speaker is temporarily stymied, with the words or phrases on the tip of the tongue.

Cognition and Hearing Impairment

The outline just presented will have reminded the reader of the huge task that faces the would-be orally communicating prelingually severely or profoundly deaf child. We now consider first some aspects of cognition in deaf children concerned with speechreading, information processing, memory, time perception, semantics and higher-level processes. We consider secondly some cognitive features of sign.

The field is difficult to conceptualise clearly because of its pragmatic orientation and historical development. The methodologies are various and there are few clear theoretical directions. For instance, most of the earlier work was done with deaf children who were educated orally, especially in Europe, while later work has involved children who are more likely to use sign in some form as their main means of communication.

Cognitive delay or cognitive difference?

An interesting model has it that the major constraint on the perception of connected speech is not so much in the nature of the available sensory data as in the extent to which a listener is versed in the interacting sets of phonological, morphological, syntactic, prosodic and semantic rules of a language. This view of speech perception predicts that even profoundly deaf individuals whose cognitive and linguistic competence is high will be able to communicate well through such residual hearing as they may have, and through lipreading. That postlingually profoundly deaf individuals generally have good levels of communication, that communication skill is only partly explained by level of hearing loss, and that lipreading and use of residual hearing are correlated with linguistic competence and knowledge of the world in the prelingually profoundly deaf is good supportive evidence for this model. Recent studies have given further weight to the argument. Lyxell and Ronnberg (1989) found no differences in speechreading ability between postlingually mildly to moderately hearing-impaired adults and hearing adults in a sentence-completion test. Rather, the use of information-processing skills was the important factor, as shown by inference-making or guessing abilities

(Burke and Nerbonne, 1978; Paniagua, 1990; Lyxell and Ronnberg, 1991).

The particular issue, then, for the prelingually profoundly deaf child is to develop linguistic competence and a high degree of associated cognitive skill when hearing loss obstructs or diverts the development of such competence and skill. It is this and related problems that we now consider.

Some earlier workers saw the cognitive processes of hearing-impaired children as normal in type. However, language development would be affected by restricted interaction with the environment and a lack of sufficient chances for learning (Furth, 1966a, b), resulting in linguistic delay. The solution, according to this view, is to provide enriched opportunities for linguistic development.

An alternative view (Myklebust, 1964) is that the diminished auditory input results not only in language delay but in different cognitive processes from those of hearing children which, in turn, compound the linguistic problems. Different cognitive mechanisms result from reliance on other sensory modalities such as vision or touch, from which hearing-impaired children develop different cognitive and linguistic styles. Adherents of this view argue for alternative methods of communication for hearing-impaired children, such as communication by sign or, to a lesser extent, by tactile signals.

Since these two extremes were first expressed, more has become known about the cognitive and linguistic processes of hearing-impaired children. However, such evidence has not clarified the situation completely in the direction of one argument or the other. Hearing-impaired children have come to be seen as a very heterogeneous group (Bamford and Saunders, 1985), differing in degree of hearing loss, age at onset of loss, motivation, familial and social background, educational environment and so on.

Environmental factors, such as social and educational background, turn out to be at least as important, and possibly more important, than the hearing loss itself. Since the child's social and educational background is all but impossible to control, the debate is likely to remain confounded. What is clear is that most, but not all, prelingually severely and profoundly deaf children do have different cognitive styles in processing linguistic material. On the other hand, in demonstrating a near-normal level of linguistic and cognitive performance, a minority of such children function as though they had been deafened postlingually.

Working in the UK, and hence at the time with mainly orally-educated hearing-impaired children, Ivimey (1977c) argued that they perform like hearing children, but show marked performance delay. Such phenomena as 'deafisms' were due to a lack of exposure to English, not hearing loss per se. Considering the processes involved in the acquisition of grammar by deaf children, Ivimey thought that they acquire grammar in the normal way, but differ from hearing children in the age of acquisition. They use their experience to form tentative grammatical rules, and generalise these rules to other situations by analogy in a sequence of stages characterised by increasing linguistic and cognitive complexity. This sequence of stages and the association of linguistic and cognitive complexity is reminiscent of a classification of the language of teachers (Blank et al., 1978), where language is ordered according to its level of cognitive demand. Although concerned mainly with teachers' questions addressed to children, the classification allows language to be scaled from low-level cognitive demand items, such as names of objects and their attributes, to higher-level demand for the relationships between objects and events. The highest level of cognitive demand in this scheme is concerned with reasoning and planning. Hence the level of demand increases from the concrete towards inference and abstraction.

The explanation for Ivimey's stages was that deaf children first learn words as individual units and in meaningful sequences, as the simplest tasks, and then proceed to the more complex forms such as noun plurals, and the more concrete prepositions identifying location such as *to* and *in*. Later come the final *s* in verbs and the dative use of *to* which may be used inconsistently. The genitive use of *s*, and the use of prepositions in a correct but less than common way ('*on* the train' as opposed to '*on* the table') are used much later, if at all. The progression illustrates increasing complexity in the underlying concepts, and involves increasing demands on cognition.

Ivimey's argument has force. Prelingually hearing-impaired children experience many similar circumstances to hearing children in understanding their environments. In acquiring language, both groups are likely to make many similar linguistic 'mistakes' as their facility with language and their accompanying cognitive processes are developing. There is no doubt that hearing-impaired children have greater difficulty, at a given age, in coping linguistically and cognitively with their environment. There may, however, be a trade-off between IQ and hearing loss in that high IQ can offset the effects of hearing loss to some degree (Gallaway et al., 1990). Hence some prelingually deaf children do manage to develop a remarkable degree of sophistication in their linguistic and cognitive development, provided that they have a supportive and educationally sophisticated environment.

Nevertheless, as Conrad (1979) and Rodda and Grove (1987) have pointed out, although the tasks involved in the perception of speech have some similarities for hearing and hearing-impaired individuals, the cognitive processes involved are not comparable in most cases. Children with hearing within normal limits, or a mild to moderate hearing loss, learn to perceive speech mainly via the auditory channel, and develop a phonological or inner speech code in processing language. On the other hand, severely and especially profoundly deaf children have limited access to the auditory channel, which may additionally distort the auditory input. They are thus denied the opportunity to develop inner speech, except in a minority of cases where speechreading can be used successfully to supplement residual hearing (Myklebust, 1964). Prelingually deaf children in the main appear to process language through a visual code (see below).

We now examine such cognitive differences in greater detail, and begin by asking what sort of memory code is used by deaf children.

Hearing impairment and memory

Memory plays a significant role in communication. As short-term memory, it is important for hearing, speaking, speechreading, writing and reading, because it is difficult to continue with communication if we are unaware of what we have just been expressing, or what has just been expressed to us.

Memory codes

In an early study of short-term visual memory (Blair, 1957), severely and profoundly deaf children were assessed on the Memory for Designs Test and the Knox Cube Test, for which the order of stimuli has to be recalled. The deaf children performed at a significantly higher level on these tests than hearing children matched for age, gender and intelligence. They also performed better, but not significantly so, on a test of object location, where they had to remember the position of everyday objects on a card. However, when they were required to recall stimuli in sequence, the deaf children performed below the level of the hearing controls. Blair suggested that the reason was that the deaf children had a problem with auditory memory, associated with their low attainment in reading. Subsequent work, discussed at length in the well known and highly influential text by Conrad (1979), confirmed this view.

Conrad (1979) set out to investigate the operation of sequential memory, which is the order in which items are organised in memory, and the use of memory codes, in a large group of deaf school leavers. The children were shown printed words, one at a time, and asked to write them down from memory in the right order. Stimulus trials used either homophone words, which sound the same as one another, or non-homophone words. The effect of hearing loss on recall errors, with scores adjusted for non-verbal intelligence, was statistically significant, but not great, when all words were scored across all trials. The effect of hearing loss was less than that of intelligence. By adjusting the scores for intelligence, and by classifying the children with a separate test for the ability to use internal speech, Conrad then showed that the hearing loss had a negligible effect on performance. More importantly, the availability of internal speech was the significant variable, and the availability of internal speech was associated with hearing loss. The original effect of hearing loss on the error scores in the memory tasks was indirect. The use of inner speech, then, was the important factor. Accordingly, the apparent relationship of error scores to hearing loss was due to the extent of use of inner speech, which was negatively correlated with hearing loss.

Conrad also showed that the children with internal speech made fewer errors in the serial recall of non-homophonous words than those without internal speech. This was to be expected. The children with internal speech, who used a phonemic code, would be less likely to confuse word items with words which would not sound the same if pronounced than those children using some other code, such as a visual one.

When errors were considered in the serial recall of the homophonous words, no difference was found for the availability or not of internal speech. The reason given was that children with internal speech produced a fairly high rate of errors as the words were phonemically confusible. For children who did not have internal speech, but who presumably used a visual code in their memory, the error rate was also fairly high, because a visual code is not effective for serial-order tasks (Paivio, 1971; Hanson, 1982).

Conrad showed, then, that hearing loss by itself had little effect on serial memory for words. He also showed that the use of a phonemic code was less likely with increasing hearing loss, even though a few profoundly deaf children appeared to use it, and that the effectiveness of the memory code interacted with the material to be memorised. A next step was to match hearing-impaired children with hearing children on the basis of internal speech, and hence use of a phonemic code. These two groups should then show the same performance in memory for words. This Conrad did, but he found a difference between the two groups of children which just attained statistical significance. On considering the possible effect of differences in intelligence between the two groups, however, he concluded that their performances were similar.

The importance of Conrad's work for communication in hearing-impaired children is that their verbal communication, whether expressed through oracy or literacy, is highly likely to be impaired when they have no internal speech, rather than because of hearing loss itself. Those hearing-impaired children who, though profoundly deaf, have access to inner speech will be good communicators in ordinary society. They are able to hold in short-term store the immediately preceding spoken or written words as an aid to understanding words that follow. Conrad also argued that the use of inner speech was of major importance not only for memory, but also for speechreading, speech intelligibility and reading.

Although several studies have shown that deaf children have particular problems with memory tasks in which verbal mediation is required, or confers an advantage (Locke and Locke, 1971; Conrad, 1972a, c, 1979; Wallace and Corballis, 1973), deaf children recall as well as or perhaps better than hearing children in tasks that involve motor or visual mediation (O'Connor and Hermelin, 1976; Siple et al., 1977). The likely explanation is that deaf and hearing children use different kinds of coding. Hearing children use a speech-like code, though young hearing children may use a visual rather than a phonemic code, as shown by their higher visual than phonemic confusions in recall tasks (Campbell and Wright, 1990). Deaf children generally seem to use a visual or spatial code. Nevertheless, some can use a speech code, and Campbell and Wright (1990) have argued that orally educated prelingually profoundly deaf children may use speech-based codes in specific situations, such as naming pictures in a serial-recall task, as well as using visual or meaning-based codes in other contexts. The next question is: how is the material to be memorised put into any given code?

Memory encoding

The usual encoding mechanism suggested is that of rehearsal, the recounting or repetition of the material as it is held in short-term memory, before it is transferred into longer-term mental storage. For hearing individuals, the memory span appears to be closely related to the internal speech rate (Standing and Curtis, 1989), implying that memory span is related to the maximum rate of rehearsal. When asked to recall items in serial order, the child aged 5–6 years typically recalls correctly fewer items than older children. Yet the younger child can improve recall performance if instructed in how to rehearse (Kingsley and Hagen, 1969; Bebko, 1979), showing that the child perceives the stimuli and can label them, but does not usually rehearse them.

Several reports have described the use of rehearsal in recall tasks by deaf children. The general finding has been that the type of rehearsal is related to the preferred method of communication. Orally well educated students tend to use verbal rehearsal, students used to the Rochester Method employ fingerspelling, and signed rehearsal is used by students in sign language and TC programmes (Beck et al., 1977; Shand, 1982; Bonvillian, 1983; Morariu and Bruning, 1984; Krakow and Hanson, 1985; Shimizu and Inoue, 1988). However, Krakow and Hanson (1985) observed that deaf signers who were college students, and deaf graduates, used a sign-based code to recall ASL signs, but not to recall English words. Hence well educated deaf signers may not translate into sign, their primary language, when the material to be recalled is in printed English.

Although deaf children encode in the mode of their familiar modality of communication, there is evidence of flexibility to use other modes, depending on experience. In a study of 58 subjects comprising six groups with different hearing levels and linguistic experience, Hamilton and Holzman (1989) showed that individuals can encode flexibly in short-term memory tasks, with the code selected being biased by the properties of the incoming stimulus: oral, manual or both modalities. Subjects with both speech and sign experience recalled simultaneous oral and manual expressions more readily than expressions presented manually or orally alone, suggesting enhanced encoding as a result of linguistic experience. The total linguistic experience affected recall accuracy rather than the selection of the code.

The problems of children with rehearsal are due to failure to make use of rehearsal, rather than in not having rehearsal available. Bebko (1984) reported findings which cast light on rehearsal strategies in severely to profoundly congenitally deaf children aged 5–15 years. Twenty-nine of these children were educated orally and 34 were educated by TC. Following the presentation of various colour stimuli there was a 15-second delay. This delay interval was either unfilled, allowing spontaneous rehearsal, or the children were induced to rehearse by demonstration, or were prevented from rehearsal by counting digits. As expected, the orally educated children tended to rehearse verbally, while those educated by TC rehearsed in sign. Both types of spontaneous rehearsal seemed to be equally effective. However, although the serial position patterns in spontaneous rehearsal (first/mid/last) were similar to those of hearing children, they were delayed in performance level by several years for both orally and TC-educated children, a delay attributed to impaired linguistic and educational experience (compare Ivimey, 1977b, c). When rehearsal was prevented or induced, the deaf recalled as well as, or better than, the hearing children. Thus the memory and rehearsal spans of the deaf children were at least as good as those of the hearing children. The difference was that the hearing children used spontaneous rehearsal effectively whereas the deaf children tended not to use the opportunity for spontaneous rehearsal to good effect. The deaf children did not have difficulty with the content, or differences in memory span per se, but their strategy for remembering was poor. This outcome is reminiscent of the writing study of Webster (1986, and Chapter 6), which indicated that the poor writing skills of hearing-impaired children were due to lack of regression, or looking back at what they had just written – another kind of strategy problem.

Bebko and McKinnon (1990) extended this work by investigating whether the language history of deaf children was related to age delay in the use of spontaneous rehearsal. Forty-one prelingually severely to profoundly deaf children aged 5–15 years and educated in a TC programme were compared with 45 hearing children aged 5–8 years in a memory-for-colours task requiring serial recall. Their language experience was defined as chronological age both for hearing children and for signing deaf children born to deaf signing parents, and as years of training in their dominant communication mode for the remaining deaf children. As with Bebko (1984), a lag of several years was found in the emergence of spontaneous rehearsal. Discriminant function analysis showed that language experience was a very good explanation of the relation between age and use of rehearsal. In other words, the use of rehearsal in serial-order recall was strongly associated with years of experience in the use of language, whether verbal, signed or mixed. Experience in the use of language provided both hearing and deaf children with an effective medium for rehearsal. The deaf children born to hearing parents took longer to make use of such a strategy because of their delayed language ability.

A similar explanation can be given for the results of earlier studies of recall in deaf subjects. For example, Koh et al. (1971) reported on the free recall of lists of words by prelingually deaf and hearing adolescents aged 13–14 years and young adults aged 18–20 years. Two types of word lists were used. The first type was mixed, for which the words were chosen at random. The second type was organised in semantic categories. Although the free recall of the hearing subjects was superior to that of the deaf, the older deaf subjects performed almost as well as the older hearing subjects, suggesting that, by 18–20 years, increased language experience permitted the use of more effective rehearsal strategies in memory. The implication is that the material to be memorised should be meaningful in terms of its potential for integration with the subjects' cognitive schemata, and should suit their long-term memory and linguistic rule-generating skills. This maxim finds support from observations (Mills and Weldon, 1983) that hearing adults who are learning sign as a second language, recall signs more readily if the signs are grouped by semantic category rather than by cheremic category. Such sign-naïve people possess a schema for semantic categorisation, but not for cheremically grouped signs (Fuller and Wilbur, 1987).

Temporal processing

Hearing has been described as the 'time sense' (Fraisse, 1964). Hearing people can detect up to 1000 interruptions per second in a white-noise signal, but only 60 flashes of bright light per second (Miller and Taylor, 1948). Beyond the sensory level, O'Connor and Hermelin (1986) have suggested that successive judgements of time depend mainly on hearing. When hearing individuals had to perform a task in which practice with auditory verbal stimuli preceded practice with a visual representation of the stimuli, they tended to repeat the auditory pattern subvocally, to improve their timing for the visual stimuli.

Earlier studies of temporal processing by prelingually deaf people suggest that they have problems with temporal order, although the findings are not very clear (Blair, 1957; Conrad, 1979; Bross and Sauerwein, 1980; Hanson, 1982). Whether or not hearing-impaired individuals have problems with temporal processing is important. In order to communicate in speech, for example, sensitivity to temporal aspects of the speech signal matters in perceiving speech sounds continuously or categorically (Liberman et al., 1967) as part of the speech code. Temporal differences are also related to cortical processing of ASL signs (Poizner et al., 1979), though temporal contrasts are more important to communication by speech than by sign (Poizner and Tallal, 1987). Indeed, the temporal order of signs is relatively less important than the order of words in verbal English, as is the case in all inflected languages.

Short-term auditory deprivation studies with hearing individuals have shown enhanced visual temporal resolution for rapidly flashing visual stimulus (critical flicker fusion frequency) thresholds (Bross et al., 1980). Hence we might suppose that longer-term auditory deprivation in the form of congenital severe to profound deafness would produce enhanced visual temporal abilities, provided that there were no visual or central visual problems. Poizner and Tallal (1987) investigated this possibility by comparing critical flicker frequency thresholds in congenitally deaf adult signers and hearing subjects. No significant differences were found, in this and related experiments. Deaf signers, then, appear to have the same sensitivity to rapid visual changes as hearing people. Further, long-term auditory deprivation, in the form of deafness since birth, does not seem to affect visual temporal processing. In other experiments on perception and memory for rapidly changing non-linguistic visual forms there was likewise no difference between deaf and hearing subjects. However, Ronnberg et al. (1989), working with mildly to moderately adult deaf subjects, found a relationship between the speed parameters of visual-evoked brain potentials and performance speed on a long-term memory non-semantic letter-matching task. They also found a correlation between performance in a complex short-term memory test and neural speed.

The results of both studies seem to be associated with visual processing speed, and suggest some relationship between hearing loss and temporal processing. It is difficult, nevertheless, to relate them. We have to conclude that this more recent work leaves the area little clearer than the outcomes of the earlier reports mentioned above.

Since hearing is the 'time sense', at another level we may expect hearing-impaired people to experience difficulties with rhythm, which depends on timing and intensity. Levine (1986), for example, suggested that congenitally hearing-impaired people will have problems in coordinating inputs from sensory pathways. Studies of rhythm production and perception in hearing-impaired children are not numerous and their implications are not very clear. One of the earlier papers was presented by Swaiko (1974) on the use of rhythm in deaf education. Asp (1984), Guberina and Asp (1981) and Rosen et al. (1981) reported on the use of methods that may aid the perception and production of the suprasegmental components of speech, which have important rhythmic properties (Darrow, 1984).

In one of the better controlled experiments, a rhythmicity-testing protocol was developed by Liemohn et al. (1990) to assess whether rhythmic performance in tapping could be improved with training and whether the stimulus modality, visual versus tactile, affected performance. The subjects, 46 children aged 11–14 years with moderate to profound hearing losses, were instructed to tap with their hands in time to various stimuli. In a pre-test an experimental group of 23 of the 46 children were trained in a variety of rhythmic activities, including locomotor tasks, manipulative tasks, dance, and hopping routines, with accompanying rhythmic stimuli such as drum beats, strobe lights, etc. A control group, consisting of the other 23 children, participated in usual physical education routines, without rhythmic stimuli. Post-test tapping in time with the original visual and tactile stimuli was undertaken after the training or control activities, when the quality of rhythmic tapping was found to be related to stimulus modality. The tactile stimulus was judged more accurately than the visual stimulus by both experimental and control groups, indicating that modality-specific encoding was in use. The effects of the training were less conclusive, though training appeared to suggest an improvement in rhythmic tapping.

To summarise, it is generally unclear whether deaf children use different temporal processing from hearing children. Given the importance of the area for the development of communication, there is obviously a need for more research.

Semantic factors and cognition

Long-term memory for the way in which the world is organised and operates has an important bearing on the considerations of semantics and is perceived as increasingly important for the development and use of communication skills (Rodda and Grove, 1987). We have seen that hearing-impaired children are more likely to take note of the spatial proximity and semantic associations of words in reading and writing tasks than hearing children, whose reading and writing take account more readily of syntax and conventional phonology and orthography (Hanson et al., 1983). It seems, then, that the knowledge of the world should help their literacy by developing and reinforcing their semantic associations.

Early studies of the development of semantics in hearing-impaired children often used the word-association approach, in which children are asked to produce words which they believe are associated in meaning with a given word. Such work showed that hearing-impaired children produced more associations of a visual kind, and produced a smaller number of associated words than hearing children (Bonvillian et al., 1973). Also hearing-impaired children were less able than hearing children to match the syntactical form of the stimulus word. This evidence confirms that hearing-impaired children have a relatively weak world knowledge, as shown by fewer word associations, and grammar as demonstrated in a lesser ability to match for syntax.

The semantic differential technique has also been used to assess semantic structures in hearing-impaired children and their knowledge of the world. Green (1974) and Green and Shepherd (1975) used the semantic differential to describe the semantic structure of 33 severely to profoundly deaf subjects aged 9–17 years.

They used a combination of scaling and association methods to present several pairs of antonymous adjectives like 'good–bad', separated on a 7-point scale. The children were given a concept, such as 'teacher', 'spider', etc., and asked to rate it on the 7-point scale. Factor analysis of the results showed the semantic system of the deaf children to contain the rather concrete Evaluation ('rich–poor') and Potency ('little–big') dimensions found with hearing children. A third dimension appeared to be related to vision and the sense of touch ('round–square'), unlike in hearing children, for whom the third dimension related to Activity ('slow–fast'). Further, the deaf children's Evaluation and Potency dimensions accounted for more of their semantic associations than found with hearing children, whose semantic structure was less restricted and contained the dimensions of Warmth ('cold–hot'), and Novelty–Reality ('new–old'), etc. Thus this study also suggested relatively limited world knowledge.

The semantic organisation of older deaf students was investigated by Tweney et al. (1975), who studied 63 deaf adolescents, aged 16–18 years, together with 63 hearing adolescents of the same age range. Subjects were presented with cards showing sound words, common nouns, and drawings corresponding to the list of noun words. They were asked to put items they did not know into a separate pile, and then to sort each of the three sets into categories of similar meaning, using as many or as few categories as they wished. Instructions were both spoken and signed. Hierarchical cluster analysis was then used to compare the semantic structures of hearing and deaf subjects. The two groups showed only minor differences for noun words and pictures. However, the deaf group did differ from the hearing subjects for sound words, for which they would have had little or no auditory experience. Even when the deaf subjects offered some category structure, it was not always semantically based. Although 'meow–bark' was clustered, so was 'whack–whine' which may have been based on similarity of lettering. The latter type of grouping was not found for noun words or pictures, suggesting that the deaf subjects used a rationale based on visual similarity when they lacked sufficient semantic reasons as a basis for categorisation.

In a second study, Tweney et al. (1975) presented stimulus words which differed in imagery but were of equal frequency of occurrence. Again, the differences between matched sets of high and low imagery words ('chair' versus 'cost') were comparable for 63 deaf and 63 hearing adolescents. The overall results of neither study supported an argument that deaf subjects are relatively more dependent on some visual mediating process than hearing subjects. The absence of an auditory mediating process such as phonological coding did not weaken the deaf subjects' performance. Tweney et al. thus argued that the subjective lexicon of deaf individuals is comparable to that of hearing people. Further, since linguistic material appeared to be organised in semantic dimensions which were independent of the receptive channel providing information to the lexicon, the central linguistic and symbolic processes of deaf individuals were seen as abstract, and not limited to concrete operations.

As indicated by Rodda and Grove (1987), this outcome contradicted the commonly held assumption that deaf individuals are relatively limited to concrete, high-imagery ways of thinking. Rodda and Grove argued that abstract verbal materials are treated in a similar way by deaf and hearing individuals when, as in the Tweney et al. study, there are no demands on syntactic skills. However, age may be an important confounding variable. There is evidence (Green and Shepherd, 1975) that younger deaf children operate semantically at a relatively concrete level, which may not persist into late adolescence. There is also evidence (Johnson et al., 1982; Liben, 1979) that, although hearing-impaired children develop networks of associations in their lexical systems, the networks are relatively weak in terms of relationships between word meanings. Further, Marschark et al. (1986) found decreasing use of lexical inventions with age.

Studies of semantics in hearing-impaired children which use such methods as closed response sets, forced choice, word associations, word sorts, picture identification and so on are open to criticism (Conway, 1990). Conway argued that these methods not only require minimal linguistic responses but preclude assessment of how the children construct word meanings and demonstrate their knowledge in definitions. He urged the use of non-restrictive methods such as open-ended questions, which would encourage the elicitation of linguistic responses to prompt search of the children's semantic systems ('Tell me about ...'; 'Tell me some more about ...'; 'What else do you know about ...?').

Conway examined the amount, type and complexity of the semantic relationships in the word meanings of two groups of prelingually profoundly deaf children differentiated by age, with a mean age of 7 years for the younger and 9 years for the older group. Employing Norlin's (1981) open-ended questions to prompt the expression of semantic relationships to ten common nouns, and using each child's preferred mode of communication, Conway found that the younger group produced significantly fewer semantic relationships than the older group. Otherwise, the performance of the two groups did not differ. However, for both groups the definitions produced were at an immature level, similar to that of younger hearing children. Studies of semantics that use non-restrictive methods can all too easily confound semantics with syntax, where the syntactic relationships provide clues to meaning (Rodda and Grove, 1987). Conway's analysis used semantic case relationships (subordinate, coordinate, purpose, attribute etc.) and does not seem to have confounded semantics with syntax in this way. Nonetheless, the situation is not clear because the more complex semantic associations may require some sophistication in syntax to express them (Watson, 1985). Clearly, more work needs to be done in this area.

Higher-level aspects

Taxonomies of levels of thinking have been devised to help analyse the processes involved in the formation and use of concepts and ideas (Bruner, 1973; Moore, 1983; Quinsland and Van Ginkel, 1990). Such taxonomies include the intellectual, knowledge, comprehension and evaluative levels among others, and may be investigated through tests of intelligence as well as purpose-designed tests.

Most earlier studies of the assessment of intelligence concluded that severely to profoundly deaf children were retarded by about 2 years or so (Pintner and Reamer, 1920). Realising the need to discount verbal reasoning abilities, Pintner and

Paterson (1923) in the USA developed a non-verbal performance scale, one of the first of its kind, involving digit/symbol substitution tests. However, here too they found a retardation in ability by some 2–3 years. A review of 22 reports by Lane (1948) narrowed the intelligence gap to less than 1 year, though a few years previously Drever and Collins (1944) using carefully devised performance tests found that the intellectual abilities of hearing-impaired children were on a par with those of hearing children. Confirmation of the latter findings was obtained by Murphy (1957) in the UK, who reported that scores for the Wechsler Performance Scales of hearing-impaired children fell within the normal range for hearing children.

Since Furth (1971), it has become generally accepted that the intellectual abilities of hearing-impaired children are of the same order as those for the hearing child, except where verbal factors have a part to play (e.g. Watson et al., 1986), though Savage et al. (1981) concluded that the data are still rather disorganised and somewhat conflicting. The reader is referred to Lewis (1968) and Quigley and Kretschmer (1982) for historical reviews.

The abilities of hearing-impaired children in the learning and use of various concepts were described by Furth (1961, 1963, 1964b). In a task for sameness, his subjects had to choose stimuli with defined properties; in a symmetry task they had to pick a stimulus showing symmetry; and in an opposition task subjects chose the opposite size stimulus to the one identified. The deaf subjects attained similar scores to hearing children on the sameness and symmetry tasks and did only slightly less well on the opposition task possibly because of weak verbal reasoning. In a pictorial choice task, deaf children were required to identify a 'part–whole' concept concealed in a confusing visual ground. Again, no differences were found between deaf and hearing children, but age and intelligence did have significant effects.

Since severe to profound hearing loss generally leads to altered cognitive function, and probably to altered perceptual function, it is likely to affect motor function in some way, especially in perceptual–motor tasks. Accordingly, it is of interest to remark that Wiegersma and Van der Velde (1983) observed lower performance in both general dynamic movement and visual–motor coordination in young deaf as compared with hearing children. Savage et al. (1981) specifically asked if deafness leads to altered perceptual organisation and hence influences aspects of motor function. They used the Minnesota Percepto-Diagnostic Test (MPDT), in which the child has to reproduce figures shown on stimulus cards, and the Digit/Symbol and Block Design Subtests from the Wechsler scales as tests of perceptual–motor function, with a sample of 55 deaf children aged 8–13 years. No significant difference was found for the MPDT between deaf and hearing children when the data were corrected for age and gender. On the Wechsler coding (digit/symbol) measure, however, deaf and hearing children differed significantly. Further, the poor and especially the very poor readers in the deaf group obtained significantly lower coding level scores than the better deaf readers. The deaf and hearing groups also differed significantly on the Block Design test. It appeared then that deafness can affect performance on perceptual–motor tasks, and that the relationship is connected with verbal ability. A similar conclusion was reached by Bolton (1971) in a factor analytic study of the communication skills and non-verbal abilities of deaf individuals. It seems likely that the use of inner speech is associated with verbal ability in some kinds of perceptual–motor tasks.

It is of interest to learn if there are differences between hearing and hearing-impaired children in higher-level cognitive processes which do not involve linguistic, and especially syntactic, mediation. Although reports in the area are few, they all point to the same conclusion. Thus, Rittenhouse et al. (1981) found that hearing loss and poor linguistic ability do not directly affect tasks involving the understanding of metaphor or tasks involving the principles of conservation. Such tasks can be undertaken using cognition alone, and in general deaf children perform them at the same level as hearing children of the same age. Any slight retardation of performance that has been noted can be ascribed to difficulties in understanding the instructions or to lesser experience of the world in general. Also, weak linguistic ability need not have much effect on the understanding of idiom, which is largely a cognitive activity. The comprehension of idioms seems to be based on memory for literal and figurative meanings in a way similar to memory for single words and single word meanings (Fruchter et al., 1984). Thus although hearing-impaired students may have difficulty in understanding idioms, they have the cognitive structures needed to understand them and can be trained to discriminate among them (Fruchter et al., 1984; Israelite et al., 1986).

The material reviewed above suggests that, provided care is taken in recognising the effects of any confounding linguistic variables, the higher-level cognitive skills of deaf children are roughly equal to those of hearing children. Although prelingually deaf children do not seem to use the same coding in their cognitive processing, such as inner speech, as do hearing children (Conrad and Rush, 1965; Conrad, 1979), this is not to say that their cognitive capacity is inferior to that of hearing children. When allowance is made for the difference in experience, especially linguistic experience, of deaf children, their cognitive performance is close to that of children who hear (Conrad, 1979). Accordingly, in a review of several papers on cognitive strategies and processes, Wolff (1985) remarked that apparent cognitive deficits in deaf subjects were generally attributable to linguistic competencies and to secondary handicaps. When such variables were taken into consideration the papers reviewed showed, on the whole, a resounding lack of difference between hearing and deaf individuals.

Such experiential differences may partly explain reports of stimulus over-selectivity in deaf children who have especially poor communicative competence, where they have not learned to focus on the relevant cues from a given complex stimulus and to ignore the irrelevant ones (Fairbank et al., 1986). Hence the specific cognitive problems experienced by some deaf children are a manifestation of a more general weakness in knowledge of the world.

Some Cognitive Aspects of Sign

Some authors (e.g. Morariu and Bruning, 1984) have commented that deaf individuals have a visual orientation, regardless of any training in sign, that leads them to develop a sign-based system of coding which predisposes them to react to sign as a familiar language. Such a position implies that deaf signers should develop a high competency in sign. Accordingly, it is to be expected that the communication ability of deaf signing children is similar to that of their hearing peers when signed performance is weighted equally with verbal performance (Arnold and Walter, 1979; Christensen, 1988).

Memory coding in deaf signers

Although the code used by many deaf children in short-term memory is spatial or visual (O'Connor and Hermelin, 1973), it may be based on fingerspelling (Hoemann, 1978a) or on signs (Bellugi et al., 1975; Shand, 1982; Bonvillian, 1983; Hamilton, 1985; Bonvillian et al., 1987). Coding by sign implies that concepts are represented by coding through the cheremes or the shape of the hand, hand position and movement, and so on. Thus, when items in a list of words have signed forms which are similar to one another we may expect them to be confused in a memory task (Poizner et al., 1981), because the coding process uses signed forms in a way analogous to the phonological coding used by hearing individuals.

We would expect to find a number of experiments that illustrate the use of a visual code in short-term memory for signs, analogous to the use of phonological coding for words, and such is the case. Bellugi et al. (1975), for instance, instructed their deaf subjects to write their responses in a serial-recall-for-signs task. Serial position effects, such as primacy and recency phenomena, were demonstrated in a similar form to those found in recall of lists of words by hearing subjects. Substitution errors occurred for items with confusable signs. The writing of English glosses for the signs may be thought to have put the deaf subjects at a disadvantage, although Klima and Bellugi (1979) argued convincingly that such was not the case.

Such issues were avoided by Kyle (1981), who both presented stimuli and permitted responses in sign or in words. Kyle described serial-recall tasks for deaf and hearing bilinguals, equally fluent in sign and spoken English. The bilingual subjects produced results similar to those obtained with English speakers, showing effects for phonological coding, such as homophone versus non-homophone differences, and verbal rehearsal superior to silent rehearsal. The deaf subjects, who preferred to recall in words, showed no overt rehearsal effect for words. Using silent serial recall of similar-sounding words, or signs with the same handshape, as a baseline for comparing the effects of overt rehearsal, Kyle found that both bilingual and deaf subjects showed similar recall effects when responding in sign, but when recalling in words, the bilingual group showed a marked advantage, due to facilitation by overt rehearsal of words. Hence effects due to 'signing aloud', the equivalent of verbal rehearsal by hearing people, seems relatively weak for deaf signers – at first thought a rather surprising result. However, this result is not so surprising when we remember that sign coding in serial recall is not found reliably in deaf people (Hanson, 1982), possibly because sign language is less order-bound than verbal language, and that hearing-impaired children can be averse to rehearsing in sign unless instructed to do so (Manion and Butcher, 1986).

If discrete coding in a given modality is employed in short-term memory, it should be possible to demonstrate it by switching the material within a memory task from one mode to another, and seeking a change in behaviour. Hoemann (1978b) used this technique in modality-switching studies with English and manual alphabets, or English words and ASL signs. Deaf students experienced in ASL and written English, and hearing adults with ASL experience, were presented with this material in short-term memory tasks. These tasks contained a number of stimulus trials, where proactive interference would build up quickly on repeated trials. On the last trial, the stimuli were switched from one modality to the other. If the modalities operated with different memory stores, then bilingual subjects who were switched to the second mode for the final trial should show increased recall scores because of release from proactive interference. Hoemann described three experiments showing just such an effect. A further study was reported by Hoemann and Koenig (1990) on hearing students beginning instruction in ASL, with 3–5 weeks' experience. The students were given a task in which proactive interference would increase rapidly with repeated trials. On their last trial, the stimuli were switched from manual alphabet to English alphabet, or vice versa. The students in the manual-to-English alphabet switch showed release from proactive interference, but those in the English-to-manual alphabet did not. Hoemann and Koenig were at a loss to explain this asymmetrical result. However, they concluded that the characters of the manual and English alphabets were coded separately in different memory stores, even with hearing people who were just beginning to learn ASL as a second language.

We saw that studies of visual short-term memory in deaf signers produced outcomes analogous to those of verbal short-term memory in hearing subjects. The results showed that the cognitive processes were similar when modality differences were taken into account. But the reader is cautioned that it is not easy to demonstrate this situation convincingly, as a study by Spencer et al. (1989) has shown.

Spencer et al. studied short-term memory in severely to profoundly prelingually deaf adolescents with lists of written words presented visually for 10s. Their 17 deaf and 10 hearing students were asked to recall the words after a 10s distraction task of adding pairs of digits. The different word lists were devised as signable with a single sign, with compound or a combination of signs, or with fingerspelling for unsignable words. Hearing students recalled significantly more words than the deaf in each of these categories. Both deaf and hearing students recalled significantly more single signable words than those in the compound/combination or unsignable (fingerspelling) categories. Differences between the latter two categories were not significant. The results showing that the hearing subjects recalled more written words than the deaf subjects were congruent with the results of previous studies, which showed that deaf individuals can recall words at the same performance level as hearing individuals when the words are signed for them rather than written (Poizner et al., 1981; Bonvillian, 1983).

Spencer et al. had hypothesised that the errors made by their hearing subjects would show use of a phonological code, and the errors of the deaf subjects would reflect a sign code, but such effects were not observed, perhaps because the error rates were low and the subjects were unwilling to guess when unsure of the correct item, though instructed to do so. This study is of particular interest in that the expected outcome was not attained, and for the methodological issues the authors raised. As they noted, many studies in this area have not used a hearing control group. Also, it is necessary to ensure that the subjects understand the task by writing, speaking or signing the instructions to them as needed, that the material is equally familiar to experimental and control groups, and that care is taken with imagery value and word-frequency effects, because the more frequently used words tend to have a single sign.

Thinking, reasoning and semantics in sign

Thinking and reasoning concern manipulations of the meanings of terms, and involve the area of semantics, where thinking, reasoning and language come together in a complex way. Furth (1966a) was one of the first to observe that the impoverished experience of deaf children was likely to show deficiencies in these areas. However, Green and Shepherd (1975, see above) found that deaf children had many similar semantic concepts to those found in hearing children, though they had an extra factor involving touch and vision, and appeared weak in structures for abstract meaning.

Developmental trends

Developmental trends in the use of sign to communicate reasoning and use of meaning in young hearing-impaired children are of special interest, since they are important for the child's education and achievement as well as everyday communication. The literature is slim in this area, but one useful report is that by Ellenberger and Steyaert (1978), who studied representation of action in a single deaf child between the ages of 3;7 and 5;11 years. In this child's learning of ASL as a first language, they found a developmental trend in the sequence: decrease in the use of gesture, pantomime or citation forms as action signs increased; gradual increase in using abstract signs while iconic re-enactments of events decreased; change from the function of actor to that of narrator in storytelling; developing ability to structure the space in which action signs moved; and increasing ability in using signs about agents in the activities described. Overall the child showed a developmental progression. Early on, the child used citation forms which were not usually modified spatially. Later, adult-like spatial structures of signs were used, illustrating a relatively advanced mastery of cognitive skills associated with semantic aspects of spatial relations.

Complex semantic representation

The notably iconic appearance of sign suggests to the unsophisticated observer that sign language has difficulty in conveying complex meanings. In fact, sign uses inflections and combinations of signs to do a remarkably good job. Bellugi (1980) explained how signs may be used to express complex semantic notions for various concepts. She also argued that there were mechanisms in ASL, used on a daily basis in conversation, which could expand the lexicon to allow for new concepts and ideas, including signed neologisms to depict advances in modern technology, such as 'genetic engineering' and 'microwave oven'. Thus the single sign glossed as LOOK could be varied to convey 'reminisce', 'sight-seeing', 'watch', 'look forward to', 'prophesy', 'look around aimlessly', 'stare', 'gaze at', and so on. The modifications or inflections to produce these various meanings involved spatio-temporal features overlaid on the basic sign. ASL processes of an inflexional kind included: Referential Indexing in the use of verbs to indicate the main actors in a sentence; Reciprocity shown by mutual action or mutual relation; Grammatical Number with verbal inflections for different plurals – dual, triple, or multiple; Distributional Aspect with verbal inflections signifying indivisible or separate action, actions occurring at certain points of time, order of occurrence of action, and relation of actions to the participants; Exhaustive Inflection shown by actions distributed to individuals in a group; Allocative Determinate Inflection in the actions distributed to individuals at specific points in time; and Allocative Indeterminate Inflection with actions distributed to unspecified individuals over time. ASL verb forms could also be inflected to convey Temporal Aspect or Temporal Focus, conveying a specific point in time or enduring activity, and Manner and Degree as in changing basic verbs to nouns or adjectives, or adjectives to nouns or verbs, etc. Further complex notions could be conveyed by the compounding of signs (GOOD + ENOUGH = JUST GOOD ENOUGH, with a different meaning from GOOD ENOUGH). Other inflections giving semantic differences have been illustrated by Klima and Bellugi (1979).

Factors associated with thinking and reasoning

Studies of thinking and reasoning among deaf users of sign language have not been numerous if we omit consideration of tests of intelligence used to determine IQ. Montgomery (1968) and Bolton (1971) used a range of tests to investigate the factors underlying communication and reasoning in deaf subjects as deaf school-leavers and rehabilitation clients, respectively. Bolton showed that both studies identified four main factors: non-verbal reasoning, oral communication, manual communication, and psychomotor ability. Arnold and Walter (1979) conducted a similar investigation on 25 congenitally profoundly deaf students with a mean age of 19 years, but included hearing controls who could sign, hypothesising that verbal reasoning would distinguish deaf and hearing signers the most. They thought, secondly, that the performance of deaf adults on non-verbal reasoning and perceptual speed tests would be similar to that of hearing people. The first hypothesis was confirmed. The deaf group had the greatest difficulty on a test of verbal reasoning. No significant difference was found for performance on tests of oral reception and manual reception, which was consistent with the second hypothesis.

Storytelling

There has been a tendency to consider sign language from a 'bottom-up' viewpoint, involving the identification of sign units followed by a consideration of how they are used (Kyle, 1983a). On the other hand, and from the psychological viewpoint, grammar, for instance, is organised through higher control processes. Syntax and propositional structures are thus controlled by higher-level semantic processing. Some kind of centrally mediated linguistic plan decides how we express our thoughts and, indeed, how we understand the language we use. Typically, storytelling has been used to illustrate the processes involved. Using the storytelling technique, Kyle (1983a) concluded that deaf and hearing individuals show differences in their accounts of a story, with deaf storytellers signing a richness in their depiction of events in a way not found in English, and with deaf storytellers tending to recall events rather than to make inferences as English speakers tend to do. Such differences do not occur necessarily because of different perceptions of the world. English speakers tend to report the events of a story in relation to the overall schema in their mind's eye, whereas deaf signers produce a version which is more directly related to the events in the story. Sign language, and presumably the thinking associated with its use, tends to be more literal in its account of events, is more imaginal in its presentation, and deviates less from the sequence of events than standard English. Sign language consequently makes use of 'mime', in re-enacting events, rather than in making great use of referential communication. In Kyle's view, sign is imaginal and uses an event structure, whereas English speech is referential and tends to modify the propositional arrangements, namely, the small units that convey items of meaning. The tendency of deaf signers to use referential devices less often than hearing individuals to communicate their meaning may explain their lower performance level in referential communication tasks (Hoemann, 1972).

The extent of use of literal presentation in sign language, however, is not clear. Everhart and Marschark (1988) compared the linguistic flexibility of prelingually, mostly severely to profoundly, deaf and hearing children from 8 to 15 years of age, in stories written and signed by the deaf, and written and spoken by the hearing children. They found for the latter group, that both written and spoken stories contained similar numbers of non-literal constructions, including figurative language, gesture and pantomime, whereas the deaf children produced significantly more non-literal constructions in their signed than in their written stories. Further, the deaf children used more non-literal constructions in their signed stories than did the hearing children in their spoken stories. The confusion may have arisen because Everhart and Marschark did not distinguish between literal ways of signing events and imaginal sign styles, such as the use of mime, for such literal presentations.

As an example of what may be observed, recall of a short silent comedy film by deaf, hearing and bilingual subjects was investigated by Kyle (1983b). Having watched the film, subjects were asked to recall the story for a deaf or hearing person who had not seen the film. After a 1-hour interval, they were asked to retell the story again. The story contained 15 main visual events which were related in time and cause. Both the deaf and hearing subjects recalled the main events equally well, but the hearing subjects kept less to the temporal sequence of the events after the time interval than the deaf subjects. The bilingual viewers' performance was in between those of the deaf and hearing subjects. Kyle (1983b) argued that the system of tenses and conditional structures in English makes it easy to refer to events out of sequence. Perhaps it was easier to present the events out of sequence to simplify the story. If so, the deaf subjects used this device less often, even though BSL, as an inflected sign language, permits a flexible approach to the construction and use of propositions, which in English most commonly occur as clauses (Kyle and Woll, 1985).

Cognitive development and signing/non-signing parentage

Although it has turned out to be a controversial topic, it has often been supposed (Brasel and Quigley, 1977; Sisco and Anderson, 1980; Zwiebel, 1987) that deaf children of deaf parents attain higher levels of linguistic, academic, communication and cognitive development than deaf children of hearing parents, because of early and continuing exposure to language through manual communication. In particular, native deaf signers are thought to present English more effectively than deaf individuals born to hearing parents, and to be more adept at code switching (Hoffmeister and Moores, 1987). One reason for such beliefs is the greater acceptance of the child's deafness by deaf parents. Noting that deaf children of deaf parents scored higher on the WISC-R (adapted for deaf children) than deaf children of hearing parents, and higher than hearing children of deaf parents, Sisco and Anderson (1980) concluded that deaf parents may be particularly suited to provide the kind of care appropriate for intellectual growth in deaf children. However, Conrad and Weiskrantz (1981), who found no superiority in the cognitive performance of deaf children of deaf parents in a study carefully devised to allow for environmental differences between deaf and hearing children, concluded that earlier investigations were lacking in their methodology. This outcome led Kyle and Woll (1985) to regard as a myth the idea that deaf children who learn sign at an early age have a cognitive advantage, even over hearing children.

However, more recent work has re-opened the issue. Zwiebel (1987) tested the hypothesis of Kusche et al. (1983) that children who were deaf for genetic reasons would show superior performance on cognitive tests, irrespective of whether their parents were deaf or hearing. He investigated 122 deaf boys and 121 deaf girls aged 6–14 years, attending regular and special educational programmes in Israel. Most (80.5%) were deaf from birth and 94.6% were deaf by 2 years of age. The great majority (85%) had a hearing loss of 70 dB or more. The children were divided into three groups: a group with deaf parents and deaf siblings ($n = 23$); a group with hearing parents and deaf siblings ($n = 76$); and a group with hearing parents and hearing siblings ($n = 144$). The groups were similar on a range of demographic and hearing-loss variables, except that the children with hearing parents and deaf siblings contained more girls and had a lower mean socioeconomic status, more children of Asian and African background, more cases of acquired hearing loss, and a greater use of hearing aids. Zwiebel found a continuum in Israeli Sign Language, the manual communication system used at home, ranging from good with deaf parents and deaf siblings to partial with hearing parents and deaf siblings, to a lack of mastery with hearing parents and hearing siblings. Findings from tests of cognition showed that the children exposed to signing gained cognitively from the exposure. Children with deaf parents and deaf siblings achieved a higher cognitive performance level than the deaf children not exposed to signing, and indeed achieved a level equivalent to that of hearing children. Comparison of the other two groups suggested that even moderate exposure to sign was of benefit in building intellectual performance.

The children with deaf parents and deaf siblings were considered to have hearing losses due to genetic factors, and used sign language. The children with hearing parents and deaf siblings had hearing losses with a genetic component and a mixed communication environment, with an emphasis towards oral communication. The children with hearing parents and hearing siblings had no overt genetic element and an oral home environment. The results of tests showed that the children using sign language scored at a higher intellectual level than those children not using sign language, and that the genetic background made no difference. Hence the hypothesis of Kusche et al. (1983) was not supported. However, the conclusions are not completely convincing, as the necessary comparison group of deaf children who used sign language, but had no genetic basis for their hearing loss – that is, signing deaf children born to hearing parents – was not available. It may also be argued that the lower scores in tests of intellectual ability of the children with hearing parents and deaf siblings could have been due to their lower socioeconomic status, rather than the genetic component, as Zwiebel appreciated, although he thought that the pattern of test performance argued against this view.

This study shows that the intellectual development of deaf children with deaf parents and siblings, and consequently using sign language, is equal to that of hearing children under certain conditions, contrary to Conrad and Weiskrantz (1981). Zwiebel concluded that the effect of early exposure to sign language on the cognitive development of deaf children is a positive one. Weisel (1988) has also shown, in a well designed investigation, that deaf children of deaf parents attained a higher level of reading comprehension, emotional adjustment and motivation for communication than deaf children of hearing parents.

Age at exposure to sign

The age at which a deaf child is exposed to sign language affects subsequent semantic processing. Mayberry and Fischer (1989) found that native and non-native sign language acquisition showed different effects on sign language processing. Their subjects were all congenitally deaf and used sign language for communication, but acquired it at different ages ranging from birth to 18 years of age. In a first study, deaf signers simultaneously watched and reproduced sign language stories presented in ASL and Pidgin Sign English, in good and poor seeing conditions. In a second study, deaf signers recalled and shadowed grammatical and ungrammatical ASL sentences. The native signers were more accurate in their tasks, understood better, and when they made lexical changes, they changed signs related to sign meaning independent of the phonological aspects of the stimulus item. Conversely, the non-native signers tended to make changes of sign related to the phonological characteristics of the stimulus independent of the lexical and sentential meaning. Semantic lexical changes were positively correlated, and phonological lexical changes were negatively correlated, with processing accuracy and understanding. This result occurred across sign dialect, seeing conditions and processing tasks. Thus the native signers processed lexical material automatically, allowing them to attend to lexical meaning and sentential meaning. The non-native signers tended to pay more attention to the identification of phonological aspects, so that they were less well able to attend to lexical meaning.

Concluding comments

We indicated earlier that recent research into semantic processes and the thinking and reasoning of deaf signers has been relatively sparse. What has become clear, however, is that our knowledge and understanding of this area may be limited, unless we concede that sign language may be quite unlike standard English, as suggested from a 'top-down' rather than a 'bottom-up' approach. Also, as with study of any natural language, we need to seek an explanation of sign language processing which can take account of discourse and reasoning. Such an explanation will need to offer a description of the relations, within and between 'sentences', which are used by the signer, and the processes by which they are derived. So, research in this area needs to study the kinds of representation which are used for discourse and reasoning. Such work would involve a study of how assumptions relate to the network of propositions in reasoning, and how attention, interpretation and inferencing are brought to bear. This field is being actively researched in verbal language (Myers et al., 1986) and hence leads are available to guide similar work in sign.

General Conclusion on Hearing Impairment and Cognition

Research into cognition and hearing impairment is both challenging and exciting. At the same time it must be agreed that some of the findings are confusing. There is little by way of consistent theoretical direction, apart perhaps from elaborations on the work of Piaget. The research methodologies also are disparate, making it difficult to compare results. There is thus a compelling need to produce clear theoretical directions to explain the salient issues concerned with cognitive processes and strategies in deaf individuals (Wolk and Schildroth, 1984) and for clear and comprehensive descriptions of subjects and research methods, to allow for closer comparison of results.

Metaprocesses

We have chosen to consider metaprocesses in this chapter on cognition as they require the application of higher-level cognitive processes, such as thinking, reflection, comparison and comprehension.

The metaprocesses (metacognition, metalinguistics, etc.) derive from work in cognitive psychology in the 1970s (Cazden, 1976; Flavell and Wellman, 1977; Brown, 1978). The field now has the status of a recognised field of inquiry in its own right, although reference to metaprocesses, in other terms, can be found in the literature going way back into the past. 'Meta' is used in the general sense of 'beyond' or 'transcending'. Thus 'metalinguistics' implies the relation between linguistics and other features of behaviour. More specifically metaprocesses, reflecting their place in cognitive psychology, have come to be associated with awareness and control in the sense of self-regulation. In reading a text in order to learn from it, for example, the effective reader needs to be aware of the logical structure of the text (Brown and Smiley, 1978), and of such possible shortcomings as ambiguities and irregular use of grammar or semantics (Harris et al., 1981).

Tunmer and Bowey (1984) have described four stages of metalinguistic awareness, thought to be particularly important in learning to read: awareness of words, phonology, pragmatics, and form. Awareness at the word level associates the spoken with the written word. Phonological awareness not only involves knowledge of phonological elements, but the ability to segment a word into its phonological parts, and the synthesis of the parts into a word. Pragmatic awareness relates to knowledge of the relationships within linguistics, between linguistics and context, and attention to a listener's knowledge. Form awareness involves the ability to reflect on the internal grammar of sentences.

The development of metaprocesses is related to proficiency in learning (Armbruster et al., 1982). Generally, younger hearing children, with less developed psychological processes, are less able to understand how the several variables involved in learning affect learning outcomes, and are less able to monitor and regulate their own abilities. Younger and poorer-hearing readers, for instance, tend to lack the two important aspects of metacognition: knowledge and control. Metaprocess training can help to overcome such problems, by bringing the learning substrate, strategies for processing it, and a knowledge of themselves as learners, to children's awareness.

Hearing children aged 7–11 years show considerable understanding of listening, although age plays a part within this range (McDevitt et al., 1990). McDevitt found that older children depended less on behavioural factors and more on comprehension in their definitions of good listening. Children felt that appropriate listening tactics depended on the situation. When confused by mothers' speech they thought it best to seek clarification directly by asking questions, but when confused by teachers, they thought that they should listen more carefully. Young hearing children tended to blame the listener if that listener could not identify an object described by a speaker, even when the description was inadequate or ambiguous (Robinson, 1981). They only ascribed some responsibility to the speaker when the nature of the problem was made explicit.

Metaprocesses and the hearing-impaired child

Hearing-impaired children frequently have problems in suiting the style of their messages to the needs of the listener, even in adolescence, resulting in breakdown of communication (Maxwell, 1980; Murphy and Hill, 1989). Such problems of adapting their behaviour to the needs of other individuals suggest that they are egocentric and non-reflective, failing to think about the consequences of their behaviour on others (Howarth and Wood, 1977). Research is needed in the metaprocesses of hearing-impaired children, so that the knowledge so acquired can be used to train them to gain insights into how they relate to others and how they themselves can help to shape their communication. We remarked earlier that research in the pragmatics of communication by hearing-impaired children leaves much to be desired. We also saw that research in the deployment of social skills by hearing-impaired children is sparse. There is also little research on hearing-impaired children's metaprocesses.

Quigley et al. (1976b) were among the first to conduct research in the area for judgements of grammaticality. Kretschmer (1982) referred to a role for metaprocesses in a discussion of decoding in reading readiness by hearing-impaired children, commenting that many teachers find that such children have problems in mapping speech elements onto their orthography. Kretschmer saw a place for metaprocesses in reading by hearing-impaired children, ranging from what the children think reading is to the use of various study skills. He drew a parallel between developed metaprocesses and an internal locus of control, noting that hearing-impaired children, whose metaprocesses seem relatively undeveloped, show behaviour characteristic of an external locus of control, associated with a reduced self-image, lack of motivation, lack of confidence, and a feeling of being controlled by the environment.

An example of the use of a metalinguistic approach is to be found in Zorfass (1981), who studied the ability of 11 prelingually severely to profoundly deaf children, aged 4–7 years, who used Signed English, to segment Signed English sentences into words. Words which did not have signs were fingerspelt. Zorfass sought to assess the children's metalinguistic abilities in segmenting sentences into words. She grouped her subjects into four classes based on four factors: class 1, sentences or groups of words not segmented; class 2, major parts of sentences segmented; class 3, major parts of sentences and some function words segmented; and class 4, whole sentences segmented. The concept of segmentation was taught with the help of toys when, for example, the tester moved a toy along a roadway in short stages, with pauses in between, and speaking segments of a sentence while the toy was moved. This task focused the children's attention on the segmentation of the sentences. In the experimental part of the study, the children increasingly omitted words as sentence length increased from two to five words. Class 1 subjects omitted two to three words in five-word sentences, while class 4 subjects omitted either no words or one word. Subjects in classes 1, 2 and 3 omitted function words and forms of the verb 'to be', but preserved content words. Zorfass suggested that such performance was associated with telegraphic information given to them by hearing teachers, who tended to delete words other than content words when presenting the signed part of Signed English (compare Marmor and Petitto, 1979). Her hearing-impaired children also omitted inflectional morphemes (-ed, plural s, and -ing), with the proportion of omissions increasing from class 4 to class 1. Zorfass ascribed such omissions to the failure of the children to use inflectional morphemes in their speech.

This study by Zorfass was a preliminary one, and did not include controls for various factors. However, her subjects showed varying metalinguistic abilities which generally increased with age and a developmental pattern similar to that found with hearing children (Ehri, 1975).

The general literature on hearing-impaired children contains allusions to the young hearing-impaired child who can listen, but who cannot integrate that listening into everyday life. The problem seems to be that the child associates listening with listening time in class, and fails to generalise classroom listening skills to listening outside the classroom. Fisher and Schneider (1986) attributed this problem to the kind of instruction, especially segmented curricula, and argued for group teaching, to indicate to the child the place of listening in a range of social contexts. However, it is also possible that the problem is a problem of metacognition. In this case, listening is not just a process in cognition, but needs for its full use in communication an appreciation and control of its functions by the child. Fisher and Schneider's hearing-impaired children were preschoolers, too young for the full development of metaprocesses. Nevertheless, Fisher and Schneider's reference to communication clarification, formulating hypotheses, explaining cause and effect, attention and awareness, suggests strongly that weaknesses of metaprocesses are part of the explanation for the effect which they described.

Wood (1991) has taken this kind of argument much further to criticise the high control by adults of both deaf and hearing children. According to Wood, such control can result in low initiative, short utterances, and a lack of speculation, hypothesis formation and imagination, leading to a meagre linguistic diet and little space in which to develop flexibility, creativity and self-expression. He suggested that difficulties in communication were a cause of this high control, which has been observed in some teachers of deaf children. Although he did not specifically address metaprocesses, it seems clear that the effects of high control will be to reduce opportunities for reflection and speculation, and thus will retard the development of metaprocesses in deaf children.

The metalinguistics of fingerspelling was investigated by Hirsh-Pasek (1987) in a study of phonological awareness related to reading ability. Phonological awareness is prerequisite to reading because it facilitates the decoding and recoding of text, and assists the identification of words and storage in short-term memory. Hirsh-Pasek assessed the metalinguistic ability of 26 congenitally deaf children of elementary and secondary school age to segment and manipulate their fingerspelt lexica. She found that metalinguistic competence in fingerspelling, shown by the children's direction of their attention to fingerspelt words, was correlated with achievement in beginning reading, even for the children of elementary school age. Metalinguistic competence in fingerspelling was not correlated with indices of intelligence, such as skill at mathematics. Training in fingerspelling helped with word identification for the words in the children's fingerspelt lexica. Since word identification is a good predictor of reading ability, this result suggests that decoding text into fingerspelling may assist beginning readers to progress to more advanced reading comprehension. Hirsh-Pasek concluded that decoding by fingerspelling allowed children who have problems with speech analysis to develop a phonological system which maps language onto print. Grapheme-to-handshape correspondences could thus help beginning deaf readers who have problems in recognising phonemes.

The use of metalinguistics in three sign systems, Signed English, Pidgin Sign English and American Sign Language, as the primary form of communication in 20 severely to profoundly prelingually deaf children aged 5–8 years was studied by Borman et al. (1988). These children, who were educated by TC, were presented with a synonymy judgement task for which they saw pairs of videorecorded sentences. They were to decide if the sentences had the same or different meanings. This task was metalinguistic because the children had to compare two sentences and judge whether their meaning was the same, thus involving attention to content and evaluation of synonymy. No differences were found between sign systems, but overall the girls' results were better than those of the boys. The children performed only slightly above chance level on the judgement of synonymy task in all three sign systems, showing that they lacked the metalinguistic awareness for judging synonymy of pairs of sentences. However, more sentence pairs with different meanings were processed correctly than synonymous sentence pairs, suggesting that gross differences could be detected before similarities could be recognised, as found with hearing children (Hakes, 1980). As the authors recognised, this study requires replication with control or comparison groups, such as older hearing-impaired children. Hearing children as direct controls would be problematical because of the different systems of communication used.

Since not much is known about how deaf learners apply cognitive strategies, the area of metacognition in the deaf may repay investigation, especially with reference to instruction and remedial education. It is thus pleasing to note that Krinsky (1990) has described an investigation into the 'feeling of knowing', an aspect of metamemory, in 40, mainly residential, moderately to profoundly deaf adolescents, aged 14–20 years, who used American Sign Language as their preferred form of communication. These subjects were asked to define words from the Peabody Picture Vocabulary Test (PPVT – Dunn and Dunn, 1981), beginning at the place appropriate for their reading level. They were then asked to rank words which they had missed for the difficulty which they would expect to experience in choosing a picture of the missing word. Thus, they were asked to make judgements of their feeling of knowing for the words which they had missed. They were then assessed with the PPVT as a test of accuracy for their ranked judgements. The results showed that the deaf adolescents were not able to judge accurately their feeling of knowing for the words missed, but control groups of hearing adolescents of the same age, and hearing children of the same reading level were able to perform this task. Krinsky explained this outcome on the basis of unfamiliarity. Familiarity, or the degree of prior learning, had been shown to affect the feeling of knowing (Nelson et al., 1982). The normative difficulty of the PPVT vocabulary items was uncertain for the deaf adolescents, although it was known for the hearing controls. These hearing controls had most probably heard all the words at some time, and were in this sense more familiar with the words than the deaf adolescents. The deaf adolescents were also less likely to guess at a solution and, when they did guess, they based their guesses on the visual appearance of words. Krinsky's findings will be interesting to therapists and teachers, since the monitoring of memory is becoming of increasing importance in research on cognition (Armbruster et al., 1982; Flavell, 1985).

Andrews and Mason (1991), mentioned earlier, pointed out that metacognitive strategies are used in fluent reading. They compared the performance of prelingually profoundly deaf high-school boys, hearing reading-disabled high-school boys and hearing boys of elementary school age in filling deleted words and phrases in expository texts. After making replacements to fill the gaps, the boys explained their decisions in sign or verbally, as appropriate. The deaf boys relied on rereading and background knowledge, whereas the hearing readers relied more on context cues in the text. Andrews and Mason recommended the teaching of metacognitive comprehension strategies to deaf students as tools to comprehend English texts, but noted that such strategies would not by themselves guarantee successful reading comprehension. For example, metaprocesses cannot take the place of seriously deficient linguistic or general knowledge. The use of learner-generated semantic mapping, in which a spatial representation or diagram is constructed of the main ideas in the text, with emphasis on active processing, looks to be a fruitful approach in developing metaprocesses in reading by deaf children, as it makes the strategy explicit (Banks et al., 1991b).

Conclusion

We have referred to reports of metalinguistic and metacognitive studies with hearing-impaired children of various ages, which have explored awareness of syntax, phonology, synonymy and pragmatics, in reading and in signed communication, a facet of memory, and strategies in reading comprehension. In view of the considerable interest in metaprocesses in other applied fields, such as language delay and learning disorders, let alone the developments on metaprocesses in normally developing hearing children, it is surprising that so little work has been done on children with hearing impairment. As there is little doubt that children's awareness of and insights into their learning are part of that learning, there is clearly a deficiency here in research with hearing-impaired children which needs to be addressed.

Central Auditory Dysfunction

Central auditory dysfunction refers to difficulties in hearing associated with the retrocochlear neurological pathways and processes, which convey sounds up to, and include, the higher cortical areas of the brain. The terms 'psychogenic' or 'functional hearing loss' are used to describe the same condition, as is the quaint 'non-organic hearing loss' beloved of otologists (Dixon and Newby, 1959). Such usages do not usually impute definite absence of physical pathology, except in cases of malingering, which are rare in children (Dixon and Newby, 1959). Rather, they describe a dysfunction for which the neurology is currently unknown or obscure (Oberklaid et al., 1989). It is usual to refer to such conditions as problems, disorders or dysfunctions, since some people with the condition show no signs of hearing loss when tested by conventional audiometry in the quiet. The disorder commonly appears when stress is placed on the auditory system (Tallal, 1980). One common technique to produce such stress is to reduce the redundancy present in speech, using such techniques as filtering or presenting the speech or other stimuli under difficult listening conditions, as in rapid switching between the ears, or in noise. Individuals with disordered auditory processing skills then have problems in reproducing the speech. Other techniques involve special psychoacoustic tests (Pinheiro and Musiek, 1985a; Tobin, 1985).

Site of lesion

There has been a continuing industry to devise audiometric tests to identify the site of a neurological lesion from sites immediately posterior to the cochlear up to and including the auditory cortex. In view of the possibility of eighth nerve tumours and similar phenomena, the importance of such tests scarcely needs comment. Because, however, the emphasis of this book is on perceptual rather than physiological or anatomical features, we make only brief mention of site of lesion here. The reader is referred to the several comprehensive chapters in Katz (1985) and Pinheiro and Musiek (1985b) for a considered treatment.

Functional aspects

A convenient synopsis of factors reportedly associated with central auditory dysfunction, or disordered auditory processing skills, was outlined by Davis and Rampp (1983). These factors, which are interrelated, include attention, auditory discrimination, analysis and synthesis, and memory and sequencing. It is apparent that problems with any of these factors will interfere with normal communication.

As regards attention, children with problems of auditory processing typically find it hard to focus their attention selectively over time on a particular task. They find it difficult to direct their attention to the salient sounds in their environment, with the result that all the sounds in the environment are treated as 'foreground' sounds. Such children are able to understand speech, especially non-complex speech, when it is presented at comfortable listening levels in the quiet, but fail to understand speech in noise, especially in speech noise. This situation may be described as one in which the children hear, but do not listen.

Most children suspected of an auditory processing disorder also have problems with auditory discrimination, sometimes assessed with the Wepman Auditory Discrimination Test (Wepman, 1975) or the Goldman–Fristoe–Woodcock Test of Auditory Discrimination (Goldman et al., 1970). Auditory discrimination is the ability to distinguish between one sound and another ('goat' vs 'coat') and hence its assessment requires tests which use such phonemic contrasts. The phonemically balanced word lists presented in the quiet, commonly used by audiologists, and often referred to as speech discrimination tests, do not use such contrasts, and hence present no special difficulty to children with auditory processing problems. A test for auditory discrimination requires the discrimination of a test stimulus from another signal. Problems with auditory discrimination can present as 'auditory distractibility', as when a child has problems in following a teacher's speech in a noisy classroom. Wepman (1960) regarded poor auditory discrimination as correlated with problems of articulation and reading disabilities. It interferes with reading and language acquisition.

Auditory analysis and synthesis are the ability to separate wholes into parts, and combine parts into wholes, as in separating sentences into words and syllables, and combining syllables and words into sentences. Tests in this area are few, but Kirk et al. (1968) have offered a sound blending test which assesses the ability to combine phonemes into words, for which the phonemes must be held in serial order and then run together to produce a common word (d-o-g = dog).

Memory and sequencing are often involved in auditory discrimination, which enables us to distinguish between sounds following one another in time, as well as distinguishing a sound from a noise background when the two occur simultaneously. Davis and Rampp (1983) have drawn attention to auditory chunking, in which the sounds to be retained are processed as combinations of phonemes (syllables), combinations of syllables (words), and combinations of words (phrases). Auditory memory is conventionally tested as memory for digits or for words and syllables, including nonsense syllables (Kirk et al., 1968). Auditory memory is typically described in age level terms. Children with auditory processing disorders frequently present with auditory memory skills 1–2 years below their chronological age.

Auditory sequencing is the ability to process auditory stimuli in serial order, a skill of relevance to English language processing, where word order is crucial to meaning. An auditory–vocal sequencing test has been described by Kirk et al. (1968), which bears some relationship to reading difficulties.

Davis and Rampp (1983) described the status of tests for auditory processing disorders as woefully inadequate. The available tests were dated and in several cases were of doubtful validity and reliability. They were often gross measures, and confounded one specific disorder with another, because they tended to assess several factors at the same time. For example, because auditory stimuli are sequential in nature, all auditory tests which involve more than one component in time necessarily involve auditory memory.

A degree of structure which escapes confounding can be introduced by separating auditory processing disorders into two classes: those which are associated with language disorders, and those which are not. Some language disorders are caused by an auditory, rather than by a linguistic or higher-order cognitive problem. In such disorders, children typically have auditory problems in discriminating between consonants presented in minimally different word pairs ('goat' vs. 'coat' mentioned above) for reasons other than sensory end-organ disorder. Tallal (1976) described a test for rapid auditory processing in which items of auditory information are presented in quick succession, which may identify auditory processing problems of the above type and problems that appear independent of any language difficulty. In the latter type of auditory processing problem, language functions assessed by conventional tests may be within normal limits, but the child may have problems of attention, memory, etc., which retard the development of skills in reading and writing.

With young children, it may be difficult to measure central auditory processing problems because of the plasticity of the central nervous system, which was considered in Chapter 2. If the functions under investigation have not become set, because of immaturity in cortical specialisation, then they will be difficult to assess. Also, it is increasingly necessary to use linguistic, or language-like, stimuli when the nervous structures associated with the central auditory processing problems are located higher along the auditory pathway. However, because language contains considerable redundancy, language stimuli presented in the quiet tend to make auditory processing too easy for test purposes. Hence we frequently find the use of time-compressed speech, filtered speech, speech in noise, dichotic listening, in which different material is presented to each ear, etc., as test stimuli. The trick is to reduce the redundancy in speech to a minimum without reducing it so far as to prevent people with normal central auditory processing functions from perceiving the content clearly. There may be objections to the use of acoustic manipulations to speech on the grounds of naturalness. A partial way round this criticism is to use statistical approximations to English, in which the syntax and semantics are manipulated to produce material which looks like some kinds of poetry ('Battle cry and be better than ever', Jerger et al., 1968).

A typical case

Because of the possible immaturity of the central nervous system in young children, and because the test materials are relatively difficult to perceive, the child typically assessed for central auditory processing problems is about 6–8 years old. He is more often than not male, underachieves academically, and yet has normal to high intelligence. However, we should note that there is generally a positive correlation between intelligence and auditory discrimination ability (Watson, 1991). The child has little or no peripheral hearing problem. He is often left-handed, as may be one or more of his close relatives. His fine and gross motor skills are usually good, and he has no apparent neurological problems.

This outline of a typical case was presented by Page (1985b), who also commented on poorly developed auditory memory as a glaring characteristic. The child may perform well when simple, straightforward directions are presented to him in quiet conditions, but appears confused when given instructions, especially instructions which contain more than one direction, in a noisy environment such as a classroom. Further, he may have problems with reading and writing. His visuospatial skills are good, so that he can draw and paint adequately. His health is good, but there may be a history of chronic middle-ear infections (compare Greville et al., 1985; Aplin and Rowson, 1990).

As far as treatment is concerned, some tests may suggest a specific lesion in the auditory pathway, which should be drawn to the attention of the neurologist or neuro-otologist. Frequently, however, these tests do not suggest a specific lesion, nor do other, neurological tests. In such a situation, the findings can be drawn to the attention of therapists and teachers, who may be able to devise remedial programmes, using carefully structured lessons given on an individual basis in quiet surroundings, to develop the child's reading, writing and related skills (Butler, 1981; Katz and Harmon, 1981; Sloan, 1986). Its seems to the author that speechreading could be helpful in therapy for some central auditory disorders but, rather surprisingly, this approach is not evident in the literature.

Some criticisms

On occasion, it may be possible to associate the functional problem with a neurological lesion, but frequently this is not possible. There remains a clear functional problem, but it is often none too clear what lies behind the problem, nor how best to treat it. 'Central auditory processing disorders', 'central auditory dysfunction', and so on, are concepts which appear 'woolly', and can be used to cloak mixed and disorderly findings of obscure aetiology.

Several authors have commented on this aspect (Sanders, 1977; Lyon, 1977) and notably Rees (1973, 1981). The auditory processing explanations, remarked Rees, are used in two different ways. On the one hand, they are used by professionals remediating children with speech, language or learning problems. These professionals tend to assume that complex communication skills can be broken down into a set of less complex subskills for assessment and remediation, hence the identification of auditory discrimination, auditory memory and auditory sequencing. On the other hand, professionals more concerned with diagnosis use a 'site-of-lesion' approach, and have developed the central auditory processing disorders emphasis. The latter group of professionals tends to focus on test development rather than on remediation.

Rees commented on the wide variety of tasks used to establish auditory processing skills, which presented a plethora of empirical endeavours devoid of any coherent or unified theory. She proceeded (1981) with a critique of efforts to identify the units to be sequenced in tests of 'auditory sequencing', citing studies which showed that phonemes, syllables, words and clauses might at different times each be the units to be sequenced. No one of these units appeared to be more salient than the others for auditory sequencing, and there was no compelling evidence for a specific problem in auditory sequencing as an explanation for failure in language and in learning. The search for units reflected associationism, the approach which seeks to reduce complex behaviour to components in order to explain it, but left us wondering about the psychological reality of the units thus identified. Rees went on to criticise the use of 'auditory synthesis' and 'auditory closure' as auditory abilities, seeing them rather as metalinguistic skills which required the child consciously to perceive words as made up of phonemic units, rather than the usual unconscious linguistic processing of the sounds of connected speech. She further criticised the use of 'auditory discrimination' for speech sounds as an 'auditory' rather than a linguistic skill involving phonological, lexical, syntactic and semantic aspects, and she was severe with the approach which treated memory as a unitary phenomenon, since it consisted of sensory, short-term and long-term aspects.

Rees was kinder in her treatment of the various tests based on reducing the redundancy of natural speech, concluding that they may be assessing functions which were more auditory than linguistic, unlike the tests for auditory discrimination, memory and sequencing. However, the relevance of tests which reduced the redundancy of speech to language acquisition and learning was not clear. The field of central auditory processing skills was, she concluded, in an exploratory state.

Conclusion

Rees performed a valuable service in subjecting the area of central auditory processing disorders to rigorous criticism. There is, however, good evidence that some children who perform poorly in tests which reduce the redundancy in speech do have problems with language, learning and reading. Devens et al. (1978) found auditory localisation problems in learning-disabled children and McGroskey and Kidder (1980) found auditory fusion difficulties among similar children. Elliott and Hammer (1988) observed long-term (3-year duration), weak, fine-grained auditory discrimination results in children with language learning problems, though Tallal (1990) has claimed that fine-grained deficits in children with language learning problems are not specific to the auditory modality nor to speech perception. Tallal et al. (1985) observed that auditory perceptual variables requiring rapid temporal analysis were highly correlated with the extent of receptive language deficit in dysphasic children. Further, in a recent report, Hartvig Jensen et al. (1989) described the administration of a battery of psychological tests, both verbal and non-verbal, to right- and to left-ear hearing-impaired children aged 10–16 years. Children with a unilateral right-ear hearing loss performed significantly worse than the left-ear hearing-impaired children, particularly in verbal tests which were sensitive to minor input or processing damage. Results from WISC Digit-Span and WISC Similarities subtests suggested that the right-ear impaired children suffered from a subtle deficit at a high cerebral level. However, Rodriguez et al. (1990), working with normally hearing and cognitively intact elderly adults, have reported central auditory processing problems without a decline in linguistic competence.

From the communication viewpoint, children with auditory processing difficulties usually communicate well enough when involved in clear, individual to individual, conversations which have a straightforward grammatical and semantic structure. However, they commonly have problems in following conversations which include complex sequencing of syntax and semantics. They often experience problems in following conversations presented against a noisy background. They have problems also with reading comprehension, especially with irregular verbs and embedded clauses and phrases. They thus may have problems with verbal communication of the more complex kind, while simpler verbal communication poses few problems. Given a normal level of intelligence, this situation can give rise to frustration for the child and bewilderment for parents who suspect a problem but cannot define it.

At the time of writing, the field remains unclear. The site-of-lesion approach continues to attract the development of sophisticated auditory tests with some success (Musiek and Pinheiro, 1987; Musiek et al., 1990), central auditory problems occurring together with cochlear loss have been studied (Speaks et al., 1985), and specific auditory perceptual dysfunction in the form of an isolated auditory-phonological processing problem has been reported (Jerger et al., 1987). Keith (1981a) emphasised that work directed to the evaluation and remediation of central auditory dysfunction needs to proceed, while the debate continues on terminology and the relationships between auditory perceptual disorders and language learning problems. His advice still holds.

Chapter 8
Individual and Social Aspects

There has been debate over the years as to whether deaf people have more than their share of psychiatric or psychological problems, and whether there is a 'deaf personality'. This chapter reviews the area, and then proceeds to consider deaf children in social contexts. Finally, an overview is presented of the emerging interest in pragmatics, the use of communication in social interaction.

In one of the earlier reviews of psychological and sociological factors associated with hearing loss, Vernon (1969) observed that for deaf and hard of hearing individuals there was an essentially normal distribution of intellectual potential and cognitive capacity. However, the hearing-impaired population was grossly below national (US) averages in educational achievement and vocational attainment. Vernon presented data on marriage patterns, organisations, mental illness and communication among the hearing-impaired community, noting inter alia that 95% of deaf people married other deaf people, that deaf individuals formed their own strong social organisations, and that most deaf employees worked in manual labour requiring varying skill levels. They did not aspire to higher levels of employment. This situation has been slow to change. For example, Sharp (1984) reported that deaf adolescents had more stereotyped attitudes than their hearing peers to gender roles and 'appropriate' occupations. They aspired to the less prestigious occupations, having limited knowledge of the characteristics of the workforce. Cole and Edelmann (1991) have recorded worries about employment opportunities and capabilities for work in British deaf adolescents, because of perceived problems with communication and employer discrimination.

Psychopathology

The greater the hearing impairment, the greater is the degree of relative social isolation, even within the most caring and sympathetic environment. Such relative isolation affects the communication behaviour of the hearing-impaired child and, in turn, this behaviour affects education and remediation (Myklebust, 1960), and might be thought to predispose to psychopathology.

First, we consider the question of whether hearing impairment is associated with a frequency of psychiatric disturbance higher than that found in the hearing population. Some earlier studies suggested that the deaf community has a relatively high population of schizophrenics, in line with a suggestion (Editorial, *Lancet,* 1981) that perceptual disturbances can cause schizophrenia. Matzker (1960) reported that, in the then Federal Republic of Germany, the incidence of deafness among a large sample of schizophrenics was unusually high. Myklebust (1964) found a tendency towards schizophrenia in a group of profoundly deaf adults as indicated by the Minnesota Multiphasic Personality Inventory. He was, however, careful to point out that feelings of isolation and detachment could have been the cause, and that his findings did not necessarily imply that deaf people suffered from schizophrenia.

Other studies have not supported a link between deafness and schizophrenia. Altschuler and Sarlin (1963) concluded that schizophrenia was no more common in deaf than in hearing people, while Kallman (1963) and Rainer and Altschuler (1971) found that schizophrenia was a little less common in psychotic deaf individuals than in hearing psychotics. Interestingly, prelingually profoundly deaf schizophrenics may experience a kind of auditory hallucination, although it is not clear that their subjective experiences are actually auditory (Critchley et al., 1981). Although they may complain of voices inside their heads (Bowman and Coons, 1990) or getting at them (Kitson and Fry, 1990), they cannot state what the voices are saying, which suggests that the hallucination is not auditory as such, but reflects visual images of people talking. Kitson and Fry (1990) concluded that, although the reliability of the data is questionable, and although the area of psychiatry and prelingual deafness has been neglected, schizophrenic psychoses are not found more frequently in deaf than hearing individuals. However, they reported that deaf schizophrenics required high doses of antipsychotic drugs, often in combination with mood-stabilising medication, to remedy their condition.

There is no reliable evidence to indicate whether or not deaf people suffer more than hearing individuals from depression or obsessional states (Moore, 1981; Evans and Elliott, 1987), even though it is sometimes said that deaf people have somewhat rigid personalities, and this rigidity constrains their communication. The one psychiatric area where there may be an association between psychopathology and deafness is that of paranoia associated with late-acquired hearing loss (Cooper, 1976). It is scarcely surprising that losing a faculty which is so important to communication and everyday living should lead to an increased incidence of paranoia in people deafened adventitiously (compare Harvey, 1989).

Although the area of deafness and psychopathology is under-researched, especially in deaf children, it seems that such children, particularly those who are prelingually deaf, are no more likely to experience serious psychiatric problems than hearing children. There is even a suggestion (Moore, 1981; Kitson and Fry, 1990) that prelingual deafness protects a child against affective disorders. However, deaf children do appear to experience a relatively high occurrence of mild psychiatric or behaviour disorders (Meadow, 1981; Prior et al., 1988) and these aspects have interested the psychoanalyst. Mendelson et al. (1960) found that the characteristics of the dreams of severely to profoundly deaf young adults were reported as vivid, brilliantly coloured and frequent. Where affect was prominent in dreams, primitive signs were reported. These characteristics were most marked in the prelingually deaf, less marked in those subjects with deafness acquired before 5 years of age, and least prominent in subjects deafened after 5 years of age. More recently, Hurst (1988) argued that communication has a peculiar dynamic in deaf people's dreams, where it is symbolically significant if interaction in a dream is spoken, signed, or represents 'pure communication', in which neither speaking nor signing are used. Thus if a deaf, signing child dreams of signing to a non-signing parent, this can indicate a wish for increased conversational exchanges. On the other hand, if the dreamed conversation occurs in speech, a desire to conform to the expectations of the hearing world is suggested.

Some unusual dream characteristics of deaf adolescents and adults have been recorded by Rainer (1976), who posed questions about their relationship to ego development and object representation. His observations led him to conclude that profound hearing loss from birth or early childhood led to a greater or lesser immaturity, a lack of empathy and stereotyped social behaviour, together with relatively shallow, short-duration, labile and detached affective responses. Rainer referred to the work of Schlesinger (1972) on the battles in communication which develop between a mother and her deaf child aged from 18 months to 3 years, as in word training, fearfulness of adult disapproval, and the pursuit of adult caring. Schlesinger stressed that parents who are afraid of the autonomy of their deaf child impose stringent measures, resulting in the child's habitual loss of autonomy and interference in the child's development of inner controls and self-concepts, as can occur also with hearing children. However, Freedman (1981) argued that young deaf children can establish a well-differentiated sense of self, and can form relationships between external objects and internal object representations if able to communicate effectively.

These extracts from the writing of some psychoanalysts may give the impression that, although deafness may not lead to psychiatric problems, it may nonetheless exert a traumatising influence on the deaf child. There is no doubt that deafness produces considerable frustrations for children, and leads to great demands on them and their parents (Brinich, 1981). There is also little doubt that deaf children show a relatively high frequency of behaviour problems, arising from difficulties in communication, which hinder the rehabilitation of their deafness. It would however be premature to conclude that the psychoanalytic view of the deaf child is a settled one. Work in the area has been relatively slight and spasmodic. Psychoanalysts seem no less prone to disagree with one another than members of the other occupations concerned with deaf children. Further, the divergent style of communication used by severely and profoundly deaf signers may make them difficult subjects for psychotherapy (Hoyt et al., 1981; Stokoe and Battison, 1981). The findings we have considered are therefore suggestive rather than conclusive.

Psychological Aspects

Given that deaf individuals can show unusual personal characteristics in childhood and in adulthood (Myklebust, 1966; Knutson and Lansing, 1990), we may ask: 'Is there a deaf personality?' or 'Is there a psychology of deafness?' (Vernon and Andrews, 1990).

A deaf personality?

Some of the earlier work in the area (Pintner, 1941; Brereton, 1957; Levine, 1960; Lewis, 1968) referred to an immaturity in deaf children of hearing parents which may appear in differences of arousal and expression of feelings. In the face of frustration such children are prone to tantrums, which seldom persist beyond infancy in hearing children, suggesting unusual personality development. Basilier (1964) described a condition of 'surdophrenia', involving emotional immaturity associated with weak ego development. Pintner (1941) and Lewis (1968) suggested that deaf children may be retarded in the way they relate to the affective aspects of language, such as the word 'mother', which releases in us all a complex emotional reaction. However (Lewis, 1968), differences in linguistic measures were clearly correlated with differences in personal and ethical traits, rather than with differences in emotional and social traits. Lewis' results indicated that the children who were the most mature in their personal and ethical development showed the greatest sophistication in features of the semantics of their language. His data support the view that a deaf child's personal development, in terms of self-confidence, initiative, determination and self-reliance influences the development of (oral) language, and hence communication.

A review and a justifiably fierce criticism of previous psychological research studies of affect in deaf people was presented by Donoghue (1968). He found that three studies described the deaf as reality-orientated, four reported them as passive in attitude, and two reported them as having hostile feelings. Attributes of rigidity in thinking featured in seven studies, impulsiveness in three, and egocentricity and insensitivity in five. One study proposed deaf neurotic symptoms, while another indicated psychosis. Three studies viewed deaf individuals as confused, and several saw the deaf as restricted in their ability to form concepts.

Donoghue concluded that because of the heterogeneity of the samples and variations in research methodology, the only reliable finding was that, as a whole, deaf individuals showed excessive rigidity. He was puzzled by the divergent findings, which ranged from serious emotional maladjustment to relatively normal social adjustment. His solution to this puzzle was to castigate the researchers for their improper approach and methodology in psychodiagnostic evaluation. Their conclusions, he argued, were at best speculations based on the questionable use of subjective reasoning and an obviously inadequate reference matrix. Few of the studies reviewed had been able, or had even attempted, to communicate with their deaf subjects to ensure a valid interchange between tester and subject. There was excessive reliance on fingerspelling and speechreading, when in many cases the preferred mode of communication by the deaf subjects was sign. With such a restricted opportunity for communication, it was not surprising to find reports of weak thinking in the abstract, rigidity, and so on. The result was a bias towards describing deaf individuals as having a constricted personality.

Donoghue ended his indictment by observing that the thinking of deaf individuals was possibly similar to that of hearing people. However, the way in which this thinking was expressed would vary with the educational and social backgrounds of the subjects. Mere professional competency in test administration needed to be complemented by an appreciation of the communication and cultural patterns of the deaf (compare Freeman, 1989).

Fortunately, nowadays a gross stereotyped view of hearing-impaired people, of the type described by the publications reviewed by Donoghue, is no longer held by professionals. Nevertheless, there is evidence of subtle and complex labelling. For example, when hearing and hearing-impaired teachers were asked to assess the behaviour of 8-year-old hearing and profoundly deaf children, on the basis of written information only, the hearing teachers were more likely to lable hearing children as behaviourally impaired whilst hearing-impaired teachers were more likley to use this label with the deaf children (Murphy-Berman et al., 1987).

In view of Donoghue's conclusions, we may wonder whether other approaches can lead to more valid results. Communication in the subject's preferred communication mode looks to be the obvious way to go, but indirect, projective methods could also be of value. Being aware of the methodological problems, Hess (1969) used a projective technique combined with non-verbal methods in a version of the Make-a-Picture Story Test – MAPS (Schneidman, 1948). The MAPS test consists of 22 background scenes and 67 figures with which to populate them. Hess found that deaf boys and girls used more, and more varied, figures than hearing children, interpreted as a leaning towards release from restrictions in the interpersonal relationships of their daily lives. Once chosen, the figures were rarely changed by the deaf children, unlike their hearing peers, suggesting that the deaf children were less flexible and realistic in interpreting their surroundings. Evidence for emotional instability and confusion was deduced from the deaf children's sorting of figures into the categories of 'happy', 'sad', etc., when the deaf attributed multiple affect to the same figure, suggesting weak concepts of emotional states. The deaf children chose significantly fewer figures as likeable, and designated more as sad and fewer as happy, than hearing subjects. Hess argued that since other investigators had found an association between accepting oneself and a tendency to look favourably on others, the deaf children felt less satisfied with themselves as they did not see their environment as particularly accepting (compare Bachara et al., 1980).

Although Hess used a projective technique, with likely uncertainties as to validity and reliability, and although it is only too easy to read into the results the interpretation which is sought, Hess's study was relatively robust because it included a group of emotionally disturbed children among the hearing controls. In general, where their performance was dissimilar to that of normal hearing children, the deaf children performed similarly to the emotionally disturbed children. Also, Hess's findings confirmed the results of an earlier study of deaf and hearing children with MAPS by Bindon (1957), who also found that differences in MAPS responses between hearing and deaf adolescents were greatest when the interactions showed the most frequent and personal relationships of daily life.

There is evidence that deaf children with different communication backgrounds differ in their personal and emotional adjustment. Weisel (1988) found that congenitally profoundly deaf Israeli children of elementary school age, born to deaf parents, performed significantly better than similar children of hearing parents in emotional adjustment, self-image, motivation for communication and reading comprehension, but not in social adjustment. Since the deafness of all the children was of genetic origin, this outcome offered support for the influence of environmental factors, such as family circumstances, and early and continuous exposure to sign language, on personal and cognitive development. Weisel's study had relatively good control over the effects of heredity, gender, age distribution and hearing loss. Its findings supported the view that the reading achievement and, more important to the present discussion, the emotional development of deaf children born to deaf parents are superior to those of deaf children born to hearing parents, as proposed earlier (Quigley and Kretschmer, 1982; Moores, 1987).

Impulsivity

The literature contains scattered reports to the effect that deaf children are more impulsive in their behaviour than hearing children. Wishing to discover the influence of such cultural factors as paternalistic practices in education, which could lead to a dependent and egocentric orientation promoting impulsivity, Altschuler et al. (1976) undertook a large-scale psychological testing of deaf and hearing adolescents in American and Yugoslavian schools. Their subjects were aged 15–17 years with IQs between 85 and 115, and with prelingual profound hearing losses in the case of the deaf adolescents. Subjects with brain damage or severe personality disorder were excluded. Altschuler et al. studied 50 Yugoslavian deaf subjects and 50 hearing controls from several states and schools, and 50 American hearing subjects and 50 deaf subjects from schools in New York. With an eye to validity, objectivity and reliability, in which they were only partly successful, they used relatively non-verbal and culture-free measures, such as assessments of long-range planning ability, impulsivity, emotional stability and flexibility versus ego-rigidity. They used the Porteous Maze test, the Draw-A-Line (DAL) test, the Id–Ego–Superego (IES) test, and the Rorschach, all of which were to have been correlated with a criterion measure of impulsivity from the ratings of two teachers. Unfortunately, the variance between the teachers was so great that their ratings had to be discarded.

Both Yugoslav and American deaf subjects showed greater impulsivity than the hearing subjects in the respective countries on the Porteous test, and on the Ego scores of the Arrow–Dot, the Picture Story Completion subtests of the IES, and the DAL test. The results of the Rorschach test were only slightly less marked. The Yugoslav subjects, whether deaf or hearing, were in general more impulsive than the American subjects. Since most findings were obtained via objective and language-free tests, they may be regarded as escaping criticisms of the type put forward by Donoghue (1968) – see above. However, for all subjects, whether deaf or hearing, the correlations between scores on one measure and scores on any other measure were close to zero, though all were devised to measure impulsivity and several clearly separated the deaf from the hearing subjects. Altschuler et al.

concluded that what is regarded clinically as impulsivity may be a final compendium which reflects a number of different personality variables.

Commenting that impulsivity continued to be a significant psychosocial problem in deaf individuals according to educators and clinicians alike, O'Brien (1987) took the concept further to ask whether the impulsivity might not only be shown by deaf individuals in their overt behaviour, but also in their underlying style of thinking. She assessed the relationship of the cognitive dimension of reflection–impulsivity to communication mode (oral or TC) and age in 71 prelingually severely to profoundly deaf and hearing boys aged 6–15 years. The Porteous Maze test, and a Matching Familiar Figures picture-matching test (MFFT), were administered to all the boys in the classroom.

The results of MFFT errors showed that the deaf boys were more impulsive than the hearing boys. On the Porteous Q scores, which were a weighted sum of errors in execution and thus related to reflection–impulsivity, there was a significant difference between the hearing and deaf TC boys. There was also a significant difference between the hearing and the deaf oral boys on MFFT responses. There were no other significant differences between deaf and hearing groups. This is not too surprising. Not all tests for emotional or personality factors used with deaf children show the anticipated findings (compare Cates, 1991). No significant differences were found between the oral and TC groups, but the older deaf and hearing groups, aged 11–15 years showed less impulsivity than the younger deaf and hearing groups aged 6–10 years. O'Brien also found some suggestion of a difference between deaf children with deaf parents and deaf children with hearing parents reminiscent of Harris (1978), who reported that deaf children with deaf parents were less impulsive than deaf children of hearing parents.

The findings of Harris (1978) and O'Brien (1987) show that the different experiences of deaf children of deaf or hearing parents affect the children's impulsivity in different ways. Possibly a greater acceptance of the child's deafness by deaf parents reduces the child's impulsive behaviour. O'Brien noted that several intervention programmes were being used to reduce impulsive behaviour in hearing children, but that only one (Kusche et al., 1987) was in progress to reduce the impulsivity of deaf children through language mediation techniques, despite the perceived need for this type of intervention programme.

Self-concept

Self-concept involves an individual's view of personal attitudes, traits and social standing. It has been argued that hearing loss leads to problems of adjustment in children, because problems with communication produce barriers to social development which are difficult to overcome. In turn, these barriers cause problems in social adjustment (Freeman et al., 1981; Schlesinger, 1978; Kusche et al., 1987) and interfere with the development of a concept of self like that of the hearing child.

In an exploratory investigation, Warren and Hasenstab (1986) studied the combination of demographic and impairment-related variables, and parental attitudes in the prediction of self-concept in 58 severely to profoundly deaf children of 5–11 years of age. The causes of deafness were congenital, illness or unknown. Almost all the parents were hearing. The children were asked to decide whether pictures showing normal home, play or school situations were happy or sad by circling faces corresponding to the pictures (the Picture Game – Lambert and Bower, 1979), a task believed to provide an index of self-concept. Parental attitudes to child-rearing were assessed with the Maryland Parent Attitude Survey – MPAS (Pumroy, 1966), to distinguish between indulgent, protecting, rejecting and disciplinarian attitudes. The parents were asked to select the different parent types, balanced for social desirability, which most reflected their views.

The results showed a clear association between the child's self-concept and parental indulgence, protection, discipline, and the child's level of language and communication at the onset of hearing loss. Warren and Hasenstab saw the results as indicating that, although the hearing parents of deaf children wish to do their best by them, most parents have problems in coping with their hearing-impaired child, and may in fact contribute to maladjusted behaviour. They argued that there was a clear need for more support for the families of deaf children.

Similar results were obtained by Loeb and Sarigiani (1986), who, in an important large-scale project, asked if hearing impairment affected children's personalities in a clear and consistent way. They studied 250 children aged 8–15 years from 33 schools with mainstream special education programmes. There were 64 hearing-impaired children, 74 children with visual impairments and 112 children with no sensory or major emotional, mental or physical impairments. Sixty of the hearing-impaired children attended schools using oral methods. The remaining four hearing-impaired children came from TC programmes. The children were assessed with the Children's Locus of Control Scale (Nowicki and Strickland, 1973) in a form which was linguistically simplified for hearing-impaired children, and which measured the extent of children's perception of their control over their life space; a Q-sort technique (Schwartz et al., 1975) requiring the children to sort into five piles 15 cards containing descriptions of human characteristics, such as 'happy', and then requiring a repeated sorting into how the children perceived they would like to be; the Children's Self-Concept Scale of Piers and Harris (1964), which is easy to read and offers a measure of self-esteem together with such components as behaviour, intellect, physical wellbeing, anxiety, popularity and happiness; a tower-building task (Loeb et al., 1980) in which they were blindfolded and asked to build two towers from irregularly-shaped blocks in a set time period; and a sentence-stem completion task, used as a projective method to indicate the issues and concerns of the greatest importance to them. Checks were made that the children understood all the tasks.

The hearing-impaired children, whose hearing losses ranged from mild to profound but were mainly moderate to severe, were lower in self-esteem (Piers–Harris' test) than the other groups, but level of hearing-impairment did not interact with self-esteem. Significant effects were found also for behaviour and popularity, with higher popularity being significantly related to later onset of hearing impairment. Girls were more anxious than boys, and black children obtained lower scores than white children on the Appearance item. The locus of control test (Nowicki and Strickland, 1973) produced no main effects. However, there was a significant interaction between race and handicap. The hearing-impaired white children showed a more external locus of control than the hearing-impaired black children. From the Q-sorts, which compared the children's ranks for items as they saw themselves and how they would have wished to be, the hearing-impaired children reported that they would have liked to be less shy and more likeable than they were. The children with later onsets of hearing loss were less satisfied with themselves than the children with early onsets. From the tower-building data, the predictions of the group of hearing-impaired children for a further tower were lower than those of the two other groups, based realistically on the lower towers they had built earlier. The height of the towers built correlated negatively with the severity of the hearing loss. From the sentence-stem completion task the hearing-impaired children appeared more often sad because of name-calling, and tended to identify a special activity or playing as most liked instead of their family or friends, unlike the children from the other groups. They were also more likely to select some aspect of their environment, such as their room, home or school, as what they would most like to change, rather than some characteristic of themselves.

Their teachers saw the hearing-impaired children as having more problems with school work, shyness, getting on with other children and adults, and lacking in confidence more than the other children. The mothers thought that their hearing-impaired children had no greater problems than the visually impaired or non-sensorially handicapped children, apart from their education, where the mothers of both the hearing-handicapped and the visually handicapped children reported more problems than the parents of the children without sensory impairments.

We have considered this report by Loeb and Sarigiani at length because of its importance in assessing a variety of self-perceptions on a large sample over several schools, with comparison groups for type of impairment and absence of impairment. Its major limitation was its restriction mainly to hearing-impaired children who were educated orally. However, it is likely that hearing-impaired children who used other modes of communication would have a similar or more pessimistic outcome in the same environment.

The results showed that orally educated hearing-impaired children in mainstreamed programmes had self-assessed problems of several kinds. They were not popular with peers, found it hard to make friends and were not often chosen as playmates. They tended to be shy, an obvious impediment to the development of communication. Surprisingly, they saw their ideal selves as less likeable than they were, and they were more interested in changing their environment than themselves, suggesting that they accepted their communication problems as a major obstacle. It appears difficult to motivate such children to develop their social interaction and their communication. They would seem, rather, to prefer to stay within the limited environment they know. However, Loeb and Sarigiani thought it encouraging that the hearing-impaired group were not more external in locus of control than the other groups. Further, from the Q-sort measure of overall self-satisfaction, the hearing-impaired children saw themselves as having a normally positive outlook, as shown also by some of the responses to the sentence-stem completion test.

In summary, this research by Loeb and Sarigiani indicates not only that hearing impairment, gender, age and race affect children's self-perceptions, but that they do so in a complex way. The differences between the children reinforce the view that each child develops self-perceptions uniquely. It is misleading to emphasise any one variable to the exclusion of the others. Having stated that, the study shows that most hearing-impaired children need special assistance to develop several personality characteristics which most people would see as desirable and which would assist their communication. In this context, the current emphasis on mainstreaming in deaf education is a cause for concern if it is not adequately supported by services. With minimal support services, mainstreamed hearing-impaired children tend to have lower self concepts (Reich et al., 1977).

As an additional comment, it is rather disconcerting that research instruments purporting to assess self-concepts or self-perceptions tend to be indirect, such as tower-building, or to have uncertain validities, as in the use of certain projective tests. Little work has generally gone into the development of personality tests for hearing-impaired people (Freeman, 1989), although Oblitz et al. (1991) have recently described a self-concept scale for older hearing-impaired children which may help to overcome some of these concerns. It is also important to estimate whether the self-concepts themselves reflect a valid situation. This situation is of particular concern since deaf individuals may have quite false self-concepts. Thus Cole and Edelmann (1991) found that some profoundly deaf adolescents described themselves as 'a bit deaf' or believed that in time they might become hearing.

Some hearing-impaired individuals may encounter special circumstances in which their personal characteristics and needs are less than sufficiently recognised. For example, problems that are incipient in the early years of life and in elementary schooling, become more obvious in the more demanding and competitive environments of tertiary education settings (Flexer et al., 1986), requiring the services of a support group. There is some indication (Israelite, 1986) that the hearing adolescent siblings of hearing-impaired children define themselves not only as individuals in their own right, but also as the siblings of hearing-impaired children. The latter definition may add to siblings' feelings of inadequacy in social situations, since adolescents do not like to appear different or deviant (Sherif and Sherif, 1964). In turn, perception of feelings of inadequacy on the part of their siblings may affect the personalities of hearing-impaired children. This is a topic for further research.

Conclusion

As regards the question: 'Is there a deaf personality?' our stance is necessarily somewhat equivocal. The test instruments used and the studies published to date have not generally been as vaild, objective and reliable as desired (Freeman, 1989). Further, hearing-impairment itself does not create personality differences as much as do the ensuing problems of communication. Such communication problems may grow less over time, as methods of communication by and with hearing-impaired people are researched and extended. Nevertheless, and for the time being, hearing-impaired individuals do seem to differ in personality from hearing people. We are content to accept the suggestion of Rodda and Grove (1987) that the concept of a deaf personality or 'surdophrenia' has some uses, provided that it is not over-emphasised or misused.

Social Aspects

In this section we consider the social interaction of hearing-impaired children outside their family. Parent–infant interactions were described in Chapter 2.

In a conference discussion on social and vocational adjustment by deaf individuals more than 25 years ago (Stuckless, 1965), it was considered that the deaf community, school and family were so active in helping deaf individuals that there was no real need for assistance from social agencies. Since 1965, not only has our knowledge of such social needs expanded, but it is also clear that much work remains to be done, both in research in the area and in the provision of services. Further, the nature of social interaction between hearing and hearing-impaired children, and between one hearing-impaired child and another, proves to be far from simple.

Some 20 years after the above conference, Hummel and Schirmer (1984) reviewed the work of programmes concerned with the social development of hearing-impaired students. There had, they thought, been a tendency to focus too much on cognitive and linguistic factors, to the exclusion of affective factors. Increased attention needed to be paid to the social development and social interactions of both handicapped and non-handicapped children. Since communication skills are acquired or learned in a social context, and since such skills need to be maximised if the child is to learn effectively, the arrangements for the education of children – hearing as well as hearing impaired – need to involve consideration of the child's development of social skills. Hummel and Schirmer commented that the existing literature in the area was relatively scanty and methodologically and conceptually weak. We might add that some of it was overly descriptive or anecdotal (e.g. Altschuler, 1974; Feinstein, 1983). The yield of the existing research did not allow Hummel and Schirmer to form firm conclusions. However, the thrust towards the integration of hearing-impaired with hearing children in educational settings was forcing more attention to be paid to well-conducted research in the area, with some promising work emerging on useful intervention strategies.

The shift, in the 1980s, towards the study of the interplay of language, cognition and social interaction, as in research on the analysis of discourse in social situations (Seewald and Brackett, 1984) and on social cognition (Peterson and Peterson, 1989), is likely to prove illuminating about the communication skills of hearing-impaired children. As regards social development itself, we begin with the review of Hummel and Schirmer, taking note of their incisive criticisms, and commenting where other, or more recent, research suggests meaningful progress.

Hummel and Schirmer (1984) remarked that, at the time of their review, much of the published research in the social development and social interaction of hearing-impaired children had been concerned with whether they had deficits in social skills. Most of this research, they observed, had taken a traditional, normative approach, involving comparisons of the behaviour of hearing-impaired with that of hearing children. It entailed estimates of the frequency with which the hearing-impaired children showed non-normal, and thus often undesirable, social behaviour, and the extent to which such behaviour was beyond norms from hearing children. Such a normative approach was criticised, first, because of insufficient standardisation of the test instruments. It was an inadequate basis for intervention, because the knowledge base was not sufficiently robust to show clearly which apparently non-normal behaviour required intervention. There were no proper test norms for hearing-impaired children. Such norms as did exist were derived from tools for describing the behaviour of hearing children. Similar conclusions were drawn by Delgado (1982). It would be preferable to have norms for hearing-impaired children and norms for hearing children of the same ages, at least until more information was forthcoming about the relation between hearing impairment and specific behaviour problems.

The second basic difficulty with the normative approach was that of judging which behaviour patterns were desirable or undesirable. It is clear in a general sense what this criticism means, but it seems somewhat unfairly levied. The judgements are not necessarily normative themselves, but reflect child conduct departing from the behavioural norms, even though some people regard conforming, or alternatively, aberrant behaviour, differently from others (Togonu-Bickersteth, 1988). There is now, however, a developing literature on the attention paid by teachers, case managers and counsellors to the social and communication skills of hearing-impaired children (Beck, 1988; Murphy and Hill, 1989; Cates and Shontz, 1990; Maxon et al., 1991).

Hummel and Schirmer stated firmly that research which shows that the behaviour in question is linked to current and/or future adjustment greatly helps the making of decisions about intervention. They referred to evidence that decreases in aggression (Feshbach, 1970) and positive peer interaction (Hartup, 1976) are desirable goals in intervention for hearing students, since these are linked with emotional adjustment, academic achievement and ethical development. A similar association was imputed for hearing-impaired children.

Peer interaction

There have been a number of reports of the social interaction between hearing-impaired children with one another and between hearing-impaired children and their hearing peers. We now outline several of these reports, following which we offer general conclusions.

The use of sociometric ratings to explore the acceptance and rejection by one another of 200 severely to profoundly deaf students aged 7–17 years was discussed by Hagborg (1987). The lowest-scoring 29 and the highest-scoring 29 students were classed as rejected and accepted groups respectively. Members of the accepted group had been enrolled in the school for a longer time, were more likely to be female, and were rated by teachers as having a more favourable behaviour adjustment than the rejected group. Thus social acceptance by peers was partly related to behavioural adjustment.

Social interactions between preschool hearing and hearing-impaired children were described by Brackett and Henniges (1976), who found that the hearing-impaired children, with a wide range of mild to profound hearing losses, began more social interactions during free play than in structured language sessions. We would expect the more linguistically competent hearing-impaired children to interact more frequently than those with weaker language skills, and this was the case. Further, the latter interacted socially with other hearing-impaired, rather than hearing children. Arnold and Tremblay (1979) obtained similar results, but found in addition that hearing children preferred to interact with other hearing children, presumably mainly because of greater ease of communication. It seems then that, where hearing and hearing-impaired preschool children play together, children with strong language ability and good communication skills, whether hearing or hearing-impaired, use that ability to choose partners in play. Otherwise, age, gender and ethnicity are the important variables in the choice of preschool deaf children's play partners (Lederberg, 1991).

For school-age children, McCauley et al. (1976) and Antia (1982) concluded that hearing-impaired children with moderate to profound hearing losses looked to teachers for positive interactions. It is not therefore surprising that the hearing-impaired children interacted at a significantly lower rate with their peers than did the hearing children. Antia (1985) suggested that, since one of the goals of main-streaming is social integration, the teacher's role needs to be considered. If teachers decrease their social interactions with the school-aged hearing-impaired children, the latter may be prompted to participate more in the play of their peers.

Hearing-impaired children are not necessarily more disposed to social interaction with hearing-impaired peers than are hearing children, as shown by Vandell and George (1981). They matched preschool children aged 14–64 months for age and gender in dyads consisting of two hearing children, two hearing-impaired children, and one hearing and one hearing-impaired child. The hearing-impaired children, who had a wide range of hearing losses, used a combination of speech and Signed Essential English. The hearing-impaired dyads began more social interactions than the hearing dyads, but these interactions were more frequently rejected or ignored by partners. Such rejection was even more marked in the mixed dyads. Hence both hearing and hearing-impaired preschoolers tended to discount the communication initiatives of their hearing-impaired partners. Also, they often began interactions which could not be perceived by their hearing-impaired partner. Accordingly, the hearing-impaired children were less likely to respond to the approaches of the other children, whether hearing or hearing-impaired.

According to Antia (1985), this study showed that lack of understanding of the needs governing the communication of hearing-impaired children was as much a barrier to interaction with peers as linguistic competence, and that the results had implications for intervention programmes for hearing and hearing-impaired children alike. The social integration of hearing-impaired children could be helped by teaching the communication skills needed to begin and to maintain positive interactions. Structured situations for positive interactions with peers would therefore increase the social acceptance of hearing-impaired children, by promoting the appropriate use of communication skills such as greetings, invitations and acceptances, asking questions about the interests of others, and turn-taking (compare La Greca and Mesibov, 1979).

Physical distance in a school playground was identified by Jones (1985) as another factor in dyadic interactions. She measured the distances between 40 hearing and 40 hearing-impaired dyads whose members were aged 6–8 years, prior to mainstreaming, when the hearing-impaired dyads were separated by about 25% more space than occurred for the hearing dyads. The effect does not seem to have been due to space needed for signing, as the hearing-impaired children were educated orally. The reason for the effect is not clear, and it may not persist with increasing age (Holton, 1978), though physical propinquity is of obvious relevance to communication. Jones thought her results could have implications for positive interactions between hearing and hearing-impaired children, if distancing formed an important part of children's interpretation of communication interchange. However, such interchange was not part of this investigation.

There is, then, an emerging literature which shows that positive peer interactions are problematical and/or different for hearing-impaired children. Their attempts at social interaction are rejected relatively often by potential hearing and hearing-impaired partners alike. In particular, their interactions will be fewer if they show poor behaviour adjustment or low levels of linguistic ability. The teaching of communication skills to both hearing and hearing-impaired children, and the opportunity to practise them in free play with limited teacher presence, could improve this situation.

However, a cautionary comment has been injected by Magen (1990), suggesting that the situation may be age-dependent. Using a questionnaire, Magen found that the intensity and frequency of interpersonal experiences were higher for hearing-impaired than for hearing adolescents. Hearing-impaired adolescents, with severe or lesser hearing losses, reported positive interpersonal experiences equally distributed between experiences with hearing-impaired and hearing individuals. It appeared that positive interpersonal experiences may be the rule, rather than the exception among hearing-impaired adolescents, though they may have had to work especially hard at developing them. However, the adolescents concerned were less than profoundly deaf. Also, the use of the questionnaires is an indirect reporting instrument which does not necessarily yield the most valid findings.

Aggression

Aggression in the social interactions of hearing-impaired children is another area where the literature is slim. In one of the few studies that reported detailed findings on aggression Maxon et al. (1991), using a self-report social awareness test, found that severely to profoundly deaf children aged 7–19 years perceived themselves differently on items relating to the verbal expression of emotion, verbal aggression, physical aggression and social interaction, when compared with hearing children. Age and gender differences were also found. The deaf children reported themselves as less verbally aggressive than the hearing children, possibly because of reduced verbal emotional expression, but they saw themselves as more aggressive physically. Overall, they saw themselves not as necessarily less or more aggressive, but as releasing their aggression in different ways. If these perceptions were true reflections of the actual state of affairs, and there is supporting evidence for this (McCane, 1980; Meadow, 1980), there are important implications for the development of positive social interactions. Initiations of social interactions could be more successful for hearing-impaired children if they were a little more verbally aggressive, and less physically aggressive, than hearing children. As Maxon et al. indicated, the problem may be greater for hearing-impaired girls, as the hearing-impaired girl who is physically aggressive will appear more socially inept than the aggressive hearing-impaired boy.

Levels of aggression may differ with the extent to which hearing-impaired children cope with feelings of frustration or inadequacy in communicating through different modes. Aggressive acts were recorded by Cornelius and Hornett (1990) in two groups of mainly lingually hearing-impaired kindergarten children, aged 5–6 years. One group attended an oral programme which used no sign. The other group used TC. Play was observed as functional play, namely, simple and repetitive muscular activity with or without objects, constructive play in manipulating objects, dramatic play in assuming a role, and social play. The groups did not differ from each other in functional and constructive play, but they varied significantly in dramatic and social play. Children using TC showed higher levels of social play, and engaged in more frequent dramatic play than the children using the oral-only mode. They touched, gestured and vocalised almost twice as much as those using the oral-only mode. Further, 17 aggressive acts were noted for the oral-only class, whereas only two such instances were observed with the group using TC. The aggressive acts were forceful, including pushing, hitting and pinching other children. Cornelius and Hornett remarked that the child's communication mode should not only allow but encourage positive play and social interaction. The introduction of sign may promote such developments for orally educated children if the reason for their aggression is frustration because of poor ability to establish communication.

Social skills training

Although there have been many recommendations for developing the social skills of hearing-impaired children, Hummel and Schirmer (1984) remarked that, at the time, there had been few reports about the implementation of such recommendations. Becker (1978) described an oral training programme conducted with 14-year-old hearing-impaired children in Montreal, designed to develop personal and social maturity, with which the staff were very satisfied. A programme of skills in attending, spontaneous interaction, communication clarification and social fluency, which were taught directly and simultaneously, at levels suitable for the age of the child, was developed by McGinnis et al. (1980). Hummel (1982) reported success in developing social skills with a structured learning approach which involved modelling of target skills, role playing, performance feedback with various methods of reinforcing children's attempts to practise the skill in daily life, and transfer of training.

Training programmes in social skills have since developed, though several

show serious design or reporting problems. There has been emphasis on appropriateness of communication, response latency, smiling, eye contact and gestures.
Lemanek et al. (1986), for example, noted an increase in such skills following the
use of a social skills training package with 11–18-year-old hearing-impaired adolescents. A procedure to increase toy sharing among five hearing-impaired children
of kindergarten age was described by Barton and Osborne (1978). Kreimeyer and
Antia (1988) drew on this work in devising a social interaction intervention programme for hearing-impaired preschool children with a wide range of hearing
losses, to increase positive peer interaction. They also wished to know whether
the taught interaction skills would generalise to free play. Positive peer interaction
was found to increase with teaching, and the taught social interaction skills could
be generalised to free play, but only when specific generalisation strategies were
used. Generalisation for interaction with peers occurred only when toys used in
the initiation of social interaction skills were offered during free play. Peer interaction did not generalise to free play on the introduction of toys which had not
been used in instruction. This outcome is reminiscent of trained skills in other
areas,which we have discussed in previous chapters. Hearing-impaired children
clearly have problems in generalising trained skills of various kinds, an issue
which begs for further research.

Situations devised by the children themselves should be particularly conducive
to social skills training. Using this approach, six profoundly deaf children aged
12–13 years were trained in a programme designed by Murphy and Hill (1989) to
improve their communication abilities. The children were trained in weekly 1.5
hour sessions over 8 weeks, using video-recorded enactments of situations by
pairs of children thought up by the children themselves. Between-session analyses
were reported to show marked improvements in communication between partners, which was generalised from one situation to another. However, no data were
given. Further, Cates and Shontz (1990) have found that role-taking behaviour
is not reliably related to some measures of social behaviour in moderately to
profoundly deaf children. The results of Murphy and Hill are therefore open to
question.

Conclusion

Despite later advances in research, including work in areas more peculiar to deaf
individuals such as signed communication (Hall, 1989), there is still a dearth of
well designed and executed studies on the development of social skills in hearing-
impaired children. Even the work on pragmatics (see below) improves insufficiently on this situation. There is no doubt, however, of the need for further
knowledge which may assist the integration of hearing-impaired children in mainstream education and elsewhere, especially given concerns that the grouping of
hearing-impaired with hearing children does not necessarily produce social interaction or social acceptance (Antia, 1985). In view of advice on techniques and
approaches, such as video-recording and analysis procedures (Johnson and
Griffith, 1985), creative drama (Davies, 1984), and the application of the Vineland
Adaptive Behavior Scale to the study of socialisation (Dunlap and Iceman Sands,

1990), we may expect to see more comprehensive and methodologically more robust future reports in this difficult and demanding area.

Pragmatics

Traditionally, analysis of the language of children with impaired hearing focused on deficits in lexical, syntactic and, to a lesser extent, phonological development. The perspective has now broadened to include the ways in which hearing-impaired children put language to use in pragmatics to attain specific goals, as in posing questions to obtain information, describing events, making promises and cracking jokes (Pien, 1985). Hence, the development of competence in communication requires mastery of stylistic variation in the use of language as well as mastery of language itself, whether in sign or verbal language (Lou et al., 1987; Mounty, 1989).

A focus on pragmatics leads to considerations of language use with fundamental implications for language assessment, intervention and teaching. A pragmatic orientation suggests change in language assessment towards evaluating various communicative functions that the child expresses. Also, the pragmatic focus suggests changes in intervention and teaching methods. The primary goal of intervention and teaching becomes the facilitation of general communicative functions, for which vocabulary, syntactic structures and phonology are tools used in context (Bates, 1976).

The relevance of pragmatics to communication is in the skills used in interpersonal communication. Conversations, for example, are conducted by means of rules which have to be learned, and the learning of the rules of pragmatics in conducting conversations is as important for communication as the learning of syntax and vocabulary. Hearing-impaired children may have difficulties in introducing a topic of conversation, or in shifting from one topic to another during conversation, because they do not sufficiently consider the needs of the listener (Moeller et al., 1983). Further, Geoffrion (1982) observed that hearing-impaired partners pass on the burden of keeping up a conversation, even in communication by teletype. Considerations of pragmatics and syntax show that relationships between the two pose special difficulties for hearing-impaired children, as when difficulty is experienced with conjunctions such as 'although' which signal a shift of topic. Also problematical for hearing-impaired children is the development of communication repair strategies (Kretschmer and Kretschmer, 1980), which require skills in pragmatics to restore a broken conversation by seeking clarification, or by repeating what is said for confirmation, or by offering additional information. Other desiderata in pragmatics for hearing-impaired children involve a readiness to seek information by repeated questioning, so that the child can continue as an effective communication partner by acquiring enough information to keep a conversation flowing, and offering prompts, as in paraphrasing, to elicit specific information.

The description of the field which follows has been divided into two main areas: Communicative Intentions and Conversation.

Communicative intentions

The study of communicative intentions, or the functions that utterances are intended to serve, are of special interest because of the relationship between intentions and linguistic forms of expression.

Skarakis and Prutting (1977) described the semantic and pragmatic components of language in the spontaneous communication of four hearing-impaired preschool children aged 2–4 years. The children had received oral language instruction, were functioning intellectually at or above their chronological age, and were severely to profoundly deaf. Data were collected by written transcript of the child's communicative acts in four different situations: free play, snacktime, and group and individual lessons, over a 4-week period. The data were analysed for semantic functions and communicative intentions. There are several advantages in using this twofold approach: first, pragmatics and semantics can be examined separately; secondly, communication skills can be studied independently of specific linguistic skills; thirdly, the children's knowledge of the world, and behaviour reflecting such knowledge, can be distinguished from their knowledge of language.

Analysis procedures were derived from Greenfield and Smith (1976) for semantic function, and from Dore (1974) and Bates (1976) for communicative intent. The communicative intent was covered by the categories Labelling, Response, Request/Demand, Greeting, Protesting, Repeating, Description and Attention. The procedures used the following evidence to determine the appropriate aspect: the relation between the child's utterance and the context; the child's utterance, gesture, facial expression, actions and body orientation; and the adult's or peer's response. In addition, physical context including the referent, events involving the child, and the prior linguistic experience of the child were considered.

Verbalisation and gesture were used by all subjects. Verbal behaviour was used predominantly by one subject, with the other three using gesture as their main means of communication. The results revealed positive implications for hearing-impaired children. First, subjects showed semantic functions and communicative intentions in spontaneous speech. Secondly, although direct comparisons were not cited, some of the communicative intentions and semantic functions were similar to those identified by Dore (1974) and Greenfield and Smith (1976) in younger hearing children. The results showed that the hearing-impaired children expressed similar semantic functions and communicative intentions to those of hearing children at the prelinguistic and one-word stage. Skarakis and Prutting thus suggested that hearing-impaired children progress through this early stage of language development in the same way as the hearing child.

A further study of the semantic and pragmatic development of young hearing-impaired children was conducted by Curtiss et al. (1979), as both an expansion and a refinement of Skarakis and Prutting (1977). A larger sample size of 12 preschool children constituted the study group, with a wider age range, from 22–60 months. Hearing impairment ranged from severe to profound deafness. Data were collected from four different environmental settings, and videotapes were used instead of written transcripts. Dore's (1974) categories were modified to facilitate the recording of behaviour of hearing-impaired subjects, resulting in 16 speech act categories. Greenfield and Smith's (1976) semantic function categories were also modified and expanded to include gestural communication. The pragmatic intention and semantic content, whether verbal or non-verbal, were recorded.

The results revealed that children of all ages used the full range of pragmatic intentions. Age was an important variable for semantic functions. Two year olds displayed limited semantic ability, but there was an increase in the expression of semantics with increasing age. Pragmatic and semantic functions expressed in combination revealed that as their semantic abilities expanded, the children were also learning pragmatics. Non-verbally, all children expressed the full range of pragmatic functions, but several categories were not expressed verbally. Individual data showed marked differences between children in the same age group. One of the most pertinent findings was that hearing loss played only a small role in non-verbal pragmatic and semantic ability. However, only individual scores were considered and statistical computations, such as correlation coefficients between different abilities, were not reported. Curtiss et al. also found that the number of combinations of pragmatic and semantic behaviours increased with age, seeing these interactions as illustrating the relational nature of communication.

A major finding of this study was that children with impaired hearing coded a variety of pragmatic intentions and semantic functions, using both verbal and non-verbal means. They showed considerable communicative ability, a finding in agreement with Skarakis and Prutting (1977). Semantic functions appeared to develop at a slower rate across all age groups than did pragmatic intention, a finding supported by a more recent report (Swanson, 1987) of the effects of self-instruction training for one profoundly deaf child, which showed that self-instruction was immediately effective on the child's signed pragmatic behaviour, with a slower effect on signed semantic behaviour. Curtiss et al. felt that the difference between the development of pragmatic and semantic functions may have been the result of difficulties, in some instances, of coding meaning through non-linguistic means. As for the effects of the hearing loss on communicative skill, Curtiss et al. pointed out that further research using aided rather than unaided loss may be a better predictor of communicative ability.

This pattern of results was continued by Day (1986) with five prelingually profoundly deaf children aged 35–42 months, who were learning Manually Coded English. Deafness did not limit the amount of communicative interaction between these children and their parents, as they communicated successfully and often with their signing hearing mothers, frequently using invented gestures beyond the sign system they were learning. The children produced highly differentiated sets of communicative intentions which were readily identified by the mothers, although the children's vocabulary and syntax were limited.

At a quite different level, in a study offering insights into communicative intentions in context for older subjects, Foster et al. (1989) investigated the meaning of communication for a group of 23 first-year hearing-impaired college students who had sustained moderate to profound hearing losses from an early age. These students, from 15 states in the USA, were interviewed in depth. They were encouraged to pursue their thoughts, though the interviews were constrained by a set of core topics about communication. The great majority of these students had some familiarity with both speechreading and manual communication. The interview transcripts were organised into categories of language-modality, affective, situational and sociopolitical. Of these, the third, situational category is relevant to the present discussion. It offers some useful insights, although because of the study design, these insights were given at a descriptive level only.

First, in the situational category, and not surprisingly, the students reported that ease of communication varied widely with the background of the communication partner. The distinction between friend and stranger was given most frequently. Friends were seen as more likely to understand the students' communication and to be more interested in keeping a conversation going. Awkward situations were seen as less likely to happen with friends and, when they did, could be handled with less difficulty.

Secondly, the purpose or topic of the conversation was seen to bear importantly on the success of the communication. Many students reported that communication was easier when the topic was of mutual interest, and that communication was more likely to fail in the absence of shared interests.

Thirdly, the environment or place in which the communication occurred was important, with environmental noise perceived as a significant impediment to successful conversation. Regional accents could also be a problem.

Fourthly, the modality of communication and situational styles were at issue. Communication was particularly difficult when the modality was unfamiliar to the students (e.g. signing versus talking), and the ability to switch between modalities was perceived as most important for handling complex communication. Support services and special equipment were seen as essential for good communication by some students. Problems could arise when equipment, such as hearing aids, could not be used, as when swimming.

Fifthly, time was mentioned as affecting all of the above, because the time expended in setting up the communication had a major influence on the quality of the subsequent relationship. Longer periods of time helped the development of communication skills and in accustoming hearing communication partners to acquire an understanding of the students' communication problems.

The purposes of communication showed a strongly social and pragmatic emphasis, as in getting a point across, sharing ideas, solving problems and so on. It was clear that the students had a very good perception of the importance of successful communication for understanding events and conditions, and for relating to other people. Their motivation and intention to succeed in so doing came through very strongly.

Conversation

A well-known and well-conducted study of language functioning in sustained communication, using video-recorded conversations between pairs of preschool hearing-impaired and hearing children engaged in play, was presented by McKirdy and Blank (1982). The hearing-impaired group, probably severely to profoundly deaf, comprised 24 children with congenital or prelingual hearing losses, whose ages ranged from 52 to 64 months. Twenty-two of the children were educated in TC programmes, with the remaining two educated orally. The hearing-impaired children were paired with hearing children of the same age, gender and non-verbal IQ. The children were arranged in same-gender dyads based on teacher's rank-order rating of preferred playmates, and placed in a room with a range of toys.

This study by McKirdy and Blank stands apart from most similar studies of its time in the use of a matched control group, and in employing statistical tests to evaluate the results. A coding system (Blank and Franklin, 1980) was used to score each participant in a dialogue, who was seen as assuming two separate roles, one of speaker-initiator; and the other as speaker-responder. As initiator, a speaker's signed and spoken utterances were judged for their level of cognitive complexity or their explicitness of demand for a response. As responder, a speaker's utterances and behaviours were judged for their appropriateness to the speaker-initiator's preceding utterance. The cognitive complexity for speaker-initiator allowed any utterance to be placed along a single continuum of complexity, divided into four levels: I Matching Experience, which involved words as symbols or labels for non-linguistic concepts already developed; II Selective Analysis of Experience, where the utterances were still tied to experience but represented a higher level of discrimination; III Re-ordering Experience, where language took on a directive function; and IV Reasoning about Experience, concerned with reasoning and problem-solving. The speaker-initiator scales also coded some pragmatic functions as to whether or not an utterance contained an explicit demand for a response. Explicit demands were termed 'Obliges' and their counterpart utterances which were not demands were 'Comments'. A scale for speaker-responder coded utterances for their appropriateness to the initiating speaker's remarks within the categories Adequate, Inadequate, No response and Ambiguous.

Communication between hearing and hearing-impaired children differed markedly. The hearing-impaired children initiated 27 conversational turns as against the hearing children's 57, reminiscent in part of Curtiss et al. (1979). Fifty-seven per cent of initiations of the hearing-impaired children's were Obliges, whereas the predominant form (57%) for the hearing children was the Comment. For both groups Obliges served to attract the partner's attention. The complexity of the interaction expressed in percentages revealed that the majority (92%) of the hearing-impaired children's initiations occurred at Level I (Matching Experience) with few occurrences at Levels II (Selective Analysis of Experience) and III (Re-ordering Experience), and none at Level IV (Reasoning about Experience). Level II accounted for 49% of the hearing children's initiations, with Levels I (29%) and III (21%) occurring in roughly equal percentages. Little use was made of Level IV (1%).

Although the percentage of responses to different levels of initiation at Levels I and II differed for hearing and hearing-impaired children, the patterns of response were similar. For both groups, Obliges were more effective than Comments in eliciting adequate responses. For example, the percentage of adequate responses to Obliges and Comments at Level I were 70% and 12% respectively for deaf children, and 65% and 34% for hearing children. The percentage of adequate responses for the deaf children decreased as the level of initiation increased from Level I to Level II, showing that the children were affected by the complexity of the formulations. Re-coded utterances, namely, utterances that were coded twice, first as responses to previous Comments, then secondly as initiations, were also examined to assess the extent to which there was a sustained exchange. Again, differences were observed. Re-coded data were obtained for all hearing children, but for only five out of the 24 hearing-impaired children, indicating the difficulty experienced by the deaf child in keeping dialogue going.

This work by McKirdy and Blank dealt with several interesting points. First, there was a difference in the rate of verbal productivity, with hearing-impaired children producing fewer messages at any one time than hearing subjects, as found by Curtiss et al. (1979). An explanation was offered that the deaf children's hands, needed for communication in sign, were occupied in playing with toys. Secondly, the range of levels in the deaf children's initiations was restricted in comparison to that of the hearing children, being limited to events and objects in the immediate present. Thirdly, the deaf children were learning their sign system, but had not proceeded very far. Instead, they relied on self-generated signs which, though adequate for signalling for attention, produced problems in coping with ideas beyond the immediate present. Fourthly, difficulties were more marked for the deaf children as speaker-responders than as speaker-initiators. They were less likely than the hearing children to respond to Comments, and offered fewer appropriate responses to Level II initiations, though the responses of deaf and hearing children to Level I initiations was similar.

As noted, a major difficulty in this study was the use of self-generated signs, which created restrictions, particularly in recording the symbolisation of ideas. The study might have achieved clearer results had children with a greater mastery of sign, such as signing deaf children born to signing deaf parents, been studied. McKirdy and Blank remarked that a pair of deaf children who were fluent in ASL had about the same initiation rate as the hearing children.

Examination of the breakdowns in conversations can provide a good indication of skills in pragmatics. Hughes and James (1985) found that TC-educated prelingually severely to profoundly deaf children aged 5–8 years were effective in dealing with communication breakdowns when the experimenter simultaneously spoke and signed: 'What?' in conversations, by revising or repeating their messages. The higher the children's grammatical skills, the more likely they were to revise their message. This use of pragmatics skills was similar to that found with the hearing child. It should, however, be appreciated that the 'What?' probe was a unitary and easily identified marker of communication breakdown. How deaf children cope with more complex breakdowns remains to be investigated.

Communication patterns in classrooms

A frequently cited study of communication patterns in classes for moderately to profoundly prelingually deaf children is that of Craig and Collins (1969, 1970). They used a modified Flanders Interactive Scale (Flanders, 1965), which contained several interactive categories, in direct observation of classroom communication.

Overall results for categories of interaction showed that in the structured areas of teaching, teachers markedly dominated classroom communication in all schools and for all ages of students. 'Questioning' and 'informing' were the categories used most frequently by teachers and students in language-dependent and specialised classes in initiating communication, though the teachers used them much more than the students. Assuming that the study was undertaken in the traditional setting where the teacher–pupil relationship is heavily structured and teacher-dominated, this finding is hardly surprising, though it is useful to have it put on record. The same comment can be made about the second overall finding, that a higher proportion of behaviour in the student 'response' category was observed when teacher 'questioning' comprised a high proportion of teacher-initiated behaviour. The very small 1% of 'confusions' showed the extent of teacher dominance. Thirdly, 'no communication' generally predominated when teacher-initiated interaction was relatively low.

Results for mode characteristics showed a predominance of the oral mode in structured situations at the primary and intermediate level classes. In language-dependent situations at the high-school level, the predominance of the oral mode continued in one school, while manual, written and combined modes were used roughly equally in another.

In the schools for the deaf investigated, limited emphasis was placed on the purpose of the students' communication, with the most obvious finding being the high level of teacher-initiated communication at all student ages. It is not clear to what extent this outcome occurred in schools for the deaf as compared with schools for the hearing, since none of the latter were included. The results of the work of McKirdy and Blank raised two main questions which their study, by design, was not able to resolve. Did the hearing-impaired students lack the ability to initiate communication? Or did they not get the chance to initiate it? Further research is required into learning under different conditions and in a variety of settings, to determine what changes in student communication would occur if differing proportions of interactions were controlled by teachers.

A subsequent investigation exploring classroom communication patterns and communication modes was conducted by Lawson (1978) to assess whether deaf students spend more classroom time on compliant, rather than self-directive, communication. Lawson adapted her method from Craig and Collins (1969), dividing it into the self-directive communications of the students and student-compliant communications. These two main categories were further subdivided to include self-directive behaviour addressed to the teacher or to another student. Lawson's study differed from that of Craig and Collins in recording exchanges not only between teachers and students but also between students themselves. However, no specific data were presented on teacher influence. Lawson gathered data from five intermediate level classrooms with student ages ranging from 10 to 13 years. One class was slow, three were average and one was advanced in achievement. Lawson offered no further information as to the degree of hearing loss of the subjects, how achievement levels were determined, or the reliability between the two observers who recorded the data. The results showed that both student-directive and student-compliant communicative behaviours occurred. The most frequent student-directive communication was 'informing', with 'following directions' being the most frequent student-compliant communication act. Students communicated during 64% of the observation period, with over half of this communication being student-compliant .

Lawson drew a number of parallels between her work and the earlier studies of Craig and Collins. First, the most frequently used category initiated by students in both studies was Informing, followed by Questioning. Secondly, there were few counts in the Development category. In order to find the extent of teacher-dominated communication, Lawson combined the categories of teacher communication with student-compliant communication for comparison with Craig and Collins' teacher-initiated communication. A large difference was found, with less teacher domination occurring in Lawson's study. Lawson suggested that this difference could be attributed to the didactic methods used with the lower grades investigated by Craig and Collins, and the possibility of changing communication involvement patterns in classrooms for the deaf, over time. However, the drawing of parallels between the two studies is questionable given the differing populations used. Further, Lawson's objective was not specifically to consider teacher dominance, since she used a category system where all teacher communications were grouped together. Combining teacher communication with student-compliant communication did not therefore necessarily facilitate a valid comparison with Craig and Collins' teacher-initiated communication category. Little information was given by Craig and Collins about the teaching methods used in their study, while Lawson provided no evidence in support of any change in communication involvement patterns in deaf classrooms. Lawson suggested that the lack of communication in the category of Development may show that hearing-impaired children do not actively integrate information into their own thinking. This view was shared by Craig and Collins (1969), but requires further investigation.

Craig and Collins' work also influenced Wolff (1977), who developed a Cognitive Verbal, Non-Verbal Observation Scale (CVNV) for in-service training of teachers in the area of cognition. This scale was used to investigate communication patterns in classes for deaf children employing different communication modes. It was based on an affective–cognitive system in which a category of communication intent, a level of cognitive implication of the communication, an indication of the mode, and a tally for the direction of communication were recorded. The CVNV schedule was based on a modified version of Craig and Collins' (1969) adaptation of the Flanders' Scale, with cognitive levels based on Piaget's levels of development. In contrast to Craig and Collins, but in line with Lawson (1978), the CVNV was able to assess student-to-student communication. However, Wolff's work differed from both in that data were provided on the cognitive levels at which the interaction generally occurred.

Limited data were provided about the population used in Wolff's study, which incorporated a wide age range of students from preschool to high-school level. No further information was given concerning the degree of hearing loss, mode of communication or classroom environment. Comparisons were drawn between traditional and cognitive classrooms, but definitions were not supplied. The lack of data and explanation in this study makes it difficult to ascertain exactly what the author was trying to achieve. The results, expressed as percentages, were compared with those obtained by Craig and Collins. Wolff, and Craig and Collins, found that 'teacher talk' comprised 47.3% and 48.5% respectively of the total talk in the primary school. At the intermediate and high-school levels, Wolff found teacher talk to be 43.4% of the total talk, while Craig and Collins found it to be 56.4% at the intermediate level, and 57% to 59% at the high-school level, depending on the subject matter. A comparison between the teachers in Wolff's study and those in Flanders (1965) and Craig and Collins (1969) at the primary level, showed that CVNV-trained teachers were 17% less immediately directive. Consequently, the students in Wolff's study showed 17% more student communication. Similar findings were reported at the intermediate level.

Taking into account the differences in the systems of analysis and the fact that teachers in Wolff's study had been trained to encourage non-directive language-supportive instruction, these results are to be expected. Wolff concluded that CVNV-trained teachers of the deaf are less immediately directive and that, as their skills improved with his training, their classes would communicate more. However, a comparison group was not used to compare direct and indirect communication, and comparisons with previous studies need to be interpreted with care. In considering the percentage of communication with cognitive intent, Wolff found that the content centred around activities involving memory and classification, with little attention paid to inference building. There was a tendency for TC classes to show more open communication than the oral classes, while those classes which employed only fingerspelling were the least open in communication. Wolff pointed out that there were differences in the three methods which could have influenced his findings about cognitive behaviour. However, whether these findings were a function of teacher style or the methodology used is unclear.

Interim summary

The studies reviewed so far showed that linguistic control of classrooms for the deaf has tended to be in the mouth and hands of the teacher, regardless of communication mode or ages of the children. However, there were indications that teachers needed to be more sensitive to the communication needs of deaf children. The studies attributed deficiencies in communication skills solely to deafness, though this conclusion cannot be fully accepted in the absence of data specifying the influence of age, IQ, hearing loss, family environment and so on. Also, several studies had design flaws, making their interpretation difficult.

Recent work with teachers

More recent work by Wood et al. (1982) examined the influence of classroom environment and the influence of the teacher in relation to deaf children's limited conversational abilities. The aim was to determine how far deaf children were capable of complying with conversational demands, and whether the ensuing conversations were governed by similar dynamic principles. Moderately to profoundly deaf children aged from 6 to 10 years from 16 different classrooms were involved.

Their non-verbal IQs ranged from 81 to 126. Data were collected in a 'news session' in which the children were asked to tell the teachers and the other children of their experiences outside school. The validity of such sessions is questionable when studying conversation, because it largely involves a monologue from the child who stands in front of the class, when a number of unconsidered child-related variables may be operating. However, an analysis of teacher talk and its relationship to averaged measures of child talk was presented. Transcripts were coded in two ways. First, the conversational moves of both teacher and child were classified into levels of control, and secondly, teacher speech was analysed in terms of the functions in each utterance. The authors were interested in the nature of the children's responses to different linguistic demands and the extent of their mean length of turn (MLT). The predictor variables were the various levels and functions of teacher moves in dialogue. A teacher power ratio was obtained from the percentage of questions and requested repetitions. Child-initiated measures were obtained from the percentage of questions, elaborations and contributions. The results were compared with an earlier study by the same authors of adult–child conversations involving young hearing children.

Initial analysis revealed that deaf children responded to the structure of teacher talk in a similar way to hearing children. Where teachers asked a high proportion of questions, children tended to display low initiative, indicating a strong effect of teacher style on the conversational capabilities displayed by children, whether hearing-impaired or hearing. In more detailed analysis, the deaf children were found to elaborate on their answers to questions only 14% of the time. They tended not to ask for repetitions or clarification, 'read' the basic force of teacher moves and seldom confused open and closed questions, and made their own contribution by developing a theme.

The relationship between moves and functions in teacher speech was also examined to reveal that some moves in teacher speech were associated with longer utterances from the children than others. This could have been a reflection of differences between the children and/or conversational style. A significant correlation was observed between MLT and hearing loss, with the least hearing-impaired children producing longer utterances. A significant correlation was also found between the frequency of move and hearing loss, where teachers tended to ask open questions of the least hearing-impaired children. It should be noted, however, that MLT does not necessarily enlighten us as to the child's conversational abilities. It could have been more informative to consider either syntactical complexity or conversational intent. Further, information about the mean number of utterances addressed to each child, the number of children in the group and perhaps even the topic of conversation is required before firm conclusions can be drawn on the correlation between teachers' conversations and hearing loss.

Continued investigations were reported by Wood et al. (1986) into why, after many years in school, most deaf children leave with low levels of linguistic and academic achievement. A summary of their conclusions, which relate mainly to orally educated children, is relevant to the consideration of pragmatics in communication. Wood et al. concluded that the disruptions, which occur for younger hearing-impaired children in mother–child and teacher–child interactions, are caused by specific difficulties in communication. An example would be the division of attention which occurs when the hearing-impaired child has to use vision to attend to both acts and objects of communication. However, adults, including teachers, may express unhelpful and even counterproductive behaviour which denies the child access to the naturally occurring non-verbal communication that helps hearing children to acquire an understanding of speech. Wood et al. concluded that the central role played by adults in guiding and promoting a child's progress through the stages involved in acquiring verbal communication is often not fulfilled for hearing-impaired children, especially where the child needs to learn how to distribute attention between communication partner and the object of the communication (compare Huntington and Whatton, 1981, 1984, 1986).

Despite the accumulating evidence of its occurrence, the didactic, overly-controlling, non-contingent ways of adult communication with hearing-impaired children continue (Lai and Lynas, 1990), though they occur more in the classroom than the home (Bodner-Johnson, 1991). Harrison et al. (1987) found, for example, that teachers interacting with four severely to profoundly deaf preschool children used labelling, modelling and correction techniques extensively. Little use was made of expansion or completion of a child's utterances, nor of reinforcement, repetition or amplification of utterances. Wood et al. (1986) were particularly critical of the question–answer exchange, which typifies many teacher–child interactions in school. This theme has been continued by Wood (1991). Wood et al. further saw teachers' language in the classroom as making no greater linguistic demands of older than of younger deaf children. The teacher's language was therefore probably not sufficiently challenging of the linguistic competence of the older children. It will be recalled that, in Chapter 2, we raised a similar query in asking whether parental language is properly 'tuned' to the linguistic abilities of hearing-impaired infants.

Nevertheless, it is unfair to single out teachers. Tests of reading designed for hearing children have also been criticised as insensitive to the linguistic abilities of hearing-impaired children, and hence poorly reflect their competencies and needs (Wood et al., 1986). Appropriate tests are important because oracy is closely involved with the development of literacy, and hence relevant tests are needed to assess both spoken and written language. The mismatch between the linguistic competence of hearing-impaired children and the demands of texts may lead to teaching strategies that teach special tactics for understanding reading material, rather than assisting the development of true literacy.

We have noted that it is sometimes said that teachers use relatively less figurative or idiomatic language with hearing-impaired children. In work by Newton (1985), communicative patterning in the classroom was investigated with a focus on the teachers' use of non-literal language as part of the linguistic environment. Newton remarked that whereas the poor English language abilities of hearing-impaired children had been attributed to impaired hearing or inadequate teaching, research was needed on the kind of language models used. He chose to study teachers' use of non-literal language because this aspect was commonly seen as deficient in hearing-impaired children. Newton compared the language spoken to hearing-impaired and hearing children to assess the influence of teachers' perceptions of the children's needs, and the influence of constraints in their children's linguistic ability on teachers' adaptations. For example, did teachers who used an oral-only approach with hearing-impaired children, use less non-literal language than teachers communicating with hearing children of comparable linguistic ability? Did teachers communicating by TC use less non-literal language than teachers using an oral-only approach when addressing hearing-impaired children?

Newton examined the use of two kinds of non-literal language: idiom ('That's kind of funny') and indirect requests ('Why don't you sit down?'), commonly used to communicate with hearing children. His subjects were 30 teacher–child dyads: 10 with hearing children; 10 with hearing-impaired children using aural/oral communication; and 10 with hearing-impaired children using TC. Each group consisted of dyads from two different programmes in two different cities. For hearing teacher–child dyads, the children were aged 2–3 years with a mean length of utterance (MLU) of at least 2.0. The teachers were those who normally worked with the child. For hearing-impaired teacher–child dyads, all children were prelingually profoundly deaf. Language matching was based on MLU data, though the hearing-impaired children had higher MLUs of at least 3.0. These children were also cognitively, physically and socially more mature, with ages ranging from 5 to 9 years. All their teachers were of normal hearing, had taught hearing-impaired children for at least 3 years, and were well-acquainted with the child in their dyad. Two tasks were assigned to each dyad – spontaneous communication and storytelling. Only the oral component of the TC teachers' language was assessed, as their greatest use of non-literal language always occurred in this oral component.

For idiomatic usage, no differences were found in the teachers' use of non-literal language between speech addressed to hearing and to oral hearing-impaired children on either task, although there was less use of idiomatic language, in both the oral and signed components, when TC was used, especially for the signed component. No significant differences were found in the oral component for indirect requests between the three groups, though few indirect requests were actually presented to the hearing children. However, only 55% of these requests were presented non-literally in the signed portion of TC.

Thus the results did not support a hypothesis of greater use of idioms by teachers with hearing than with oral hearing-impaired children, but the expected difference between oral- and TC-educated hearing-impaired children was found. For the hearing-impaired children educated via TC, their teachers seldom used idiomatic structures, and when they did, about two-thirds were not signed for the children to observe. Teachers used no more indirect requests with the older and cognitively and socially more mature hearing-impaired children. The explanation is unclear, as the maturity variables between hearing and hearing-impaired children were not adequately matched.

In conclusion, both the earlier studies (Craig and Collins, 1969, 1970; Wolff, 1977; Lawson, 1978) and the more recent reports (Wood et al., 1982; Newton, 1985; Wood et al., 1986; Wood, 1991) reveal an inappropriate, overly directing orientation in teachers of the deaf towards their students, which Wood (1991) has ascribed to the effort involved in coping with individuals who have weak communication skills. This style seems universal where there is a large mismatch in communication between hearing adult and deaf child. It may partly explain why similarities are found in the approaches to coping with classroom conversations in hearing-impaired and learning-disabled children (Weiss, 1986).

It would be informative to discover if overly directing approaches by native deaf signing teachers of the deaf do not occur towards native deaf signing students, who would communicate well in sign. There is some evidence that this is the case. Observations by Mather (1989) suggested that, of two teachers, one who was a native deaf signer encouraged wh- questions, risk-taking, role-playing, etc., in her deaf preschool students more than a hearing teacher using signed English. Also, Murphy and Hill (1989) and Musselman and Churchill (1991) have concluded that communication by TC, with its sign component which puts hearing teachers and deaf children on a more even communication footing, is effective in developing pragmatics skills in deaf children, allowing the children to obtain more conversational styles or more conversational control. However, the results of Newton (1985) are grounds for scepticism about such a conclusion. TC may have the potential to assist the development of skills in pragmatics, but this potential may not be realised.

Interactive communication patterns

The next group of studies to be reviewed consider the interactive communication patterns of hearing-impaired children, beginning with work on referential communication, which relates globally to pragmatics.

We start with the study by Hoemann (1972), in which the accuracy and quality of peer-to-peer referential communication in prelingually profoundly deaf children who used sign was compared with that of hearing children using spoken English. Half the subjects had a mean age of 8 years and half of 11 years. Half were hearing and half were deaf. The reader is referred to Chapter 5 (page 112) for other details of design and methodology.

Receiving scores were higher than sending scores for all four samples. As this finding was most marked in the 8-year-old deaf subjects, it suggested that their low communication accuracy score was due more to poor messages than to poor receiving skills. The hearing subjects manifested two achievements lacking in the deaf children, namely, establishment of a social contract over whose perspective to take, and description of pictures in left–right trials according to the receiver's right or left hand. In the task of explaining the rules of a game, results were recorded both before and after prompting, and classified as adequate, fair or deficient. Little difference in deaf subjects was noted before and after prompting, whereas the hearing children were able to add rules they had omitted. Younger and older deaf subjects with deficient explanations behaved inappropriately. However, all 40 deaf subjects were able to teach their peers how to play the game when permitted to demonstrate the rules in action, suggesting that although they knew the rules, they were unable to communicate them manually to their peers.

Whilst Hoemann's study indicates that deafness was a handicap in peer-to-peer communication, there are other aspects to be considered. Was the poor performance of the deaf children due to the channel properties of sign? Hoemann noted some instances where gestural communication presented special difficulties, but it is unclear whether they were sufficient to account for a generally deficient performance. He hypothesised that a general experiential deficit could account for the handicap, presenting evidence in the form of overlapping contributions of scores, in which some deaf subjects did as well as their hearing peers. Further, the role of experience in developing communication was indicated by the improvement with increasing age. There are several other factors which need to be investigated before accepting this explanation. Previous experience with similar tasks needs consideration, as does the developmental stage of an individual's manual communication skills. Also questionable is the extent to which formal referential tasks may have restricted the use of non-verbal modes of communication (Chapter 7). Hoemann's study provided an interesting basis for further work on interactive communication patterns of deaf children. However, it was limited in terms of furthering our knowledge of deaf children's communicative competence in social communication.

Similar remarks can be passed on the work of Jordan (1983), who studied pairs of hearing-impaired children ranging in age from 3 to 15 years, and a hearing group, pairing the children by age. They were asked to describe 25 pictures to an age-matched listener, so that the listener could identify the picture from a picture set. Differences were found with age in communicative accuracy across age groups of hearing-impaired subjects and between hearing-impaired and normally hearing children, but statistical evaluations were not reported.

Other workers, however, have not found differences between hearing and hearing-impaired children on referential communication tasks. Thus, Breslaw et al. (1981) compared groups of hearing-impaired children with a mean hearing loss of 88 dB and a mean age of 8 years, from different educational backgrounds, with groups of hearing children. Each child had to place coloured blocks on a board and tell a listener about it, so that the listener could perform the same task. The performances of the hearing-impaired and the hearing children were generally not significantly different.

It is of interest to enquire further into whether communication mode affects the conveying of information in referential communication. This question can be answered by comparing the performance in the same task of hearing-impaired children who communicate in different modes. For instance, message-formation skills involved in referential messages from differently communicating hearing-impaired children to their mothers were studied by MacKay-Sorota et al. (1987). The children were aged 6–10 years, and came from oral or bimodal, namely, oral plus manual programmes. They were tested in two tasks. In the first task, the children described a specified picture in a set of four, so that the mothers could identify the referent from the alternatives. In a second task, the children viewed a single picture, and subsequently had to identify it from a set of four related pictures. Nevertheless, although their hearing losses were greater, the bimodally educated children produced more differentiated messages than the orally educated children. They also gave better reformulations of messages that at first were inadequate. Although the mothers of the orally educated children received inferior messages, they were as successful as the mothers of the bimodally educated children in selecting the correct referent. This result is odd. It suggests that the picture-description task was too simple to be a good test of differences in modality in conveying the information as compared with forming it. Both groups of children were near-perfect on the picture recognition task, showing that the differences in the first task were due to differences in skill at message formation rather than differential visual perceptual processing of the task materials.

More detailed research is needed in the area of referential communication with hearing-impaired children to answer the several queries which we have raised. The results outlined are insufficiently clear, and conflicting.

We now consider a selection of other work on interactive communication, to illustrate further interactive communication patterns.

Interactive communication in group work has been described by Pendergrass and Hodges (1976), who observed children involved in group problem-solving. Six groups, comprising 4–6 severely to profoundly deaf children each, were brought together to solve a problem presented to them by the examiner. The Bates' (1950) Interactive Process Analysis (IPA) procedure was used to evaluate the quantity and quality of communicative interactions. The IPA has a standardised set of 12 categories, and interaction can be considered in a number of ways – in relation to the 12 categories, the four major areas into which the 12 categories can be grouped, and/or pairing specific categories with each pair representing a typical problem in group interaction.

The six groups were divided so that four contained younger, 6–9-year-old, children with limited formal communication skills. The other two contained older, 11–13-year-old, children with more refined skills. Two problems were presented. The first was a puzzle, and the second involved unscrambling letters to form words that matched pictures of animals. Pendergrass and Hodges stated that the problems could be solved for the most part with limited formal communication skills, but they encouraged maximum communication between students. Data were recorded in relation to the child initiating the interaction, the child being addressed, and the category of communication.

While the distribution of communication activities among the 12 categories revealed the use of all categories, few interactions were recorded in a 'questioning' category, implying that these deaf children lacked the general ability to ask for information, make suggestions, provide orientations, or seek clarification of the opinions of others. Interactions within the four major categories saw 'attempted answers' ranking the highest, followed by 'positive social–emotional areas'. 'Questions' ranked the lowest. A comparison of positive and negative social emotional areas for each group found little difference between them, in the groups of younger children. However, a higher percentage of interaction in the positive area was found in the groups of older children. This may indicate that, with maturity, the deaf child becomes more task-orientated.

Without a comparison group of hearing subjects, it is not clear whether the degree of interaction between the hearing-impaired subjects would differ significantly from that for hearing subjects. Whether the problems presented actually encouraged interaction is also questionable. Considered with the other studies reviewed above, problem-solving tasks by pairs or larger groups present some difficulties in their application to informal social communication. They do, however, permit not merely an estimate of how well a message was communicated or received, but also a systematic analysis of communicative intent and social interaction.

It is of special interest to study the pragmatics of communication in deaf infants in their first few months of life, before the emergence of recognisable language. We need to know, for instance, how early prelingual communication patterns develop so that we can interpret the mapping of communication through verbal or sign language on to prelinguistic forms. A longitudinal study which offered insights into this process was conducted by Scroggs (1983) on the communicative interactions between hearing-impaired infants and their parents. Four hearing-impaired infants identified in their first year were video-taped for half an hour once a month in play sessions with their parents. Observations concentrated on the communicative strategies used by the children and their parents. The preliminary observations involved the behaviour used by the parent or child to initiate 'conversations', the simultaneous and sequential turn-taking behaviour used to sustain conversation, and the procedures used to end them.

The first observation was that rhythmical behaviour occurred when the parent and infant were communicating. This behaviour played an important role in engaging the infant's attention, in cueing the infant into a familiar play sequence, in checking the infant's interest in a particular game, and in continuing the conversation through imitating the infant's behaviour. In addition, a coordinated rhythmic behaviour was observed, which served as a turn-taking strategy. The infant became familiar with a behaviour pattern and would wait until the mother had finished before taking his turn. This rhythmic behaviour was seen as playing a fundamental role as the basis for successful communication. The communicative strategies used by deaf infants and their parents differed little from those of hearing infants. Vocalisations were not the major factor in conversations, which may explain why the auditory component does not, at this stage of development, cause serious disruptions to communication, and also why deafness in infants is not easily suspected by parents at early developmental stages. Scroggs did not, however, point out that the parents' knowledge of their child's deafness may have influenced some or many of the interactions observed.

All too often the education of hearing-impaired children has emphasised the acquisition of vocabulary and syntax, without an equal and necessary emphasis on the use of language for interaction in communication (compare Duffy, 1984; Giorcelli, 1985). Facilitation of interactive communication patterns was investigated by Antia and Kreimeyer (1985), who introduced social interaction routines to assist peer interaction in preschool hearing-impaired children. They devised a programme consisting of a number of social skills and social interaction routines. The programme was administered to three groups of preschool children, with 3–5 children in each group. The children were aged 3–5 years, with normal IQs and mild to profound hearing losses. All wore hearing aids which were checked daily. Two groups used oral communication while the third used signed English. The programme was conducted for 20–30 minutes each day over 1 year.

Data were collected from observation of the frequency of peer interaction, and from a questionnaire for parents and teachers, on which they rated the children on changes in interaction skills at home and in class. The data showed that positive interactions increased from an average of 6% to 12% of recorded intervals before the programme to 30–38% during the programme. Questionnaire data indicated increases in Praising and Cooperating for some 80% of children and increases in Sharing and Assisting for 70%. Teachers reported no change in negative behaviour for 80% of the children, while parents reported a decrease for about 70%.

Like several others in the field, this study of Antia and Kreimeyer was not designed so that the effectiveness of the programme, which looks impressive, could be validly assessed. There was no matched control group which did not receive the programme, nor were data offered about the progress which might be expected over 1 year by hearing children of similar age. The results are therefore more indicative than compelling.

Summary and conclusions

Analysis of the communication of hearing-impaired children has, in the past, focused on the linguistic aspects of vocabulary, syntax and, to a lesser degree, phonological development. However, with a growing emphasis on pragmatics, in the fields of normal and specific language impairment, researchers have begun to broaden their perspective to include pragmatics in considering how hearing-impaired children put language to use. The available literature is small and has to date made little use of pragmatic theories and systems of analysis.

Our review has examined the research in two main areas – communicative intentions and conversation. There are few general conclusions that can be drawn from the research, for several reasons. First, research in this area is scanty (Foster et al., 1989). Secondly, the majority of studies used a research design which had lacunae in one or more of the following:

1. Did not draw on benchmark measures, which could have been obtained by incorporating control groups.
2. Did not assign children randomly to experimental and comparison (control) groups or, where matched groups were used, did not use appropriate matches.
3. Made limited use of statistical methods to test the reliability and significance of results.
4. Omitted to measure or record salient subject variables.

In fairness we should note that such design issues are not limited to work on the pragmatics skills of hearing-impaired children. They are to be found also in other areas (Beisler and Tsai, 1983; Prinz and Ferrier, 1983; Damico et al. 1984).

Investigations of the functions that utterances serve revealed that hearing-impaired children code a variety of communicative intentions. The work of Skarakis and Prutting (1977), Curtiss et al. (1979) and Scroggs (1983) showed that hearing-impaired infants and young children express similar semantic functions and communicative intentions to those of hearing children at the prelinguistic and one-word stage. For older individuals, the interviews conducted with college students by Foster et al. (1989) suggest practical contexts where future work may be undertaken to advantage. All these studies have implications for assessment and remediation. Analysis procedures could be used as assessment tools. Parallels drawn between hearing-impaired and hearing subjects can provide the language teacher with guidelines for the content and sequencing of language remediation programmes. Results illustrating the interdependence of semantics and pragmatics also hold implications for remediation. It may be worthwhile, for example, to teach the use of a particular semantic function with a number of different pragmatic intentions. In addition, it could be shown that one feature in pragmatics can be used to express a variety of semantic functions. The extent to which the hearing-impaired differ significantly from hearing individuals in this area is not clear and further research is needed for the planning of adequate remediation programmes.

McKirdy and Blank (1982), who evaluated language within a communication framework, pointed out that past discussions of language programmes have seldom concerned communication or the multiple roles that communication demands. The assumption had been that if a suitable linguistic system was available to the child, it would invariably be followed by the ability to communicate through that system. Their study showed that this is not necessarily so. In conversation, their hearing-impaired children functioned both as initiators and responders, but their pattern of performance differed in quantity of conversational turns, and the quality and complexity of the interaction. The data showed that communication ought not to be considered as inevitably following from given language abilities.

Work which considered communication patterns in the classroom indicated that the degree and type of communication used by the students was heavily dependent on the teacher. There were a number of limitations in each of these studies, and differences across groups and methods of analysis did not enable adequate comparisons to be drawn between the studies. However, the reports provided information on measuring instruments, such as the instrument devised by Craig and Collins (1969), modified by Lawson (1978), and by Wolff (1977). The reports also contained implications for investigating teaching methods. Some suggestions for further research have been indicated.

The rationale within our schools for the deaf is to provide not only academic training, but also language-supportive and language-stimulating instruction. Granted these goals, there are clear implications for reassessing teaching methods. The degree to which hearing-impaired children in the classroom have the opportunity to initiate and engage in interactive communication should be queried (Wood et al., 1982, 1986; Wood, 1991). Further research is thus required into learning in different communicative roles and in a variety of settings. This research would determine the degree of change in student communication when faced with varieties of teacher talk.

A weaker performance by hearing-impaired children, in comparison with hearing children, was found by Hoemann (1972) and Jordan (1983) in the accuracy and quality of peer-to-peer communication, though Breslaw et al. (1981) found otherwise. Whether it is hearing loss that causes this possible handicap, and/or the manual method of communication, and/or other factors, requires further investigation. One means would be to conduct studies with children who are proficient in manual communication, or those using an alternative means of communication. In this context, Newton's (1985) report suggests strongly that the use of idiom is restricted by normal forms of communication.

The study by Pendergrass and Hodges (1976), which considered interactive communication patterns through a group problem-solving task, showed that deaf children were limited in their ability to question and that, with increased maturity, the deaf child became more task-orientated. This study may help educators of the deaf with teaching group problem-solving tasks. It is implicit that small group analysis provides a structured tool for the identification of specific strengths and weaknesses of pragmatics skills in hearing-impaired children. The findings suggested that for educators to help hearing-impaired children in these skills they may need to devote more time to intensive training in questioning skills, in reinforcing social maturation by teaching positive social skills in group problem-solving situations, and in training the skills needed for attention to tasks. The findings of Antia and Kreimeyer (1985) pointed in the same general direction.

Some of the fundamental groundwork for the understanding of the pragmatics skills of hearing-impaired children has been laid. The continuation of research in this area is important not only for the understanding of communication in hearing-impaired children, but for the ongoing development of remedial programmes. The studies reviewed raise a number of issues to which more fundamental research can now be addressed.

By way of final comment, we note that no published studies have focused on the development of pragmatics skills in young cochlear implantees. Given that certain pragmatics skills in communication are known to precede the use of language in hearing infants, this is astonishing. Some of the procedures currently used in the rehabilitation of young implantees should benefit from increased attention to the pragmatics of communication, rather than concentrating quite so much on the use of hearing and aural rehabilitation in the narrow sense. Techniques of the type described by Tait and Wood (1987), covering the progression from non-verbal communication to language, and involving visual attention-sharing and turn-taking, suggest some paths to be explored.

Chapter 9
Management of the Hearing-impaired Child

This chapter outlines selected 'milestones' seen as historically important in approaches to the management of the deaf child. It then considers a number of issues of a practical nature which bear on education and therapy. The chapter concludes with a consideration of the options available to parents with young severely to profoundly deaf children, and remarks on several areas about which there is continuing debate.

Up to about the 1960s, the approach taken towards the rehabilitation of hearing-impaired individuals was based on the defectology model. Hearing-impaired people, especially those deafened before acquiring verbal language, were regarded by and large as 'defective' (Garrison and Tesch, 1978; Murphy-Berman et al., 1987). Although such individuals could gain from rehabilitation and education, it was generally believed that their communicative abilities remained problematical, and they could not attain the life styles of hearing individuals. Nor should they aspire to do so. A particularly moving account of the experiences of deaf individuals in such a climate is given by Petkovsek (1961), and a very readable collection of the varied experiences of deaf people can be found in Taylor and Bishop (1991).

Negative attitudes towards deaf individuals among professionals have changed, but they have far from changed elsewhere, in both children and adults (Dengerink and Porter, 1984; Sacks, 1989). Attempts to modify these negative attitudes meet with mixed success (Strong and Shaver, 1991).

Some Milestones

Professional attitudes towards hearing-impaired individuals and their rehabilitation have been subject to fashion and change no less than other topics in human affairs. As a result, certain areas in the treatment of deaf people have varied in prominence over the years. We comment now on several, not necessarily directly connected, topics which have affected the management of hearing-impaired children over the last few decades.

Linguistic deviancy

Some expressions produced by hearing-impaired children have been represented as 'deafisms', a kind of linguistic deviancy, most marked in commentaries about the attempts of deaf children who are trying to grasp verbal language. Such deafisms have been ascribed to children with the more severe hearing handicaps, especially the profoundly deaf. This topic is important. The implications are weighty if deafisms are so pervasive as to constitute a deaf communication system or language (deaf English), because it will be hard to develop communication skills if the linguistic base is obscure to others (see below).

Linguistic deviancy can be associated with various impairments besides deafness. Hence, if deafisms are unique, it must be shown that their linguistic divergence differs qualitatively, or shows marked quantitative differences, from other deviances. It is easy to confound linguistic deviancy with language delay, as when a certain expression appears to be deviant at first sight, given the age of the child, but on inspection is seen to be due to delayed rather than divergent language development. If deafisms are uniquely divergent, they should occur uniquely in the language of hearing-impaired children and not occur in the early development of hearing children or elsewhere.

Deviancy is, by definition, difficult or impossible to analyse with the conventional tools used in language analysis. Such a situation will at once alert us to a possible deviancy. However, we will need several instances of such deviancy if we are not to regard it as an idiosyncrasy or slip of the tongue, or as an unwitting error or lacuna in writing. We also need to be careful lest the apparent deviancy represents an accepted local form, for example: 'She's having a maggot' – a seeming semantic deviancy, used by a hearing-impaired child in Oxfordshire, UK, to describe to the writer's colleagues a picture containing an obviously annoyed woman.

Fusfeld (1955) saw the deviances of hearing-impaired individuals as a state of non-language, because the words were not aligned in an orderly way. Myklebust (1964) gave instances of linguistic deviancy, but did not seek any systematic characterisation among them. As he remarked, we need to know not only whether hearing-impaired children have reduced linguistic skills, but whether their errors show characteristic patterns. Brannon (1968) studied the picture-elicited spoken language of hearing, partially hearing and profoundly deaf children with a mean age of 12;6 years. He found a marked decrease in the number of words used as hearing loss increased. He also found that of 14 parts of speech analysed, the partially hearing differed notably from hearing children only in the use of adverbs, pronouns and auxiliaries, in which the deaf children were the most deficient. These deaf children used all classes of words, except conjunctions, less than the hearing children. Brannon confirmed Goda's (1964) previous finding that the speech of profoundly deaf children contained relatively fewer 'function words' (auxiliaries, prepositions, etc.) than the speech of hearing children. However, because of the method of analysis, the distinction was presented quantitatively, and hence the observed differences were of degree rather than kind, even though the speech of the deafer children seemed 'telegraphic' (Goda, 1964).

Similar findings were obtained by Pressnell (1973) for the comprehension and spoken syntax of 47 profoundly deaf and partially hearing children with an age range of 5–13;3 years, using the Northwestern Syntax Screening Test (Lee, 1969) with a set of pictures. While analysis showed that the performance of the older was superior to that of the younger hearing-impaired children, further analyses of spontaneous utterances, scored according to Lee and Canter (1971), showed that the children had the greatest difficulty with compound verbs. Relatively little difficulty was found with uninflected verbs and the copula. The results revealed particular difficulties with auxiliary verbs and morphology, but again the differences were in degree rather than in kind.

Wilcox and Tobin (1974) used a sentence-repetition task to assess the spoken language of hearing and hearing-impaired children. Special attention was paid to verb constructions. Results for their 11 congenitally mildly to severely deaf children, of mean age 10 years, and 11 hearing children of the same mean age, showed that verb constructions were significantly poorer for the hearing-impaired than for the hearing group. Wilcox and Tobin concluded that the performance differences across the verb forms were distinguished in quantity rather than in quality, since the patterns of scores were similar for both groups. However, they remarked that there was a marked divergence in performance for (*have* + *en*) and negative passive. Use of the negative passive in particular showed a considerable difference between the groups. These instances suggested a difference in kind, tantamount to a qualitative difference. Also, the relatively marked difficulty with (*have* + *en*) was similar to the findings of Pressnell (1973) – see above – indicating that hearing-impaired children have a characteristic difficulty with this verb form.

Ivimey (1976) commented that evidence of deviant skills abounded in the literature and, in reviewing studies such as those described above, asked if the many defects and deviances in the language of the deaf were sufficiently consistent and widespread to justify classing them as a system that is the only one of its kind, namely, a peculiar language that differs to a greater or lesser extent from normal English. This is an interesting question because, if the language of the deaf is different in kind from normal language, then deaf people will have qualitatively distinct communication skills. Ivimey thus asked whether the language of deaf children was systematic and, if so, whether it was congruent with the language of hearing children. If not, was it to be considered a deviant subsystem or as a language in its own right?

To answer such questions requires the analysis of a large corpus of material from a large representative sample of deaf children, because the need is to show whether the majority of deaf children exhibit the linguistic behaviour in question. The effort involved in such a task is so great that it has not been attempted on the scale desired. Rather there are a number of relatively small-scale or individual studies. One such study was that described by West and Weber (1974) for a partially hearing girl aged 4 years, who produced a number of non-standard English forms, such as bound morphemes like 'badboy', in addition to conventional English. Other interesting reports include that of Davis (1977), who found that one group of hearing-impaired children with moderate hearing loss, and another group with severe to profound hearing loss, had difficulty with linguistically advanced forms. Since the hearing-impaired children studied by Davis and the other workers cited above had problems with the more difficult linguistic constructions, it is not clear that their language was deviant. Rather, it could be argued that the language was retarded.

Most of the quoted examples of deviancy in the literature have been obtained from written rather than spoken examples. One of the few large-scale studies of spoken language from hearing-impaired children was reported by Bamford and Mentz (1979). They found no syntactic deviancy in a detailed grammatical analysis of picture-elicited speech in a sample of 263 children aged 8–15 years with mild to profound hearing losses. However, their sample overall comprised partially hearing rather than profoundly deaf children.

The studies outlined so far were mainly concerned with grammar. Studies of semantics in hearing-impaired children are relatively rare, although this area overlaps that of cognition, which has received considerable attention. Investigations that show semantic deviancy are even rarer. One such investigation, noted in Chapter 8, was recorded by Green and Shepherd (1975), who explored the adjectival semantic structure of the language of 33 severely to profoundly deaf children, aged 9–18 years with performance IQs of 80–125, with the semantic differential technique as adapted by Di Vesta (1966). The data from 28 scales were subjected to factor analysis, yielding six factors. The first two factors reflected the Evaluative ('good–bad') and Potency ('weak–strong') dimensions respectively, as seen also in the semantic systems of hearing children. However, the hearing children's Activity dimension ('slow–fast') was displaced by a dimension involving sensory judgements associated with visual and tactile modalities ('wet–dry', 'round–square'). Other factors found in the semantic systems of hearing children were missing. Hence Green and Shepherd found an unusual pattern of semantic factor structures with this group of deaf children.

More recently, Schaefer (1980), who was interested in the semantic relationships underlying the categories which capture verb meaning, prepared videotapes of situations encoded by the categories 'cut', 'break', and 'open', which were arranged as expected- and unexpected-choice pairs. Various groups, including deaf and hearing children, matched as the 'same' one choice from a pair to a video-taped sample of the expected category. The choices for the children, as compared with adults, showed that unexpected choices were preferred as a match, with the choices of younger and older hearing children following a developmental pattern. Although the basis for their choices was not clear, the deaf children did not fit this pattern. Their performance may have been associated with problems of developing meanings for words as independent entities (Lewis and Wilcox, 1978). More studies of this type, concerning boundary features of words, which minimally constrain judgements of 'sameness', would be of value.

Commentaries on linguistic deviancy in the spoken language of deaf children have fallen away in recent years, though Bamford and Saunders (1985) observed that even if 'deaf English' was denied as a system, deafisms were still commonly found. In part, the reduced emphasis on deafisms is due to an emerging realisation that hearing-impaired children do not form as homogeneous a group as originally thought. Hearing loss is only moderately positively correlated with linguistic development, and other factors such as age, intelligence and auditory perceptual and cognitive processes need to be considered. For the present, a convincing case, based on substantial data and thoroughgoing analysis, has yet to show that the language of deaf children, or of any well identified deaf subgroup, contains linguistic deviancy to such a degree as to confirm the existence of a deaf verbal language. The language of hearing-impaired children generally approximates to standard verbal language, though it is characterised by difficulties with linguistic forms more complex than simple SVO constructions (Leslie and Clarke, 1977; Tate, 1980).

For some hearing-impaired children these problems will be temporary. They will go on to master the more complex forms in due course. For others, there will be a level beyond which they will find it difficult to proceed (compare Charrow, 1975). We have considered some of the reasons for this situation in previous chapters. It is particularly disconcerting to have to remark that the cause of unusual language in deaf children is repeatedly ascribed not so much to deafness itself, but to the ways in which the deaf child's education has been managed (Arnold, 1978; Gormley and Franzen, 1978; Wood, 1991).

Advent of hearing aids

The development of the wearable hearing aid, in the years leading to and following the Second World War, did much to reveal to administrators, educators and therapists, and hearing-impaired people themselves, that hearing-impaired individuals could be divided broadly into two groups. The majority had usable residual hearing in the region of mild to severe hearing loss. For most of the individuals in this partially hearing group, the fitting of a hearing aid made the speech of others accessible. Even though distorted, as the hearing aids of the time were rather crude audio-amplifiers, and given also the distorting effects of inner-ear hearing loss, access to the speech of others allowed the child to communicate fairly well. Although partially hearing children with prelingual hearing loss experienced difficulties in language development, and even those children who became hearing-impaired postlingually had real problems, they were nonetheless generally able to acquire language and speech. They were hence able to communicate at levels not too different from those of their hearing peers, especially when given sufficient therapeutic and other support. One result was that a large proportion of hearing-impaired children formerly regarded as 'defective' could be seen as more like hearing children, though the obvious clumsily packaged body-worn aids of the time continued to mark them as different.

Conventional hearing aids were, and are, of much less help to the child with profound hearing loss. Although high-gain and other sophisticated aids give the child a perception of the rhythms of speech, and can assist with the discrimination of some speech sounds, it was and has remained generally the case that many, if not most, children with profound prelingual deafness do not acquire sufficient speech, let alone intelligible speech, despite the strenuous efforts of parents, teachers and therapists.

Part of the problem is that hearing-impaired children, particularly those who are born profoundly deaf, have problems in generalising from one stimulus situation to another. Although a given communication skill, such as distinguishing one phoneme from another, may be learned, it proves difficult for the child to translate the skill to other phonemic contexts. Also, while a particular approach to the perception of speech may be taught and learned sufficiently thoroughly for a given purpose, it is not transferred to other parts of the programme (Fisher and Schneider, 1986). We noted similar problems in our discussion of social skills in Chapter 8. It is as though the child comes to regard what is taught in a given situation as specific to that situation, and not to be used, or not of use, outside it. The problem may arise from the approach taken to the child's remediation or education, where segmented teaching produces segmented communication skills. Or perhaps it is a characteristic of deaf children, who have problems in understanding the value of listening (Smith and Richards, 1990).

Various authors have remarked on ways to overcome the difficulty (Ling, 1976; Fisher and Schneider, 1986), but further research is required. Increased use of group discussion in the classroom, which is designed to allow the practice of skills taught to children individually, and which forces the use of a variety of communication skills if the child is to contribute, may be one way forward. Even so, and although there were, and continue to be, remarkable exceptions (McCartney, 1986), generally the profoundly deafened ear yields aided hearing which is too limited or too distorted for the acquisition of speech and language, and hence severely reduces opportunities for everyday communication (Maxwell, 1989).

Aided hearing is improved only modestly by speechreading. As noted in Chapter 3, only about half of the phonemes can be perceived visually. Only about eight can be identified without ambiguity, and that under good seeing conditions such as short distance, good illumination and limited angle of regard (Erber, 1979). These conditions are not easy to meet in the classroom. Given that speechreading often has to take place in less than good seeing conditions, that only some phonemes can be perceived visually, that most prelingually profoundly deaf children do not have well developed skills for coding speech, and have a weak verbal language which makes it unproductive for them to guess, it is scarcely surprising that the use of speechreading and what little residual hearing they may have is often ineffective (Conrad, 1979).

Where the use of speechreading appears to be efficacious, the perception of the speech may be due more to a lack of control for gestures and to the level and use of residual hearing, which is such that the child is severely rather than profoundly deaf. Erber (1972, 1979) has shown that the contribution of speechreading to speech perception in hearing-impaired children is relatively small, and is about the same for profoundly and severely deaf children. Younger postlingually profoundly deaf children are in only a moderately more advantageous position as regards aided hearing, depending on the extent to which they could recognise speech sounds before the deafness occurred. Although then, the advent of wearable hearing aids may have helped to remove the stigma of defect from partially hearing children by improving their verbal communication, it did less to help children who were profoundly deaf.

Recognition of sign language

Profoundly deaf individuals who communicate by sign continue to be seen as in some way defective. The use of sign marks them as very different from hearing people. Historically, because hearing people have not understood sign, they have held it in contempt (De l'Epée, 1784). The recognition of sign as language was also held back because the field of linguistics was insufficiently advanced and because those who used it as their first language, namely deaf signers, did not have the academic background to research it. However, in the 1960s, the work of Stokoe and his colleagues (Stokoe, 1960; Stokoe et al., 1965) began to change the perceptions of professionals about sign and its users. The earlier perceptions that the gestural means of communication used by profoundly deaf people was less than an accepted language began to alter. Although there are dissenters (see Chapter 5), it is now generally accepted that deaf sign language is a language in its own right (Lane, 1988). Its native users are increasingly seen as different rather than deficient, which can only assist in the management of the deaf child.

Sign language is increasingly used in schools for the deaf, although it has yet to be used extensively in deaf education (Woodward and Allen, 1987). An impressive token of its acceptance in the community is that sign language is now offered to hearing students in schools and colleges as a second language (Chapin, 1988; Selover, 1988).

Diversity in communication ability

Research over the last 20 years or so has shown that, within limits, hearing loss or deafness is not the sole determinant of difference. Nor does it make sense any longer to lump together all individuals with a given degree of loss, such as severe or profound deafness. Research has shown that deafness leads to cognitive and linguistic differences which are the proximal causes of several communication problems, with hearing loss itself being the distal cause. There is, for example, particular diversity in communication ability in children who are severely deaf. Some severely deaf children behave like other children with lesser degrees of hearing loss, and communicate orally. Others operate more like the profoundly deaf child who prefers to sign. The difference is probably associated with the child's development of inner speech (Conrad, 1980). However, even profoundly deaf children seem to have at least some elements of coding for inner speech (Geers et al., 1984), perhaps developed through residual hearing, speechreading or kinaesthetic stimulation, while hearing individuals, who operate on the basis of inner speech can also acquire coding processes for signs (Crittenden, 1974). As we have seen, there is conflict in research findings on the oral and manual communicative abilities of severely and profoundly deaf children. This conflict is often a reflection of the considerable diversity in communicative abilities found among hearing-impaired individuals of all ages, even within narrow ranges of hearing loss.

Acknowledgement of diversity in communication, the increasing recognition of sign as a language, the development of combined communication methods such as TC and cued speech, the use of signed forms which approximate the syntax of spoken English, and research showing the limitations of the oral approach, have dealt severe blows to the former dominant position of oralism in deaf education and therapy. It is all the more surprising, in view of the displacement of oralism, that the movement towards integration or mainstreaming of hearing-impaired children into normal schools was prosecuted with such vigour and resolution in the 1970s and 1980s. It is, however, clear that the impetus to mainstreaming is here to stay, though not all would have it so (Branson and Miller, 1989). The advent of combined methods helped to promote such mainstreaming but, more importantly, the move to decentralise deaf education was the result of new thrusts in political philosophy (Trybus, 1987). Drives towards social equity and equal opportunity in access to society's resources have included hearing-impaired individuals in a trend which accepts difference and diversity, but not separatism. Whatever the merits or disadvantages of mainstreaming for education or remediation, one positive effect is that of providing for recognition of diversity and hence reducing the stigma of defect associated with separatism.

'Deaf power'

A further force to challenge oralism, with obvious implications for the management of communication for the deaf child, is the movement to promote deaf–mutism in the form of deaf culture – 'deaf power' (Nash and Nash, 1981; Sacks, 1986, 1989; Rutherford, 1988). This movement is characterised by its own institutions, attitudes and ways of socialisation, in addition to striving to raise the status of sign language (Humphries, 1991). The deaf culture movement has become very active in recent years, notably among and for the severely and profoundly deaf. The origins of this increased activity stem largely from the notions of equity discussed above, but also from a rejection by deaf pressure groups of the paternal orientations of institutions for the deaf. These institutions have usually been administered by hearing individuals, and many have tended to perpetuate, sometimes insensitively, their own practices and agendas rather than those of their clientele (Schowe, 1979; Lane, 1990). The deaf culture movement is notable for the emphasis it has given to the recognition of sign language which 'belongs' to the deaf community, and which the movement has promoted as a communication mode to be recognised as having a rightful place of its own.

In understandable zeal for its recognition as a linguistic minority using sign, the deaf culture movement has opposed the promotion of medical technology where the technology aims to assist the deaf to communicate by hearing, and especially against research in and application of cochlear prostheses. Such has been the vehemence of this clash that some members of the deaf culture movement see the advent of the cochlear implant prosthesis as threatening to eliminate deafness and hence the very existence of deaf culture, in a kind of genocide (National Union of the Deaf Steering Committee, 1982). It is presently too early to ascribe such a threat to cochlear implant programmes, for the reasons given in Chapter 3, though the situation could change quickly with developments in technology.

Lane (1990) was particularly critical of implant programmes. He argued that the increases in speech perception and production gained with a cochlear implant are modest; that about one in 30 implants develops surgical complications; that a partially successful implant may be worse than none at all as it may hinder or delay the acquisition of sign language on which the implantee will have to fall back; and that there were insufficiently considered ethical issues. Among these ethical issues was the likely rejection by signing deaf adults of an implant were they to be offered one (Evans, 1989), and hence a possible wish by implantees, later in life, that they had not been implanted as children. Wilbers (1988) mused that, if a cure could be found for all deafness, some hearing-impaired people would choose not to avail themselves of the remedy, while nearly all would lament the break-up of a close-knit community. The view here is that the deaf community is defined by a common language, a common means of communication in sign and a common culture, and not by a handicap. The difficulty is that there are no clear and unambiguous rules for deciding how to separate diversity from deviance (Lane, 1990).

Practical Issues Affecting Management

This section discusses some practical issues closely related to hearing for the child with mild to moderate, and severe to profound hearing loss. Next follows consideration of some social aspects of practical relevance, such as involvement of the family in assessment and remediation, the relationship of child and family with professionals, and the relationship of the hearing-impaired child alone with professionals. This then leads to an outline of mainstreaming (integration) activities.

Mild to moderate hearing impairment

The child with a mild to moderate hearing loss will communicate with parents and peers, and embark on programmes of instruction at school via hearing. Such children usually develop and progress in ordinary ways, although their language development and academic achievements may be retarded. The identification of these children is frequently made around the age of 1–5 years or so, when slowness in language development and other behavioural milestones leads to a check of their hearing status. Preschool and school-age hearing screening programmes also identify large numbers of children with mild to moderate hearing losses.

A few of these children will have inner-ear losses, but the greater number will have a middle-ear problem. A high proportion of these middle-ear problems, especially in the case of mild hearing losses, will resolve themselves as they are caused by a cold or other upper respiratory tract infection, which is of short duration and remits spontaneously. Mild losses due to transient infections are very common – so common, indeed, that it is preferable to check for their continued presence some 4–6 weeks after the first detection, rather than to make immediate referrals for medical treatment, unless there are clear signs of pathology such as suppuration or inflammation. Persistent mild to moderate hearing losses of middle-ear origin should, however, be referred for treatment without undue delay. There is evidence that a persistent, or fluctuating hearing loss delays the acquisition of language and academic progress (Bamford and Saunders, 1985). If untreated, the condition may develop into the more serious problem of secretory otitis media or other sequelae.

Where, following medical treatment, there continues to be a mild to moderate conductive or inner-ear hearing loss, and where there are no medical contraindications of serous otitis or otherwise, the fitting of a hearing aid may restore the hearing threshold to normal. However, the fitting of aids may not be very helpful with mild losses, if the child spends much time in noisy surroundings. In any case, the child will continue to acquire information orally, though parents and teachers should be advised on management techniques which will minimise the effects of the hearing impairment on communication and learning. Children with unilateral hearing losses, even if quite severe, will also learn to communicate orally, though they will experience communication problems, especially in noisy environments, which are likely to compromise their educational development (Bess and Tharpe, 1984).

Severe to profound hearing impairment

The situation is very different when we consider children with severe to profound hearing losses. Fortunately, the greater the hearing loss, the easier it is to detect (Upfold and Isepy, 1982). Thus children with marked hearing losses are usually identified fairly early. The proportion of such children in the general population has declined considerably since the late 1960s, due in large part to the success of rubella immunisation and other programmes (Upfold and Isepy, 1982). Yet although the incidence of congenital moderate to profound hearing impairment is reduced nowadays, children with such degrees of impaired hearing continue to be found. Services to assist in the development of their communication skills are constantly required.

For reasons considered earlier, there is a very considerable difference required in the management of the prelingually and postlingually hearing-impaired child. A postlingual hearing loss, occurring after the age of 2 years or so, and certainly by the age of 3–4 years, means that the child will usually have acquired sufficient language through hearing and sufficient inner speech to continue with oral education. There is no doubt that the education will at times be very difficult, but generally there will be a firm base in oral language and communication from which residual hearing and speechreading can be used to make significant progress. For the prelingually hearing-impaired child the situation is quite dissimilar, especially where the child is born to signing parents, as we have seen.

Granted the very considerable diversity across many variables among prelingually deafened children, which has been a recurring theme in this book, a child's inclinations towards oral, manual or combined communication can be reinforced from an early age, by taking a cue from the child's preferred means of communication (Conrad, 1980). A problem arises, however, when the approach is not limited to the supportive or remedial, but becomes what Lewis (1968) has called prophylactic – when we foster the child's tendencies in a direction which *we* prefer. Then there arises the question of which communication method to teach.

At this point, we need to review our previous consideration of early intervention and its effects (Chapter 2). We saw that all, or almost all, reported early intervention programmes included some aspect of oral training, even in programmes where manual communication was fostered, and all, or almost all, such programmes fitted hearing aids. Early intervention programmes which relied entirely on a manual means of communication were very rare or non-existent. This is to be expected in the case of deaf children born to deaf parents: manual communication is their natural communication mode. The children themselves are the experts, and early manual-only intervention would be a nonsense. There is, however, a case for the early teaching of a gestural form of communication to deaf children born to hearing parents, and to the parents themselves, whether to supplement the use of residual hearing, as with cued speech, or to enable such children to learn a sign system or language to communicate with deaf peers. Such signed intervention is worth considering because most deaf children born to hearing parents learn sign language from other deaf children, and hence their learning of sign is impoverished and parochial (Stokoe, 1983).

Irrespective of mode of communication, the great majority of prelingually severely to profoundly hearing-impaired children do not develop verbal language and academic skills appropriate for their age, as shown time and again in the literature (McConckey Robbins, 1986). Yet the studies of early intervention reviewed in Chapter 2 suggest that significant gains can be made in language development over various periods by the young hearing-impaired participants in these programmes. Thus, although early-intervention programmes may produce important gains, almost all the hearing-impaired children who participate in such programmes still show delays in verbal language and academic achievement throughout their development. Although they may follow the same path as hearing children, their progress is slower and there is some evidence of deviancy. As a result, continuing attention is being paid to the identification of the relevant factors and their manipulation in management strategies and educational curricula (Cole and Mischook, 1985; Mischook and Cole, 1986). Until such research provides more illuminating information than is currently available, it is premature to close off the options for communication mode, by arguing exclusively for one mode versus others.

As the field develops, new and sometimes disturbing findings emerge concerning some of the effects of early intervention. For example, we saw that listening skills, involving hearing, attention and understanding, may be learned in task-specific situations, but frequently fail to generalise to daily life. The problem could be due to a failure in management to teach listening skills in settings which promote communication as a social activity. We also saw that educational practice has been criticised for teaching language, especially syntax and vocabulary, by overly formal techniques. It now appears that similar criticisms can be levelled at some early intervention activities (Fisher and Schneider, 1986). Socialisation begins from birth, and accompanies the development of communication in hearing children until they are able, on entering school, to divorce the social aspects of communication from the academic ones. By school age, hearing children have a sure social, language and communication system which supports the more abstract levels of language learning offered in school. However, younger hearing children acquire their linguistic and communication skills in the strong social context of the family. It therefore seems clear that language and communication need to be taught in a socially relevant way in early intervention programmes, especially while the rudiments are being learned.

Family involvement

For the severely to profoundly deaf child born to deaf signing parents, the child's signing family environment is most probably the normal communication environment. This situation is implied by the almost complete silence on the topic in the literature, though that very silence makes us cautious about being too dogmatic on the subject.

For hearing parents, the discovery that their child is deaf or has a severe hearing loss often results in a period of extreme stress (Moores, 1987). Ogden (1984) and Ogden and Lipsett (1982) have described a sequence of reactions through which parents pass: shock; recognition; denial; acknowledgement; and constructive action. Some parents may stay indefinitely at one stage in this sequence, without proceeding through all the stages.

Parents' usual initial reaction is one of shock when told that their child has a serious hearing impairment. This reaction may extend over a few hours or a few days, and is characterised by a stunned withdrawal. After the initial shock there follows a period of recognition, in which the parents begin to explore the implications of their child's hearing impairment, and to learn about the medical, social, educational and communicative aspects. At this stage, the parents may experience feelings of anger, frustration, guilt, blame and grief. As they realise the demands which will be placed on them and their child in coping with the hearing impairment, they may attempt to deny the fact of the child's hearing loss. Nevertheless, they usually come to acknowledge the existence of the problem, and discuss it with their relatives and friends. Finally, they set themselves to learn more about the child's hearing impairment and participate in the child's rehabilitation and education. In such a sequence of stresses, parents need support and advice in the management of their child. Indeed Luterman (1979) has argued that, to begin with, the parents need more attention than the child. As Mischook and Cole (1986) have pointed out, the parents are not to be seen as intruding on the management and rehabilitation of the child. Although their initial reactions of shock, confusion and so on may not be in the best interests of the child, it is of great importance for therapists and teachers to resolve such emotional responses in order to recruit the parents to work for the child's remediation.

As they begin to overcome their emotional reactions, parents feel daunted by the task of assisting in the development of their child's communication, and especially by the effort involved in teaching language. They may feel inclined to back off, though achieving reciprocity in parent–child interaction is seen as highly important for the child's social progress and the development of communication skills (Hadadian and Rose, 1991). At this stage, professionals need to be competent to explain the nature of the task, to facilitate decisions about which communication mode to use, and to promote the child's development. Parents and other family members can be encouraged to start by observing and recording the child's efforts to communicate. Such observations and records will not only help the family to adjust to the problem, but will greatly assist the work of the professional. They will also help to orient the family, and especially the mother, who usually takes the lead in deciding on the communication method to be used (Kluwin and Gaustad, 1991), towards managing the child's communication, rather than relying too heavily on professional help. The professional then becomes the adviser to the family, rather than being the immediate agent for change.

Cole and St Clair-Stokes (1984) presented a procedure for video-recording and analysing those caregiver–child interactions which can facilitate or hinder the child's communication. Video-recording can be introduced from an early stage, as soon as the parents are ready to accept and use it. As a guide, the literature contains several papers (Bromwich, 1981; Blennerhassett, 1984; Matey and Kretschmer, 1985; Nienhuys and Tikotin, 1985; Connard and Kantor, 1988; Plapinger and Kretschmer, 1991; and others) describing communicative behaviour between caregiver and child for hearing, hearing-impaired and other children, from infancy to school age. Video-recording techniques can be used (Cole and St Clair-Stokes, 1984) to illustrate such desiderata as talking in a normal way within the range of the child's hearing ability; using normal gestures appropriate to the topic and the child's age; avoiding the use and elicitation of single words; using connected speech with the appropriate length and level of complexity, depending on the child's age and ability; allowing the child to take a turn; keeping up with the interests of the child for a significant part of the time; responding to all, or almost all, of the child's attempts to communicate; talking about people and objects in the immediate context; and using various strategies to maximise hearing. This list implies an oral approach. However, it may be adapted where the communication mode is manual, or where some auditory/manual combination is used.

The use of video-recordings helps to involve other members of the family in the rehabilitation of the child, gives them a feeling that they can make useful contributions, and guides them in matching their communication behaviour to levels and activities which suit the child. At the same time, those aspects of the communicative behaviour of members of the family which do not help the child can be identified, and discouraged in further interaction. The use of video-recording in this way is somewhat similar to that of keeping a diary of caregiver–child interactions (Pearson, 1984). However, video-recording provides for replays of detail in ways that a diary cannot.

The understanding of the child's message in response to parental communication requires concentration and guessing. Further, whereas the parents of hearing children can continue with other activities while talking to their child, these other activities have to stop when communicating with the hearing-impaired child. Parents cannot take it for granted that their messages will be received by their hearing-impaired child and need to check on message reception and understanding. The availability of radiofrequency hearing aids assists only a little in coping with this situation. Communication between parent and hearing-impaired child needs to be explicit. As the child develops, parents and other family members become concerned with issues other than communication, such as concepts in ethics and morality, for example. Getting across to the child such abstract concepts as moral behaviour involves a considerable effort (Ogden, 1984). Much research is needed in this area.

Although many publications suggest that the quality of interaction between hearing-impaired children and their families is of considerable importance, there have been few well designed empirical studies in the area. Bodner-Johnson (1985) described some activities and interactions between families and their pre-adolescent hearing-impaired children. In this study, the parents of 125 prelingually severely to profoundly deaf 10–12-year-old children were interviewed in their homes. Parents' responses were factor-analysed to produce representative dimensions, which were subsequently used in a discriminant analysis to investigate those dimensions in the family environment that distinguished the children's levels of achievement in reading comprehension and mathematics. Children with high levels of achievement in reading and mathematics had parents who were attuned to their child's hearing loss and pressed the child to achieve.

Interestingly, family involvement in the child's academic learning was less important in attaining levels of achievement than the parents' acceptance of the hearing impairment and their thrust for the child to achieve. These parents reported that they had accepted their child's hearing loss early on, and had integrated the childs' needs, including special communication needs, into the family routine. They tended to use methods of simultaneous communication and were permissive, rather than over-protective, in their child-rearing. They praised the child's school work, had made plans for the child's future education, and had relatively high expectations for the child's further education and occupation. The parents viewed their child's hearing loss as a personal characteristic of the child rather than as a handicap. They had also dealt with each crisis in a rational way, while recognising their own emotional responses. They saw their lives as a sequence of more or less difficult stages, and recognised the difference. In their treatment of the child, they gave similar supervision to that expected for a hearing child. They did not so much change their rules for their hearing-impaired child's behaviour, as modify their style to take account of the hearing loss.

In work on the parental experiences of mothers of severely to profoundly deaf adolescents aged 12–18 years, Morgan-Redshaw et al. (1990) interviewed five hearing mothers who were willing to share their experiences, from a pool of about 50. At a first interview, the mothers were allowed as much time as needed to relate their experiences as mothers of deaf children. There followed an interval of 2–3 weeks, during which the mothers kept a record of their further thoughts and feelings, and incidents during the interval which related to mothering. They were then interviewed again and, when offered additional information, they elaborated on responses to some points raised in the first interview, and discussed the themes in the first interview.

The main themes were several: the mothers' personal growth, which was extended by their experiences; the mother–child relationship, which showed more dependence of the child on the mother than occurs for hearing children;

parent–professional relationships, which included a mix of positive and negative aspects; school programmes, some of which were highly praised while others were described as unpleasant, non-challenging or non-facilitating; fluent communication, where fluency in communication was seen as more important than the method of communication; and sources of support. These sources were multi-faceted, with hearing siblings being generally supportive but not always so because, particularly in the earlier years, the hearing-impaired child needed much of the mother's time, and the siblings had to assume additional responsibilities because of the needs of the deaf child.

The five mothers participating in this study were a small group, but represented a range of parental experiences. A major methodological drawback was that the mothers were selected for their willingness and ability to share their experiences, and were possibly non-representative of mothers of hearing-impaired children as a whole. However, the study has value in showing that the mothers' varied experiences could be represented in six main themes, which were identified and discussed. It is reassuring to note that the mothers were fond of their hearing-impaired children, generally thought of them highly as individuals, and had managed to establish satisfactory communication. However, the mothers found the absence of a cure, and their inability to prepare the children for a full life painful and frustrating. Although as the child grew older these negative feelings grew less, they continued to surface occasionally.

Hearing-impaired children, families and professionals

A variety of recent research reports referred to the roles of various professionals (e.g. Harvey, 1989; Erlbaum, 1990): factors associated with the selection of modes of communication in various settings (Caccamise et al., 1983; Raimondo and Maxwell, 1987), the communication skills of professionals in sign language (Caccamise et al., 1990), the effects of different ethnic backgrounds (Cohen et al., 1990), competencies for teaching (Luckner, 1991a) and the attitudes of deaf adults to sign systems used in classrooms (Kautzky-Bowden and Gonzales, 1987). With the placement of hearing-impaired children in schools catering mainly for hearing children – the mainstream or integration approach, reviewed for its history by McCartney (1984) and more recent developments by Schildroth (1988) – many papers have dealt with factors guiding parents and others about placements (Jones, 1984; Bunch, 1987; Goldberg et al., 1989), the classroom participation of mainstreamed hearing-impaired students (Saur et al., 1986, 1987), and reverse mainstreaming, which involves bringing hearing children into classes for hearing-impaired students (Dean and Nettles, 1987). These papers raised a plethora of stimulating findings and equally stimulating questions, which we cannot cover here.

Of immediate interest, however, is the way in which hearing-impaired children, their families, and the therapists, teachers, and other professionals interact. Since the information that their child has a hearing impairment is so often stressful for parents, some earlier workers suggested that a professional discipline be formed for parent counselling (Whetnall and Fry, 1964; Northcott, 1975). Such calls have not been made in recent years. Most families seem to get over an initial crisis and, as with Ferguson and Watt (1980), who found no more anxiety in mothers of severely mentally handicapped children than in mothers of normally developing children, continuing maladjustment to the child's hearing handicap was probably never of frequent occurrence.

Nonetheless, parent counselling needs to be handled sensitively. The way in which parents of hearing-impaired children saw how they were informed of their child's hearing loss and how they were advised in coping with the situation was investigated by Williams and Darbyshire (1982). They interviewed 25 families with severely or profoundly deaf children under 11 years of age who were educated in a variety of placements. The parents, who covered a wide range of social backgrounds and came from predominantly rural and small town areas in Canada, had little or no contact with other parents of hearing-impaired children. Their experience is probably typical of parents in rural areas in other countries also.

The age at which parents first suspected a problem ranged from 4 months to 6 years, with a mean of 28 months, but the responses of family physicians led to the postponement of diagnosis of hearing impairment. Eighty per cent of the family physicians appeared to disagree with or dismissed the parents' suspicions. The mean age of the child at diagnosis was 48 months, following several steps of professional involvement (physician, otologist, audiologist etc.), but the diagnosis, rather than the delay, caused severe negative reactions in 80% of parents. Most (84%) were unable to understand all the information given at diagnosis.

Only a minority of the families received professional in-home training. Although parents accepted the value of home training, they themselves did little of it, except for the parents of deaf preschoolers who had experience of the government's peripatetic preschool teaching programme. The service offered by the preschool visiting teacher was praised consistently, though not more than one-third of the sample had experienced it. Parents commonly complained that they did not know of the services available. Also there was little follow-up by the professionals who had made the diagnosis. Eighty-eight per cent of the parents stated a need for more factual information about hearing impairment, what the hearing loss meant for their child, the future prospects for the child, child management problems, and correspondence courses. Few parents realised that they could be the main agents for change in managing their child. This situation seems unfortunately to have been all too common up to the 1970s and, in predominantly rural areas, up to the 1980s.

The provision of family therapy is worth considering for families in which there are hearing parents and at least one deaf child whose preferred mode of communication is manual. The provision of family therapy in such situations, together with the use of an interpreter for communicating in sign, was proposed by Harvey (1984a). The therapist was seen as knowledgeable about the psychosocial and cultural aspects of deafness, and should preferably be able to communicate in sign language and signed English, although it was not feasible for the therapist to interpret for all the family while providing treatment. Harvey thought that the use of an interpreter went beyond the facilitation of communication between family members who used spoken English and the deaf child who preferred manual communication. The interpreter could help the therapist to modify family rules that denied the implications of deafness and forbade the use of sign. The interpreter could also help to modify the balance of power in a family threatened by allowing the child to communicate, through the interpreter, in sign, and to encourage parents to bring to awareness their emotional responses by projecting, transferring or displacing to the interpreter their feelings about their deaf child.

Scott (1984) took issue with aspects of Harvey's approach. Scott viewed the approach as condescending towards the families, who were seen as incompetent without the therapist's intervention, blaming of the families for compounding the deaf child's problems, overly focusing therapy on the disability and on communication at the expense of other family problems, sidestepping the family's natural pace of transactions in order to communicate at the speed that the therapist thought was adequate, and antagonistic towards the family rather than encouraging it to develop its resources. In a spirited defence, Harvey (1984b) referred to the controversy pervading the provision of psychological services to deaf individuals. He saw the controversy as rooted in communication, namely, how and to what degree communication takes place between deaf and hearing people. His case for the use of interpreters was for families whose deaf child preferred manual communication when hearing members of the family communicated verbally. Such families commonly, though not always, prohibited the use of sign. Harvey listed specific points for family therapy: it was impossible to do therapy and be an accurate interpreter at the same time; the therapist must respect each individual's model of the world, and preferred mode of communication; and the therapist must be a competent family therapist and be knowledgeable about deafness. He saw no need for condescension or lack of respect.

Hearing-impaired individuals and professionals

A short review of communication between health care professionals and deaf individuals, primarily as hospital patients, was published by Ludders (1987). He saw most hospital staff as knowing little about deafness and how deaf people communicate. The first encounters with hospital staff caused deaf patients to experience a high degree of anxiety. The problems may have dated back to the deaf patient's early family experiences as a sick child, when all communication took place between the usually hearing parents and the physician. No one may have made the effort to explain the illness to the child (Di Pietro et al., 1981). Ludders suggested a role for social workers as advocates for deaf patients. Such social workers would not be expert about deafness, but should be trained to be sufficiently knowledgeable in identifying and resolving communication problems between deaf patients and health care professionals.

The counselling of families of hearing-impaired children by Australian and United States audiologists was investigated by Martin et al. (1989), using a questionnaire approach. Audiologists reported parental denial of hearing loss more frequently than the parents themselves. It is thus interesting to note that parents in both countries appreciated 'honesty' in the audiologist. For both countries also, many parents gave sorrow as a typical subsequent response. There was a suggestion that many audiologists did not realise how long a parent's sorrow about their child's hearing loss may persist. Most parents and audiologists in both countries found it helpful for parents to watch the assessment of the child's hearing ability. A similar proportion of parents in both countries stated that they had received the same kinds of information about the child's hearing impairment at diagnosis, with a high proportion of parents remarking that they wanted details of the hearing loss at diagnosis. However, several parents' wished to receive details later when they felt less emotional, or to receive written information for later perusal. Martin et al. recommended that, because parents' reactions were so varied, audiologists should follow parents' leads in presenting factual information. Referral to a parental support system was strongly recommended.

The importance of parental counselling, support and case management of the hearing-impaired child continues to be recognised by audiologists. However, audiologists are divided on the issue of how much responsibility they should assume for case management, with many realistically seeing this responsibility as shared with other professionals, such as the classroom teacher (English, 1991).

As hearing-impaired children attain school age, they could themselves be asked how they perceive the approach used by the professionals responsible for their development. It would be of particular interest to learn how hearing-impaired children feel about their experiences during the difficult time of transfer from home or preschool to primary school. There have been reports of this transition, and the transition from school to community, which refer to family issues, both for children with hearing-impairment only and for children with hearing-impairment and other disabilities (Elliott and Powers, 1988; Davis and Bullis, 1990). However, little is known specifically about the children's views.

There is a considerable literature on the attitudes of teachers to students and to their work with them, teachers' views of their own abilities, and to the views of older students of their teachers' and interpreters' instructional ability (e.g. McKee and Dowaliby, 1985; Murphy-Berman et al., 1987; Foster and Brown, 1989; Mertens, 1991). In one such study, differences were found by White (1990) in the way in which teachers of hearing-impaired children perceived their ability to teach speech, their own ability to understand deaf speech, and the ability of hearing-impaired children to use speech. Not surprisingly, teachers from schools which differed in the communication mode taught to hearing-impaired children differed in expectations for the children to attain speech. As also expected, teachers with greater oral experience held higher expectations for a child's speech than teachers with experience of TC. Teachers with oral experience also had the most confidence in their ability to teach speech, and placed the greatest importance on the use of speech. However, some teachers who used an oral approach in a residential school were less confident about the children's potential to achieve speech than teachers in oral day schools.

White argued that, although they may have held a good opinion of their abilities to teach speech, their work in a residential school gave them a different, and lesser, expectation of the children's speech potential. He also argued that variables associated with the attitudes of teachers to speech development were among the most important variables involved in speech instruction. He felt that significant gains might never be made in developing speech in hearing-impaired children until there was a fuller appreciation of the emotions underlying the teaching and learning of speech. In this sense, the social environment in which the child is managed may be as important for speech development as knowledge about speech, and the effort put into its teaching. There is evidence to support this view showing that the social environment created by teacher expectations has a significant effect on a child's performance (Martinek, 1980; Ryan and Levine, 1981).

Mainstreaming (integration)

In the 1980s, teachers in schools for hearing children became increasingly concerned with the education of a variety of handicapped children who had moved from special schools and institutions to normal schools. The mainstreaming, or integration, of these children greatly stretched and expanded the skills of teachers. Initially there was much comment from the teachers themselves and in the media about the strains that integration imposed on the teachers and on the handicapped children, despite some obvious benefits such as the decrease in stigma associated with handicap, as hearing individuals became more aware of handicapped children.

The management of the hearing-impaired child in the normal, or regular, classroom is difficult because the hearing child learns largely through speech, and spends about half of the time at school in listening (Berg, 1987). On the other hand, effective teaching of hearing-impaired children is generally best attained by the use of more visual, pictorial material supplemented with spoken information (Waldron et al., 1985). Even so, hearing-impaired children need to be able, in a mainstreamed setting, to operate their hearing aids, to change the batteries, and to use such messages as: 'I can't hear you'; 'I don't know'; 'Please say it again'. Deaf children often just shrug their shoulders when addressed, making it difficult for the teacher to follow what is meant (Cochrane, 1991).

We saw that the attitudes of teachers can have significant effects on the achievements of their charges, and Strong et al. (1987) have remarked that in some cases, the teacher's willingness to accept hearing-impaired children into classes hitherto designed for hearing children has been a factor in the children's placement (compare Salend and Johns, 1983).

Chorost (1988) asked: what were the attitudes of such teachers who were relatively or absolutely untrained for teaching hearing-impaired children; did their attitudes change when hearing-impaired children were placed in their classes; what support services did they think were helpful; and what could be achieved to make the placements a more positive experience? Chorost studied the integration into regular classroom settings of six children with congenital mild/moderate to profound hearing losses, ranging in age from 3 to 12 years. Support was provided by special materials and access to a teacher of hearing-impaired children. From a survey of teachers' initial feelings on learning that they would be teaching hearing-impaired children, five of 15 teachers surveyed were negative or very negative, and eight were positive or very positive about the forthcoming experience. Two were neutral. All teachers expressed initial anxieties. At the end of the school year, only one teacher rated her feelings as very negative as compared with three teachers who had given very negative initial ratings. Eight teachers rated their experience at the end of the year as very positive, whereas only two teachers had given initial ratings of very positive. Four teachers felt the same at the end as at the start of the year, but the remainder felt more positive. Thus there was an important overall shift towards positive feelings by the teachers between the start and end of the year, but not by all teachers. Importantly, no teacher felt more negative at the end than at the start of the year.

Sixty per cent of the teachers felt that the placement was appropriate for the children, especially given a support structure. However 40% thought the opposite, indicating that a given child was so far behind classmates that little mainstreamed academic learning took place, and that too much of the teacher's time was taken up by such a child, to the disadvantage of the hearing children. The teachers reported different experiences on the amount of extra time spent with the hearing-impaired children, ranging from an extra 5–15 minutes, up to an extra 1–2 hours per day. Eight of the 15 teachers became comfortable with the child in their class during the first month, while two more teachers took 1–3 months. One-third of the teachers never felt comfortable with the hearing-impaired child placed in their classes. The teachers used the support resources to different extents. On being asked what else could have helped, they cited observations of other classes with integration children, extended use of a class aide, more visual and manipulable teaching aids, and advance notice of the child's characteristics, including secondary handicaps.

Chorost concluded that, although much extra time and effort was generally demanded of the teachers, most thought that the time and effort was well spent and saw the experience as a positive one. The teachers of the younger children, from kindergarten age to grade 2, felt less positive than the teachers of the older children in grades 3–6, perhaps because the older children were able to work more independently. It is not clear whether the younger children were among the more severely hearing-impaired, which could also account for this result. However, Chorost did indicate that children with mild or moderate hearing losses could be viewed more positively by teachers than children with severe to profound losses. The lack of information and adequate preparation of teachers found by Chorost has been reported by others (Hull and Dilka, 1984; Martin et al., 1988). It is a severe criticism of the lack of planning by employing authorities.

The overall situation has been assessed very recently by Luckner (1991b). He sent a questionnaire to members of three organisations for teachers of the hearing-impaired, who were asked to pass it on to normal education teachers who had a hearing-impaired child in their classrooms. A 58% response rate ($n = 354$) was obtained from teachers working with hearing-impaired children aged 4–18 years. The 16 questions in this survey were adapted from Chorost (1988) and addressed teachers' attitudes to working with hearing-impaired children, the amount of extra time entailed, the type of administrative support received, the type of help given by teachers of the hearing-impaired, their perceptions of the functioning of the hearing-impaired student in the normal classroom, their perceptions of how they might be better prepared, and any suggestions they had for teachers of hearing children who had hearing-impaired children in their classes.

Most respondents stated that when mainstreaming began, they felt positive or very positive towards the forthcoming experience. Only 6% recalled negative feelings, while 31% were of neutral outlook. At the end of the year, 89% felt positive to very positive and wished to continue with another hearing-impaired child. They also replied (86%) that they felt comfortable with the hearing-impaired child in less than 1 month, and that the child needed only an extra 5–15 minutes attention each day. The teachers received only minimal administrative support, and consulted the teacher of the hearing-impaired less than six times per month. Almost all (95%) of the teachers regarded the placement of the hearing-impaired children in their classrooms as appropriate. The perceived socialisation of the hearing-impaired children was variable. About 12% did not socialise well or worse, some 26% had adequate socialisation skills, about 28% had good socialisation abilities, and about 34% showed high socialisation skills.

Generally, then, the teachers participating in this survey felt positive about working with integration hearing-impaired children, on whom they did not spend a great deal of extra time. They saw the children as appropriately placed in their classes and often socialising well, implying that the placements were suitable for the educational management of the children, and that the children were able to develop and use communication skills with their hearing classmates (Ross et al., 1982; Saur and Stinson, 1986). However, the teachers lacked appropriate preparation and assistance. Also, plans specifying objectives for placements, programmes and services were not sufficiently delineated, and systems for evaluating the progress of the hearing-impaired children were insufficient. Powers (1990) has expressed similar concerns. Further, the effects of the changes caused by integration programmes on teachers of the hearing-impaired, who often acted in a consulting role, had yet to be considered in detail. Luckner recommended that teachers of the hearing-impaired should be instructed, as trainees, in the role of collaborative consultants for teachers in integration classes.

Luckner's work is reassuring in many of its findings, apart from the weaknesses reported above by the respondents. However, it would have been informative if the paper had given some indication of the effects of age and hearing loss of the child on the teacher's perceptions. It is also rather worrying that the response rate was only 58%. The reader is left wondering whether a large proportion of the 42% of non-respondents did not reply because of mainly negative experiences of integration. Finally, as Luckner himself pointed out, positive perceptions by the teachers does not necessarily mean that the educational needs of the children were being met, or that they were making adequate educational progress. To address the latter issue requires a longitudinal study with controls, and hence a long-established programme. No such experiment is known, but one study without controls has been desribed by Saur et al. (1986), in which path analysis was used to investigate the contribution of academic performance, mainstream experience and employment concerns in a model of the relationships of mainstreaming and achievement. The level of mainstreamed experience was moderately positively correlated with measures of academic achievement, but around zero with job satisfaction. The most interesting outcome was that hearing loss was not significantly related to the other variables.

Without controlled longitudinal studies, the efficacy of mainstreaming for academic achievement and career prospects remains obscure. However, some investigators have shown that deaf students in secondary and tertiary education experience limited interaction with hearing peers, both in and out of school (Ladd et al., 1984; Brown and Foster, 1991), implying that mainstreaming amounts to physical placement rather than integration. Hearing-impaired mainstreamed college students may be lonely, though no difference in loneliness was found between hard of hearing and profoundly deaf students by Murphy and Newlon (1987).

Conclusion

The approach to the management of hearing-impaired children has changed considerably in recent years. Formerly, the child would be put into the charge of a teacher or therapist, with little parental involvement. From the 1970s, parents have been actively encouraged to participate in the management of their child in both educational and therapeutic settings. Increasingly, parents are accepted as members of a team which plans for the education of the child and devises programmes for therapy (Crickmore, 1988), though progress towards a team approach varies from one country to another. It is likely that parental involvement of this kind has been accelerated in those countries which have introduced integration programmes, since for most of these programmes the specialist professional functions more as a consultant and less as the main day-to-day agent for change. This distancing of the specialist professional forces increases reliance on everyday resources and thus promotes the involvement of the child's family. The involvement of parents and family may be all the more important since deaf children in mainstreamed programmes do not seem to socialise well with hearing students.

As hearing parents were becoming more involved in the management of their hearing-impaired child, and as hearing-impaired students were increasingly placed in mainstreamed environments, events elsewhere took another turn. Profoundly deaf adults concerned for the education of their young deaf children, and for the acceptance of the deaf signing culture by the hearing community, began to argue forcefully that their children should be taught sign language, and should otherwise be taught in sign by deaf adults who had sign as their first language. Prelingually profoundly deaf children born to deaf parents represent only 5–10% of the profoundly deaf population (Arnold, 1985), and therefore represent only a very small proportion of the overall population. However, the strength of the movement should not be underestimated.

Options for Parents with Deaf Children

This section considers possible approaches to the management of the deaf infant and child in the current climate where, as we have seen, the complex, diffuse and sometimes conflicting findings of recent research have made few management choices easier than hitherto. It is stressed that the material which follows attempts only to provide some thoughts for deliberation; it does not present firm prescriptions for management. We have repeatedly emphasised the diversity to be found among hearing-impaired children, even within narrow ranges of hearing loss. Such diversity, together with the complex and sometimes perplexing outcomes of research, make it foolhardy to be dogmatic over management. The emphasis is therefore on options and not on rules.

Deaf parents with a young profoundly deaf infant will usually choose for their child to use sign language as a means of communication. They seem very unlikely to opt for use of residual hearing and speechreading. To opt for sign by no means implies that the child's development will be impoverished. We have seen that deaf children of deaf parents can do better academically than deaf children born to hearing parents, who communicate orally, via a combined method, or signed English. There is also evidence that deaf children born to a fluent signing family develop higher intelligence than deaf children born to hearing parents, presumably because fluent communication aids cognitive development (Conrad, 1979: Zwiebel, 1987).

Unfortunately, the integration movement has complicated the issue of communication for deaf children born to deaf parents. Although communication by sign within the family and among the deaf community appears to be generally accepted as the way for them to go, problems arise when signing deaf children encounter mainstreaming on entering school. Present integration policies impose on the child some kind of bilingualism, such as the additional learning of signed English or a combined method, unless the parents can arrange for the education of their child at separate, signing classes for the deaf.

Despite such problems, the deaf child born to hearing parents presents more complex issues. So, what advice is to be given to the hearing parents of an infant who has been newly diagnosed in the first 2 years of life as profoundly deaf?

Auditory assistive devices

One option is to fit a hearing aid and to begin an aural rehabilitation programme, though the parents should appreciate that this approach requires much time, advice, effort and skill, and hence is likely to be directly or indirectly costly if it is to succeed. Having started, if the infant appears to make good use of the aid, then the use of the aid can be continued. Some infants seem to do well with this approach, especially if they have intensive rehabilitation from an early age, well motivated parents, and are of above average intelligence. Others, however, will perform poorly. Evidence suggests that the less bright child born into the lower socioeconomic groups may have problems. There is thus a wide range of individual differences (Brookhouser and Moeller, 1986), and unfortunately, the extent of progress in language and communication will not usually become clear until the infant is in the 3rd or 4th year.

If the infant does not appear to benefit from the aid, a further option is cochlear implantation, not necessarily right away, but after the parents have considered the issues, if the child is thought to be of suitable disposition, and when the child is considered ready to withstand the stress of hospitalisation. Some factors considered to be associated with successful implantation have been described by Hellman et al. (1991) and Beiter et al. (1991).

The best that can presently be achieved with cochlear implantation is the substitution of something like severe deafness in place of the profound deafness. Since what is achievable is most often something between the two, parents need to realise that implantation is not likely per se, to change the situation all that much for the child or for themselves, as compared, say, with the use of hearing aids, unless the child is profoundly to totally deaf. One advantage of implantation is that it holds the promise, but not the certainty, of indicating to the child what may be perceived with residual hearing, a perception which may be more difficult for the non-implanted child who is fitted with a conventional hearing aid. Another advantage is that implantation extends the promise, but not the certainty, of easier integration into mainstreamed schooling, by modestly improving residual hearing, though special training programmes will be needed both for the child and for teachers (Robbins, 1990; Moog and Geers, 1991). Some readers will see at once that cochlear implantation could result in a revival of oralism, since there is usually some improvement in residual hearing with implantation. However, the improvement at present ranges from none to modest, so that any fresh impetus to oralism will be rather weak.

Screening for oral skills

If not implanted, the child will continue to be profoundly deaf. Also, a minority of cochlear implantees seem to obtain little or no advantage from the implant. Where do we go from here? The USA Commission on Education of the Deaf (1988) has recommended, among other things, that the facilitation of vocal, visual and written English language is a paramount concern, and that positive action should be taken to enhance the quality of education for children with limited proficiency in English whose native language is American Sign Language. This suggests that deaf children should be screened for oral skills before their method of instruction is set. We saw that this topic has been addressed (Northern and Downs, 1984; Geers and Moog, 1987), but such evaluation cannot be done until the child has entered the postlingual years. It will not help the hearing parents of a newly diagnosed deaf infant. Although there is some prospect that ability for speechreading may be assessed by measuring averaged visual evoked responses (Samar and Sims, 1983), more work remains to be done in this area with young children. The technique may give parents a pointer towards their child's likely success with an oral approach, but it is not routinely available.

Bilingual approaches

Faced with this situation, how do we begin to advise hearing parents with a deaf infant? Conrad (1980), from his research with English deaf school-leavers, argued for a close association between the degree of hearing loss and speech intelligibility. In turn, speech intelligibility was associated with the likelihood of using internal speech, namely of thinking verbally or orally. The use of speechreading and residual hearing proved to have been a very poor way of learning language for Conrad's population of deaf school-leavers, and severe retardation in reading was a result. His findings held with but few exceptions for his prelingually profoundly deaf school-leavers, and for a substantial proportion of his partially hearing children, though these findings may have been somewhat pessimistic (Chapter 6). Conrad's solution was to leave the choice of communication method to the children, when they were old enough to make that choice, and not to wait until they had failed with the oral method they were currently using. He argued for an early bilingual approach, allowing the child to use speechreading and residual hearing for verbal English language, and sign for the other language, as suggested earlier by Wolff (1973). There are some problems with this approach (Maxwell, 1990). For example, one problem is that lip and facial movements may be used in sign as well as verbal English. It is also by no means clear which sign language or system should be taught. Fluent communication in sign language is very difficult for hearing parents or teachers to learn, which is why sign language alone is not generally recommended. It may also be queried when the child has sufficient maturity to make the choice (see below).

The family of sign systems known as signed English use the syntax of English, not that of native sign languages, although they are contrived systems which result in impoverished communication when compared with native sign languages. Conrad did not see this as a daunting problem. He thought that use of signed English would suit in the early stages, when only a relatively simple syntax and a small vocabulary would be needed, though deaf infants would need plenty of practice in it. Since parents already know the syntax, they would only have to learn a vocabulary of signs. These signs are for the most part the same in signed English and sign language, so that the child would not have to learn a new sign vocabulary if sign language was subsequently chosen as the preferred means of communication. Further, signed English, but not native sign, would facilitate simultaneous communication, as the spoken and signed versions would be largely isomorphic.

Any problems occurring with such an approach to the early development of communication would, Conrad implied, be greatly outweighed by the advantages. His approach has much to commend it, but considerable research remains to be done. Since this bilingual approach offers a relatively straightforward solution to a complex problem (Moores, 1991), it is surprising that it has only very recently received more serious consideration. A particular advantage is that, where there is uncertainty, a bilingual approach appears to keep the communication options open, and would seem to insure against failure with any one choice. The child will be too young to appreciate such an advantage, but it could be attractive to parents, especially if the child is likely to be enrolled eventually in a mainstreamed educational programme, and needs to communicate with deaf and hearing children.

What should be done for the deaf child in preschool or beginning primary school? Here, the question of which sign approach to use has generated yet more choice and controversy. Gustason (1981) among others concluded that young deaf children using Signing Exact English in TC attained improved English language, though such findings have not always been supported (Nix, 1983). Similar criticisms have been addressed by Rodda and Grove (1987), with the conclusion that the sign system to be chosen is the one which allows the greatest degree of isomorphism between signed English and sign language, which seems reasonable enough. Few other authors, however, have accepted Conrad's (1980) suggestion that signed English could be followed by a transition to sign language at the appropriate time, if the child so chooses. If such a choice were not made, bilingualism would continue to be a communication option. The child needs to become comfortable with the communication approach if it is to be used successfully (Palmer et al., 1990).

Debates continue

Given the diversity among deaf children and research findings, it is not surprising that debates about the preferred approach to communication continue, largely because of insufficient well designed studies in the area (Pudlas, 1987; Lou, 1988). The debates were given a further stimulus from proposals that American Sign Language should be the primary language for American deaf children in bilingual programmes. Lieberth (1990) presented a detailed and powerful criticism of this movement, arguing that the curriculum should be one which allows access for deaf children, and there is no one best way, at present, for deaf children to learn to communicate. In addition, she pointed out that considerably more research is needed on the appropriateness of applying the principles of bilingual education in the following topics: the effects of offering two languages in different modalities; the effects of changing from a visual–gestural to an auditory–verbal language; the development of competency in English through writing; the way in which ASL is learned or acquired; the degree of competency in sign required of parents; the relationship between child and parents; the heterogeneity of deaf children; and so on. Stuckless (1991) shared some of these concerns. Some of the necessary research is being put in hand, especially as regards the acquisition of grammar and the learning of writing (e.g. Jackson, 1989; Davies, 1991).

There are also findings of equipotentiality between gestural and vocal modalities in deaf and hearing infants around 1 year of age, with gestures and vocalisations both going through decontextualisation to become signs and words early in the first year. The choice between the two modalities eventually depends, if the child has a choice, on the efficacy of the linguistic input which the child receives (Volterra and Caselli, 1986). It would seem wise, however, not to allow the child to make such a choice until there is good evidence that the child has attended assiduously to both modalities and has the maturity to make a considered and reasonably informed decision. This area needs urgent research.

In view of our discussion of the diversity of deaf children, the definition of 'best' is at present as much a political and socioeconomic issue as an argument about the effectiveness of communication. The problem is, of course, that once professionals and deaf people themselves have invested considerable time and effort in a given approach to communication, they feel obliged to defend it. This seems especially true when a condition is made the subject of an infirmity model (Lane, 1990). In this context the education and training of the professionals should repay study.

Chapter 10
Concluding Comments

This short concluding chapter summarises several of the points made in the preceding pages and reinforces the emphasis on communication.

The material reviewed in the areas of oracy and literacy, the debate over the status of sign as language, the contentions about method or mode of management or instruction, the discussion of individual and social aspects, and the current concern for the rights of deaf people point to deafness not only as a problem of impaired hearing but also as an issue in communication (Schuchman, 1988). To be deaf is to communicate differently from hearing people. It is this situation, as much as lack of hearing, which affects the daily life of deaf individuals.

Until quite recently, 'ownership' of the concept of deafness was the preserve of hearing professionals, especially medical practitioners and other clinicians, educators and psychologists. These hearing professionals developed models of deafness which attempted to explain what was seen as inadequate, defective or deviant behaviour resulting from the pathology of sensory impairment (Gregory and Hartley, 1991). Deafness as an issue of communication was downplayed until the work on sign in the 1960s and the advent of more recent insights, such as the suggestion that speech may be amodal, forced the acceptance of a broader view. Somewhat more emphasis is now placed on communication as the paradigm to direct work in the field though, as we have seen, the study of communication in deaf individuals has a long way to go. It seems that although many professionals in the field would not be unhappy nowadays to be described as involved in the area of disordered communication, allegiances to individual professional disciplines can still obstruct the recognition of such a broader view.

With the discussions of multiculturalism in the wider community and the 'discovery' of the deaf community as a cultural minority, there has been some increase in recognition of a place for deaf culture in pluralist society. On the other hand, the alternative movement towards cultural assimilation, as seen in integration or mainstreaming programmes, has diminished the significance of deaf culture. Each of these two developments has increased the familiarity of hearing people with the characteristics of hearing impairment, as the adherents of each position have indulged in public discussion which has brought issues affecting deafness to popular attention. Unfortunately, however, such debates have at times been shrill.

One result has been to sharpen the awareness of many parents of deaf children to issues of management, without ameliorating management dilemmas. These dilemmas are of very real concern to hearing-impaired children and their parents, as shown in the preceding chapter.

Problems in this area are essentially to do with communication, because they are intimately bound up with the role of the deaf child as a communicating individual in the complex world of modern society. Presentation of the alternatives of speech, sign and the various combined methods, as *choices about communication*, and the skills needed to develop that communication, should help hearing-impaired children, their parents, and professionals to organise their thinking on how to conceptualise the numerous issues involved.

Using the concept of communication to provide the framework will offer a greater unity of approach and reduce apprehension about the fragmented and perplexing nature of the field. To start from a basis of communication should ensure consideration not only of face-to-face interaction, which tends to dominate initial concerns, but also the part to be played by literacy, by cognitive styles and by the various social and environmental factors. The concept of communication can also provide a useful framework for considering the often confusing outcomes of research studies, which amply illustrate the complexities of hearing impairment, but which at present cannot direct our approaches to education and therapy as well as could be desired.

By way of final comment, attention is again drawn to the diversity in abilities and performance found among hearing-impaired children, which has been one of the recurring themes in this book. Such diversity means that 'controlled group experiments' can only go so far in informing us about the complexities involved. A good argument can be made for more work on case studies, especially case studies of treatments (Leutke-Stahlman, 1984). This is not to say that the purely descriptive case study is necessarily the way to go. Properly conceived experiments of the single-case design type would seem to offer more exact intelligence.

Treatments in education and therapy for hearing-impaired individuals, and others, are concerned with serially correlated behaviour over time. It is therefore puzzling that so little use has been made of the techniques of time series analysis (Gottman, 1981; Kendall and Ord, 1990) in evaluating these treatments. Perhaps the mathematical complexities of time series analysis have proved off-putting, or the emphasis on controlled group experiments has crowded out such an approach. However, neither reason should obstruct the pursuit of well-designed single case studies of changes in behaviour with time, to complement the more traditional controlled group work. Such studies using time series analysis should be of particular value to the practising teacher or therapist.

Glossary

adventitious
accidental, acquired (as opposed to hereditary)

ambient
environmental, surrounding

American Sign Language (ASL)
native sign language in the USA

audiometry
measurement of hearing, normally with electro-acoustic apparatus

auditory training
instruction in the use of hearing, especially in listening, and the use of hearing aids and similar devices

aural
related to hearing

aural rehabilitation
treatment or therapy in the use of hearing

Australian Sign Language (Auslan)
native sign language in Australia

binaural
involving hearing with both ears

brainstem evoked response audiometry (BSER)
assessment of sound-evoked computer-averaged electrical responses from the brainstem, sometimes known as auditory brainstem response audiometry (ABR)

British Sign Language (BSL)
native sign language in the United Kingdom

central auditory dysfunction
malfunction of processing of sound stimuli in the higher centres of the brain

cerebral dominance
priority taken by one side of the brain over the other

chereme
manual analogue of phoneme

closure
making up the whole from the presentation of a part

cochlea
spiral organ of hearing in the inner ear

cochlear implant
surgically-implanted device which stimulates the cochlea directly and electrically with an external signal received at the ear, processed by a body-worn unit and transmitted to an induction coil inserted under the skin near the ear

cognition
thinking, knowing or apprehension, in contrast to emotion or impulse

combined method
use of speech, speechreading and fingerspelling (compare Rochester Method and Simultaneous Method)

conductive hearing loss
hearing loss associated with pathology of the outer and/or middle ear

confounding
forgoing information in failing to separate the effects of two or more variables

contralateral
on the opposite side of the body or head

cued speech
natural English speech accompanied by hand movements next to the lower part of the face, especially to indicate speech which cannot be seen on the lips

dactylic
related to the fingers, as in fingerspelling

decibel (dB)
a level of measurement on a ratio scale, for which the reference may be specified or implied

dichotic
relating to each ear separately

diotic
relating to each ear identically

discriminant analysis
statistical technique to maximise the difference between groups relative to the spread of scores within groups

distinctive feature
property which distinguishes a given phoneme from other phonemes

distortion
perversion of a sound or waveform resulting in false reproduction

dyad
pair functioning as a unit (e.g. mother–child)

dyslexia
disability in learning to read and spell

electroacoustic
interface involving electrical and acoustic properties

electrotactile
use of electrical signals to stimulate the sense of touch or vibration

factor analysis
statistical technique to determine how many distinct attributes can be ascribed to data, and to find the relationship between these attributes and the data

filter
device, usually electrical, which passes some frequencies and attenuates others

fingerspelling
manual communication where letters of the alphabet are shown by the position of the fingers

formant
energy peak in the spectrum of a phoneme

free field
area with acoustically unimportant or non-reflecting perimeters

frequency
number of times a signal repeats itself in a given time interval

frequency modulation (FM)
variation of frequency as used in varying a carrier wave to convey information

gain
amount of amplification

gloss
explanation or translation (of a sign)

grammar
syntax and morphology

handicap
disadvantage

hard of hearing
mildy to severely hearing-impaired (21–90 dB HL)

hearing level (HL)
level relative to the hearing threshold of young, normally hearing adults

hearing threshold level (HTL)
see hearing level

homograph
word which is written the same as another, but pronounced differently (e.g. present and past tenses of 'read')

homophene
word which appears the same on the lips as another word (e.g. 'fat', 'vat')

homophone
word which sounds the same as but is written differently from another (e.g. 'due', 'dew')

impairment
diminished function or structure

impedance
resistance to the flow of alternating electrical or acoustic energy

incidence
number or proportion of new cases of a condition over an interval of time in a given population

inner ear
cochlea and related structures

intelligibility
degree to which speech is understood

intensity
energy per unit area per unit time

interaural
between the ears

intonation
modulation of the pitch of the voice

ipsilateral
on the same side of the body or head

lacuna
gap or hiatus

language
complex generative code for conveying information

latency
period between stimulus and response

lateralisation
sensation or perception of a stimulus within one ear or within but to one side of the head

learning disability
want of ability in learning, not associated with sensory impairment

lesion
wound or injury

lexicon
all the words in a vocabulary or language

Linguistics of Visual English (LOVE)
sign system emphasising English morphemes and speech rhythms

localisation
perception of the locus of a stimulus in space

mainstreaming
placement or integration in a class in a normal school

Manually Coded English (MCE)
any one of several systems where signs represent the more important aspects of English (e.g. SEE_1, SEE_2)

masking
suppression of the perception of one sound by another

mental handicap/mental retardation
condition associated with low intelligence

middle ear
cavity containing ossicles which transmit sound from the eardrum to the oval window in the cochlea

mildly deaf
hearing loss of about 20–40 dB HL

modality
any primary method of sensation or communication

mode
see modality

moderately deaf
hearing loss of about 40–70 dB HL

monaural
involving hearing with one ear

monotic
relating to one ear only

morpheme
smallest meaningful linguistic unit

morphology
study of morphemes

noise
unwanted sound or signal

oralism
method of perceiving speech using residual hearing and speechreading

otitis media
inflammation of the middle ear

outer ear
pinna and ear canal, terminating at the eardrum

partially hearing
see hard of hearing

performance–intensity function
plot of speech correctly identified versus the relative intensity of the speech

phoneme
smallest unit of speech distinguishing one speech item from another

phonetic balance
pattern of phonemes which simulates the phonemic pattern of everyday speech

Pidgin sign English
attenuated communication system using signs or fingerspelling in the word order
of English

postlingual
after the development of language (after 2–3 years of age)

prelingual
before the development of language (before 2–3 years of age)

prevalence
number or proportion of cases of a condition at a given time in a given population

profoundly deaf
hearing loss greater than about 90 dB HL

prosody
intonation, stress of speech

psycholinguistics
study of the interaction of linguistics and behaviour

psychometric
related to the measurement of intellectual abilities

pure oralism
method of speech perception using speechreading only

redundant
that which can be lost without decreasing the information

rehabilitation
therapy to improve impaired function

residual hearing
usable hearing of a hearing-impaired individual

retrocochlear
posterior to the cochlea, especially relating to the auditory nerve

Rochester Method
communication by speech and fingerspelling

Seeing Essential English (SEE$_1$)
modification of ASL to resemble English word roots and affixes

semantics
the field concerned with meaning

sensorineural hearing loss
hearing impairment associated with lesions in the inner ear

sequela
after-effect, consequence

severely deaf
hearing loss of about 70–90 dB HL

sign language
language conveyed by gesture and facial expressions

Signed English (Siglish)
sign system using ASL signs for English words

Signing Exact English (SEE$_2$)
modification of ASL to resemble English words, with sign markers to denote English grammar

Simultaneous Method
use of speech, speechreading and sign

sound pressure level (SPL)
level of sound relative to 20 mPa or 0.0002 dyn/cm^2

spectrum
range of frequencies

speechreading
lipreading plus monitoring of facial expression and gestures, often including use of hearing

suprasegmental
variation in voice pitch, intonation, stress etc. (see prosody)

syntax
relation of words to one another, especially in word order

total communication (TC)
rationale in which all means of communication are allowed

transducer
device which changes one form of energy into another form

verbotonal method
use of residual hearing, tactile sensation and body movements to perceive speech

vibrotactile
using touch to sense vibrations

viseme
smallest unit of speech which can be seen on the lips

vocoder
device which transposes the frequencies of speech into some equivalent signal, such as vibratory stimulation

References

ABDELHAMIED, K., WALDRON, M. and FOX, R.A. (1990). Automatic Recognition of deaf speech. *Volta Rev.* 92, 121–130.

ABEL, S.M. and TSE, S.M. (1987). The Nucleus implant: rehabilitation and results. *J. Otolaryngol.* 16, 295–299.

ABKARIAN, G.G., JONES, A. and WEST, G. (1990). Enhancing children's communication skills: idioms 'fit the bill'. *Child Lang. Teaching Ther.* 6, 246–254.

ABRAHAM, S. and WEINER, F. (1985). Efficacy of word training vs. syllable training on articulatory generalization by severely hearing-impaired children. *Volta Rev.* 87, 95–105.

ABRAHAM, S. and WEINER, F. (1987). The effects of grammatical category and syntactic complexity on articulation of severely and profoundly hearing-impaired children. *Volta Rev.* 89, 197–210.

AD HOC COMMITTEE ON COCHLEAR IMPLANTS (1986). Report of the Ad Hoc Committee on Cochlear Implants. *ASHA* 28, 29–52.

AFFOLTER, F. (1985). The development of perceptual processes and problem-solving activities in normal, hearing-impaired, and language-disturbed children. In: Martin (1985).

AKAMATSU, C.T. and ARMOUR, V.A. (1987). Developing written literacy in deaf children through analyzing sign language. *Am. Ann. Deaf* 132, 46–51.

AKAMATSU, C.T. and STEWART, D.A. (1989). The role of fingerspelling in simultaneous communication. *Sign Lang. Stud.* 65, 361–373.

ALATIS, J.E. (Ed.) (1980). *Current issues in bilingual education.* Washington, DC: Georgetown University Press.

ALCANTARA, J.I., WHITFORD, L.A., BLAMEY, P.J., COWAN, R.S.C. and CLARK, G.M. (1990). Speech feature recognition by profoundly hearing-impaired children using a multiple-channel electrotactile speech processor and aided residual hearing. *J. Acoust. Soc. Am.* 88, 1260–1273.

ALCORN, S. (1932). The Tadoma Method. *Volta Rev.* 34, 195–198.

ALLEN, G.D., WILBUR, R.B. and SCHICK, B.B. (1991). Aspects of rhythm in ASL. *Sign Lang. Stud.* 72, 297–320.

ALLEN, T.E. (1986). Patterns of academic achievement among hearing impaired students: 1974 and 1983. In: Schildroth and Karchmer (1986).

ALTSCHULER, K. and SARLIN, M. (1963). Deafness and schizophrenia: a family study. In: Rainer et al. (1963).

ALTSCHULER, K.Z. (1974). The social and psychological development of the deaf child: problems, their treatment and prevention. *Am. Ann. Deaf* 119, 365–376.

ALTSCHULER, K.Z., DEMING, W.E., VOLLENWEIDER, J., RAINER, J.D. and TENDLER, R. (1976). Impulsivity and profound early deafness: a cross cultural inquiry. *Am. Ann. Deaf* 121, 331–345.

AMERICAN NATIONAL STANDARDS INSTITUTE (1969). *American National Standards Institute. Specification for Audiometers.* New York: ANSI s3.6.

AMERICAN SPEECH AND HEARING ASSOCIATION (1974). The audiologist: responsibilities in the habilitation of the auditorily handicapped. *ASHA* **16**, 68–70.

AMERICAN SPEECH AND HEARING ASSOCIATION (1990). Aural rehabilitation: an annotated bibliography. *ASHA Suppl. No. 1*, 1–30.

AMMON, P. (1981). Communication skills and communicative competence: a neo-piagetian process-structural view. In: Dickson (1981).

ANASTASIOW, N.J. (1986). *Development and Disability: A Psychobiological Analysis for Special Educators.* Baltimore, MD: PH Brooker.

ANASTASIOW, N.J. (1990). Implications of the neurobiological model for early intervention. In: Meisels and Shonkoff (1990).

ANDERSON, G.B. and WATSON, D. (Eds) (1987). Innovations in the habilitation and rehabilitation of deaf adolescents, Proc. Second Nat. Conf. on the Habilitation and Rehabilitation of Deaf Adolescents, University of Arkansas.

ANDERSON, R.W. (Ed.) (1981). *New Dimensions in Second Language Acquisition Research.* Rowley, MA: Newbury House.

ANDERSON, R.W. (1983a). Introduction: a language acquisition interpretation of pidginization and Creolization. In: Anderson (1983b).

ANDERSON, R.W. (Ed.) (1983b). *Pidginization and Creolization as Language Acquisition.* Rowley, MA: Newbury House.

ANDREWS, J.F. (1988). Deaf children's acquisition of prereading skills using the reciprocal teaching procedure. *Except. Child.* **54**, 349–355.

ANDREWS, J.F. and MASON, J.M. (1991). Strategy usage among deaf and hearing readers. *Except. Child.* **57**, 536–545.

ANGELOCCI, A.A. (1962). Some observations on the speech of the deaf. *Volta Rev.* **64**, 403–405.

ANGELOCCI, A.A., KOPP, G.A. and HOLBROOK, A. (1964). The vowel formants of deaf and normal hearing eleven to fourteen-year-old boys. *J. Speech Hear. Disord.* **29**, 156–170.

ANTHONY, D.A. (1971) *Seeing Essential English.* Anaheim, CA: Anaheim Union High School District.

ANTIA, S. (1982). Social interaction of partially mainstreamed hearing impaired children. *Am. Ann. Deaf* **127**, 18–25.

ANTIA, S. (1985). Social integration of hearing-impaired children: fact or fiction? *Volta Rev.* **87**, 279–289.

ANTIA, S.D. and KREIMEYER, K.H. (1985). Social interaction routines to facilitate peer interaction in hearing-impaired children. *Aust. Teacher of the Deaf* **26**, 13–20.

AOKI, C. and SIEKEVITS, P. (1985). Ontogenetic changes in C 3'-5' monophosphate stimulatable phosphorylation of the cat visual cortex proteins, particularly of microtubule-associated protein 2 (MAP 2): effects of normal and dark rearing and of the exposure to light. *J. Neurosci.* **5**, 2465–2483.

APLIN, D.Y. and ROWSON, V.J. (1990). Psychological characteristics of children with functional hearing loss. *Br. J. Audiol.* **24**, 77–87.

ARGYLE, M. (1972). *The Psychology of Interpersonal Behaviour,* 2nd edn. Harmondsworth: Penguin.

ARMBRUSTER, B.B., ECHOLS, C.H. and BROWN, A.L. (1982). The role of metacognition in reading to learn: a developmental perspective. *Volta Rev.* **84**, 45–56.

ARNOLD, D. and TREMBLAY, A. (1979). Interaction of deaf and hearing preschool children. *J. Commun. Disord.* **12**, 245–251.

ARNOLD, P. (1978). The deaf child's written English – can we measure its quality? *J. Br. Assn. Teachers of the Deaf* **2**, 196–200.

ARNOLD, P. (1981). Recent research on the deaf child's written English. *J. Br. Assn. Teachers of the Deaf* **6**, 174–177.

ARNOLD, P. (1985). Experimental psychology and the deaf child. *J. Rehab. Deaf.* **19**, 4–8.

ARNOLD, P., CROSSLEY, E. and EXLEY, S. (1982). Deaf children's speaking, writing and comprehension of sentences. *J. Aud. Res.* **22**, 225–232.

ARNOLD, P. and WALTER, G. (1979). Communication and reasoning skills of deaf and hearing signers. *Percept. Mot. Skills* **49**, 192–194.

ASHER, S.R. and ODEN, S.L. (1976). Children's failure to communicate: an assessment of comparison and egocentrism explanations. *Devel. Psychol.* **12**, 132–140.

ASHER, S.R. and WIGFIELD, A. (1981). Training referential communication skills. In: Dickson (1981).

ASLIN, R.N. (1981). Experimental influence and sensitive period in perceptual development: a unified model. In: Aslin et al. (1981).

ASLIN, R.N., ALBERTS, J.R. and PETERSEN, M.R. (Eds) (1981). *The Development of Perception: Psychobiological Perspectives.* New York: Academic Press.

ASP, C.W. (1984). The verbo-tonal method for establishing spoken language and listening skills. In: Perkins (1984).

ATKINSON, R.C., HERRNSTEIN, R., LINDZEY, G. and LUCE, R.D. (Eds) (1988). *Stevens' Handbook of Experimental Psychology.* New York: Wiley.

BABBINI, B.E. and QUIGLEY, S.P. (1970). *A Study of the Growth Patterns in Language, Communication, and Educational Achievements in Six Residential Schools for Deaf Students.* Urbana, IL: Institute for Research on Exceptional Children.

BACHARA, G.H., RAPHAEL, J. and PHELAN, W.J. (1980). Empathy development in deaf preadolescents. *Am. Ann. Deaf* **125**, 38–41.

BADDELEY, A.D. (1979). Working memory and reading. In: Kolers et al. (1979).

BAIN, A.M., BAILET, L.L. and MOATS, L.C. (Eds) (1991). *Written Language Disorders: Theory into Practice.* Austin, TX: Pro-Ed.

BAKER, C. (1980). Sentences in American Sign Language. In: Baker and Battison (1980).

BAKER, C. and BATTISON R. (Eds) (1980). *Sign Language and the Deaf Community: Essays in Honor of William C. Stokoe.* Silver Spring, MD: National Association of the Deaf.

BAKER, C. and PADDEN, C. (1978). Focusing on the non-manual components of American Sign Language. In: Siple (1978b).

BAKER-SCHENK, C. (1985). The facial behavior of deaf signers: evidence of a complex language. *Am. Ann Deaf* **130**, 297–304.

BALL, V. (1991). Computer-based tools for assessment and remediation of speech. *Br. J. Disord. Commun.* **26**, 95–113.

BALL, V., FAULKNER, A. and FOURCIN, A. (1990). The effects of two different speech-coding strategies on voice fundamental frequency control in deafened adults. *Br. J. Audiol.* **24**, 393–409.

BALLANTYNE, J. (1977). *Deafness.* 3rd Edn, Edinburgh: Churchill Livingstone.

BALLGE-KIMBER, P.J. and GIORCELLI, L.R. (1989). The perceptions and attitudes of hearing teachers towards sign language: an Australian study. *Aust. Teacher of the Deaf* **30**, 54–73.

BALOW, F., FULTON, H. and PEPLOE, E. (1971). Reading comprehension skills among hearing-impaired adolescents. *Volta Rev.* **73**, 113–119.

BALOW, I.H. and BRILL, R.G. (1975). An evaluation of reading and academic achievement levels of 16 graduating classes of the California School for the Deaf, Riverside. *Volta Rev.* **77**, 266–276.

BAMFORD, J.M. and BENCH, J. (1979). A grammatical analysis of the speech of partially-hearing children. In: Crystal (1979).

BAMFORD, J. and SAUNDERS, E. (1985). *Hearing Impairment, Auditory Perception, and Language Disability.* London: Edward Arnold.

BAMFORD, J.M. and MENTZ, D.L. (1979). The spoken language of hearing impaired children: grammar. In: Bench and Bamford (1979).

BAMFORD, J.M., WILSON, I.M., ATKINSON, D. and BENCH, J. (1981). Pure tone audiograms from hearing-impaired children, II: predicting speech-hearing from the audiogram. *Br. J. Audiol.* **15**, 3–10.

BANG, C. (1980). A world of sound and music: auditory training of hearing-impaired pre-school children. *Scand. Audiol. Suppl.* 10.

BANKS, J., GRAY, C., FYFE, R. and MORRIS, A. (1991a). An investigation of story schemata in deaf children using a new picture arrangement test. *J. Br. Assn. Teachers of the Deaf* **15**, 9–19.

BANKS, J., MACAULAY, M. and GRAY, C. (1991b). The use of semantic mapping and cloze inferencing in the reading instruction of deaf children: an exploratory study. *J. Br. Assn. Teachers of the Deaf* **15**, 46–59.

BANNISTER, M. and BRITTEN, F. (1982). Linguistically based speechreading assessment. *J. Commun. Disord.* **15**, 475–479.

BARTAK, L., RUTTER, M. and COX, A. (1975). A comparative study of infantile autism and specific developmental receptive language I: the children. *Br. J. Psychiat.* **126**, 127–45.

BARTON, E.J. and OSBORNE, J.G. (1978). The development of classroom sharing by a teacher using positive practice. *Behav. Modif.* **2**, 231–249.

BASILIER, T. (1964). Surdophrenia. *Acta Psychiat. Scand. Suppl.* **40**, 362–374.

BATES, E. (1976). *Language and Context: The Acquisition of Pragmatics.* New York: Academic Press.

BATES, E., MacWHINNEY, B., CASELLI, C., DEVESCOVI, A., NATALE, F. and VENZA, V. (1984). A cross-linguistic study of the development of sentence interpretation strategies. *Child Devel.* **55**, 341–354.

BATES, R. (1950). *Interaction Process Analysis: A Method for the Study of Small Groups.* Cambridge: Addison-Wesley.

BATKIN, S., GROTH, H., WATSON, J.R. and ANSBERRY, M. (1970). The effects of auditory deprivation in the development of auditory sensitivity in albino rats. *EEG Clin. Neurophysiol.* **28**, 351–359.

BATTISON, R. (1978). *Lexical Borrowing in American Sign Language.* Silver Spring, MD: Linstock Press.

BEAUPRE, W. (1985). Phonetics for the hearing-impaired university student: an alternate strategy. *Volta Rev.* **87**, 345–348.

BEBKO, J.M. (1979). Can recall differences among children be attributed to rehearsal effects? *J. Psychol.* **33**, 96–105.

BEBKO, J.M. (1984). Memory and rehearsal characteristics of profoundly deaf children. *J. Exp. Child Psychol.* **38**, 415–428.

BEBKO, J.M. and MCKINNON, E.E. (1990). The language experience of deaf children: its relation to spontaneous rehearsal in a memory task. *Child Devel.* **61**, 1744–1752.

BECK, B. (1988). Self-assessment of selected interpersonal abilities in hard of hearing and deaf adolescents. *Internat. J. Rehab. Res.* **11**, 343–349.

BECK, K., BECK, C. and GIRONELLA, O. (1977). Rehearsal and recall strategies of deaf and hearing individuals. *Am. Ann. Deaf* **122**, 544–552.

BECKER, S. (1978). An approach to developing personal and social maturity. *Volta Rev.* **80**, 105–108.

BEDROSIAN, J.L., WANSKA, S.K., SYKES, K.M., SMITH, A.J. and DALTON, B.M. (1988). Conversational turn-taking violations in mother–child interaction. *J. Speech Hear. Res.* **31**, 81–88.

BEGGS, W.D.A. and BRESLAW, P.I. (1983). Reading retardation or linguistic deficit? (III): a further examination of response strategies in a reading test completed by hearing-impaired children. *J. Res. Read.* **6**, 19–28.

BEGGS, W.D.A., BRESLAW, P.I. and WILKINSON, H.P. (1982). Eye movements and reading achievement in deaf children. In: Groner and Fraisse (1982).

BEISLER, J.M. and TSAI, L.Y. (1983). A pragmatic approach to increase expressive language in young autistic children. *J. Autism Devel. Disord.* **13**, 287–303.

BEITER, A.L., STALLER, S.J. and DOWELL, R.C. (1991). Evaluation and device programming in children. *Ear Hear. Suppl.* **12**, 25–33.

BELLACK, A.S. and HERSEN, M. (Eds) (1979). *Research and Practice in Social Skills Training.* New York: Plenum.

BELLUGI, U. (1980), How signs express complex meanings. In: Baker and Battison (1980).

BELLUGI, U. and FISCHER, S. (1972). A comparison of sign language and spoken language: rate and grammatical mechanisms. *Cognition* **1**, 173–200.

BELLUGI, U. and KLIMA, E. (1976). Two faces of sign: iconic and abstract. In: Harnad (1976).

BELLUGI, U. and KLIMA, E.S. (1975). Aspects of sign language and its structure. In: Kavanagh and Cutting (1975).

BELLUGI, U. and KLIMA, E.S. (1978). Structural properties of American Sign Language. In: Liben (1978).

BELLUGI, U., KLIMA, E.S. and POIZNER, H. (1988). Sign language and the brain. *Res. Publ. Assoc. Res. Nerv. Ment. Dis.* **66**, 39–56.

BELLUGI, U., KLIMA, E.S. and SIPLE, P. (1975). Remembering in signs. *Cognition* **3**, 93–125.

BELLUGI, U., POIZNER, H. and KLIMA, E.S. (1989). Language, modality and the brain. *Trends Neurosci.* **12**, 380–388.

BELLUGI, U. and STUDDERT-KENNEDY, M. (Eds) (1980). *Signed and Spoken Language: Biological Constraints on Linguistic Form.* Weinheim: Verlag Chemie.

BENCH, J. (1970). On the implications of the critical period concept for early diagnosis. Proc. Internat. Congr. Educ. Deaf., Stockholm. 128.

BENCH, J. (1978). The basics of infant hearing screening: why early diagnosis? In: Gerber and Mencher (1978).

BENCH, J. (1979). Auditory deprivation – an intrinsic or extrinsic problem? Some comments on Kyle (1978). *Br. J. Audiol.* **13**, 51–52.

BENCH, J. and BAMFORD, J. (Eds) (1979). *Speech–Hearing Tests and the Spoken Language of Hearing-Impaired Children.* London: Academic Press.

BENCH, J., BAMFORD, J.M., WILSON, I.M. and CLIFFT, L. (1979). A comparison of the BKB Sentence Lists for children with other speech audiometry tests. *Aust. J. Audiol.* **1**, 61–66.

BENCH, J., COLLYER, Y., MENTZ, L. and WILSON, I. (1976a). Studies in infant behavioural audiometry, I: neonates. *Audiology* **15**, 85–105.

BENCH, J., COLLYER, Y., MENTZ, L. and WILSON, I. (1976b). Studies in infant behavioural audiometry, II: six-week-old infants. *Audiology* **15**, 302–314.

BENCH, J., COLLYER, Y., MENTZ, L. and WILSON, I. (1976c). Studies in infant behavioural audiometry, III: six-month-old infants. *Audiology* **15**, 384–394.

BENCH, J., DOYLE, J. and GREENWOOD, K.M. (1987). A standardisation of the BKB/A Sentence Test for children in comparison with the NAL-CID Sentence Test and the CAL-PBM Word Test. *Aust. J. Audiol.* **9**, 39–48.

BENCH, R.J. (1968). Sound transmission to the human foetus through the maternal abdominal wall. *J. Genet. Psychol.* **113**, 85–87.

BENCH, R.J. (1971). The rise and demise of the critical period concept. *Sound* **5**, 21–23.

BENCH, R.J. and MENTZ, D.L. (1975). On the measurement of human foetal auditory response. In: Bench et al. (1975).

BENCH, R.J., PYE, A. and PYE, D. (Eds) (1975). *Sound Reception in Mammals.* London: Academic Press.

BENNETT, C. (1978). Articulation training of profoundly hearing-impaired children: a distinctive feature approach. *J. Commun. Disord.* **11**, 433–442.

BENNETT, C. and LING, D. (1973). Discrimination of the voiced–voiceless distinction by severely hearing-impaired children. *J. Aud. Res.* **13**, 271–279.

BENNETT, R., RAGOSTA, M. and STRICKER, L. (1984). *The Test Performance of Handicapped People: Report No. 2: Studies of Admissions Testing and Handicapped People.* Princeton, NJ: Educational Testing Service.

BERG, F.S. (1975). Evaluation section. In: Clark (1975).

BERG, F.S. (1976a). Programming beginning during infancy. In: Berg (1976b).

BERG, F.S. (1976b). *Educational Audiology: Hearing and Speech Management.* New York: Grune and Stratton.

BERG, F.S. (1987). *Facilitating Classroom Listening: A Handbook for Teachers of Normal and Hard of Hearing Students.* Boston, MA: College Hill Press.

BERGER, K.W. (1972). *Speechreading Principles and Methods.* Baltimore, MD: National Educational Press.

BERGMAN, B. (1983). Verbs and adjectives: some morphological processes in Swedish language. In: Kyle and Woll (1983).

BERNSTEIN, J. (1977). Intelligibility and simulated deaf-like segmental and timing errors. *Proceedings of the IEEE International. Conference on Acoustics, Speech and Signal Processing* 25, 244–247.

BERNSTEIN, L.E., GOLDSTEIN, M.H. and MASHIE, J.J. (1988). Speech training aids for hearing-impaired individuals: I. overview and aims. *J. Rehab. Res. Devel.* 25, 53–62.

BESS, F., FREEMAN, B. and SINCLAIR, S.J. (Eds) (1981). *Amplification in Education*. Washington, DC: Alexander Graham Bell Association.

BESS, F.H. and THARPE, A.M. (1984). Unilateral hearing impairment in children. *Pediatrics* 74, 206–216.

BEST, C.T. (Ed.) (1985). *Hemispheric Function and Collaboration in the Child*. Orlando, FL: Academic Press.

BEVER, T.G. (1970). The cognitive basis for linguistic structures. In: Hayes (1970).

BEVER, T.G. (1973). The influence of speech performance on linguistic structure. In: Flores d' Arcais (1973).

BEYKIRCH, H.L., HOLCOMB, T.A. and HARRINGTON, J.F. (1990). Iconicity and sign vocabulary acquisition. *Am. Ann. Deaf* 135, 306–311.

BILGER, R.C., BLACK, F.O., HOPKINS, N.T., MYERS, E.N., PAYNE, J., STENSON, N., VEGA, A. and WOLF, R. (1977). Evaluations of subjects presently fitted with implanted auditory prostheses. *Ann. Otol. Rhinol. Laryngol. (Suppl. 38)* 86, 1–76.

BINDON, M.D. (1957). Make-A-Picture Story (MAPS) test findings for rubella-deaf children. *J. Abnorm. Soc. Psychol.* 55, 38–42.

BINNIE, C.A., JACKSON, A.P. and MONTGOMERY, A. (1976). Visual intelligibility of consonants: a lipreading screening test with implications for aural rehabilitation. *J. Speech Hear. Disord.* 41, 530–539.

BISHOP, D.V.M. (1988). Can the right hemisphere mediate language as well as the left? A critical review of recent research. *Cognit. Neuropsychol.* 5, 353–367.

BISHOP, M., RINGEL, R. and HOUSE, A. (1973). Orosensory perception, speech production and deafness. *J. Speech Hear. Res.* 16, 257–266.

BLACKWELL, P.M. (1983). Training strategies in functional speech routines. In: Hochberg et al. (1983).

BLAIR, F.X. (1957). A study of the visual memory of deaf and hearing children. *Am. Ann. Deaf* 102, 254–263.

BLAIR, J.C., PETERSON, M.E. and VIEHWEG, S.H. (1985). The effects of mild sensorineural hearing loss on academic performance of young school-age children. *Volta Rev.* 87, 87–93.

BLAMEY, P.J. (1990). Developments in tactile devices. Tutorial Day Notes, Proc. SST-90 Conf. Melbourne: Australian Speech Science and Technology Association.

BLAMEY, P.J., COWAN, R.S.C., ALCANTARA, J.I. and CLARK, G.M. (1988). Phonemic information transmitted by a multichannel electrotactile speech processor. *J. Speech Hear. Res.* 31, 620–629.

BLANK, M. and FRANKLIN, E. (1980). Dialogue with pre-schoolers: a cognitively-based system of assessment. *Appl. Psycholing.* 1, 127–150.

BLANK, M., ROSE, S.A. and BERLIN, L.J. (1978). *The Language of Learning: The Preschool Years*. New York: Grune and Stratton.

BLENNERHASSETT, L. (1984). Communicative styles of a 13 month old hearing-impaired child and her parents. *Volta Rev.* 86, 217–228.

BOCHNER, J.H. (1982). English in the deaf population. In: Sims et al. (1982).

BOCHNER, J.H., SNEIL, K.B. and MCKENZIE, D.J. (1988). Duration discrimination of speech and tonal complex stimuli by normally-hearing and hearing-impaired listeners. *J. Acoust. Soc. Am.* 84, 493–500.

BODE, D. and OYER, H. (1970). Auditory training and speech discrimination. *J. Speech Hear. Res.* 13, 839–855.

BODE, D.L., TWEEDIE, D. and HULL, R.H. (1982). Improving communication through aural rehabilitation. In: Hull (1982).

BODE, L. (1974). Communication of agent, object, and indirect object in signed and spoken languages. *Percept. Mot. Skills* 39,1151–1158.

BODNER-JOHNSON, B. (1985). Families that work for the hearing-impaired child. *Volta Rev.* 87, 131–137.

BODNER-JOHNSON, B. (1991). Family conversation style: its effect on the deaf child's participation. *Except. Child.* 57, 502–509.

BOLTON, B. (1971). A factor analytic study of communication skills and non-verbal abilities of deaf rehabilitation clients. *Multivar. Behav. Res.* 6, 485–501.

BOND, G.G. (1987). An assessment of cognitive abilities in hearing and hearing-impaired preschool children. *J. Speech Hear. Disord.* 52, 319–323.

BONVILLIAN, J.D. (1983). Effects of signability and imagery on word recall of deaf and hearing students. *Percept. Mot. Skills* 56, 775–791.

BONVILLIAN, J.D., CHARROW, V.R. and NELSON, K.E. (1973). Psycholinguistic and educational implications of deafness. *Hum. Devel.* 16, 321–345.

BONVILLIAN, J.D., NELSON, K.E. and CHARROW, V.R. (1980). Languages and language-related skills in deaf and hearing children. In: Stokoe (1980).

BONVILLIAN J.D., ORLANSKY, M.D. and NOVAK, L.L. (1983). Developmental milestones: sign language acquisition and motor development. *Child Devel.* 54, 1435–1445.

BONVILLIAN, J.D., REA, C.A., ORLANDSKY, M.D. and SLADE, L.A. (1987). The effect of sign language rehearsal on subjects' immediate and delayed recall of English word lists. *Appl. Psycholing.* 8, 33–55.

BOOTHROYD, A. (1968). Developments in speech audiometry. *Sound* 2, 3–11.

BOOTHROYD, A. (1972a). Audiological evaluation of severely and profoundly deaf children. In: Fant (1972).

BOOTHROYD, A. (1972b). Sensory aids research project – Clarke School for the Deaf. In: Fant (1972).

BOOTHROYD, A. (1978). Speech perception and sensorineural hearing loss. In: Ross and Giolas (1978).

BOOTHROYD, A. (1984). Auditory perception of speech contrasts by subjects with sensorineural hearing loss. *J. Speech Hear. Res.* 27, 134–144.

BOOTHROYD, A. (1985). Evaluation of speech production of the hearing-impaired: some benefits of forced-choice testing. *J. Speech Hear. Res.* 28, 185–196.

BOOTHROYD, A. (1989). Developing and evaluating a tactile speechreading aid. *Volta Rev.* 91, 101–112.

BOOTHROYD, A., ARCHAMBAULT, P., ADAMS, R.E. and STORM, R.D. (1975). Use of a computer-based system of speech training aids for deaf persons. *Volta Rev.* 77, 178–193.

BOOTHROYD, A. and HNATH-CHISHOLM, T. (1988). Spatial, tactile presentation of voice fundamental frequency as a supplement to lipreading: results of extended training with a single subject. *J. Rehab. Res. Devel.* 25, 51–56.

BORMAN, D.L., STOEFEN-FISHER, J.M., TAYLOR, N., DRAPER, L.M. and SCHMIDT-NEIDERKLEIN, L. (1988). Metalinguistic abilities of young hearing-impaired children: performance on a judgment of synonymy task. *Am. Ann. Deaf* 133, 325–329.

BORNSTEIN, H. (1973). A description of some current sign systems designed to represent English. *Am. Ann. Deaf* 118, 454–463.

BORNSTEIN, H. (1979). Systems of sign. In: Bradford and Hardy (1979).

BRRILD, K. (1972). Cued speech and the mouth–hand system. A contribution to the discussion. In: Fant (1972).

BOSHOVEN, M.M., MCNEIL, M.R. and HARVEY, L.O. (1982). Hemispheric specialization for the processing of linguistic and non-linguistic stimuli in congenitally deaf and hearing adults: a review and contribution. *Audiology* 21, 509–530.

BOUSE, C. (1987). Impact of a cochlear implant on a teenager's quality of life: a parent's perspective. *Hear. J.* Sept. 24–29.

BOWMAN, E.S. and COONS, P.M. (1990). The use of hypnosis in a deaf patient with multiple personality disorder: a case report. *Am. J. Clin. Hypnosis* **33**, 99–104.

BOWMAN, S.N. (1984). A review of referential communication skills. *Aust. J. Hum. Commun. Disord.* **12**, 93–112.

BRACKETT, D. (1983). Group communication strategies for the hearing impaired. *Volta Rev.* **85**, 116–128.

BRACKETT, D. and HENNIGES, M. (1976). Communicative interaction of preschool hearing impaired children in an integrated setting. *Volta Rev.* **78**, 276–285.

BRADEN, J., BOOTH, K., SHAW, S., LEACH, J.M. and MACDONALD, B. (1989). The effects of microcomputer telecommunication on hearing-impaired children's literacy and language. *Volta Rev.* **91**, 143–150.

BRADFORD, L.J. and HARDY, W.G. (Eds) (1979). *Hearing and Hearing Impairment.* New York: Grune and Stratton.

BRAGG, B. (1973). Ameslish – Our American heritage: a testimony. *Am. Ann. Deaf* **118**, 672–674.

BRANNON, C. (1961). Speechreading of various materials. *J. Speech Hear. Disord.* **26**, 348–354.

BRANNON, J.B. (1964). *Visual Feedback of Glossal Motions and Its Influence on the Speech of Deaf Children.* Evanston, IL: Northwestern University: unpublished Doctoral Thesis.

BRANNON, J.B. (1966). The speech production and spoken language of the deaf. *Lang. Speech* **9**, 127–136.

BRANNON, J.B. (1968). Linguistic word classes in the spoken language of normal, hard-of-hearing and deaf children. *J. Speech Hear. Res.* **11**, 279–287.

BRANSFORD, J., SHERWOOD, R., VYE, N. and RIESER, J. (1986). Teaching thinking and problem solving: research foundations. *Am. Psychol.* **41**, 1078–1089.

BRANSON, J. and MILLER, D. (1989). Sign language, oralism and the control of deaf children. *Aust. Hear. Deaf Rev.* **6**, 19–23.

BRASEL, K.E. and QUIGLEY, S.P. (1977). The influence of certain language and communication environments in early childhood on the development of language in deaf individuals. *J. Speech Hear. Res.* **20**, 95–107.

BRERETON, B. le G. (1957). *The Schooling of Children with Impaired Hearing.* Sydney: Commonwealth Office of Information.

BRESLAW, P.I., GRIFFITHS, A.J., WOOD, D.J. and HOWARTH, C.I. (1981). The referential communication skills of deaf children from different educational environments. *J. Child Psychol.* **22**, 269–282.

BRIMER, A. (1972). *Wide-Span Reading Test.* London: Nelson.

BRINICH, P.M. (1981). Application of the metapsychological profile to the assessment of deaf children. *Psychoanalyt. Study of the Child* **36**, 3–32.

BROMWICH, R. (1981). *Working with Parents and Infants: An Interactional Approach.* Baltimore, MD: University Park Press.

BROOKHOUSER, P.E. and MOELLER, M.P. (1986). Choosing the appropriate habilitative track for the newly identified hearing-impaired child. *Ann. Otol. Rhinol. Laryngol.* **95**, 51–59.

BROOKS, P.L., FROST, B.J., MASON, J.L. and GIBSON, D.M. (1987). Word and feature identification by profoundly deaf teenagers using the Queen's University tactile vocoder. *J. Speech Hear. Res.* **30**, 137–141.

BROSS, M., HARPER, D. and SICZ, G. (1980). Visual effects of auditory deprivation: common intermodal and intramodal factors. *Science* **207**, 667–668.

BROSS, M. and SAUERWEIN, H. (1980). Signal detection analysis of visual flicker in deaf and hearing individuals. *Percept. Mot. Skills* **51**, 839–843.

BROWN, A.L. (1978). Knowing when, where and how to remember: a problem of metacognition. In: Glaser (1978).

BROWN, A.L. and SMILEY, S.S. (1978). The development of strategies for studying texts. *Child Devel.* **49**, 1076–1088.

BROWN, P.M. and FOSTER, S.B. (1991). Integrating hearing and deaf students on a college campus: successes and barriers as perceived by hearing students. *Am. Ann. Deaf* **136**, 21–27.

BROWN, R. (1973). *A First Language: The Early Stages*. Cambridge, MA: Harvard University Press.

BROWN, S.C. (Ed.) (1974). *Philosophy of Psychology*. London: Macmillan.

BROWN, W.S. and GOLDBERG, D.M. (1990). An acoustic study of the intelligible utterances of hearing-impaired speakers. *Folia Phoniat.* **42**, 230–238.

BRUNER, J. (1983). *Child's Talk: Learning to Use Language*. Oxford: Oxford University Press.

BRUNER, J.S. (1973). *Beyond the Information Given*. New York: WW Norton.

BRUNER, J.S., JOLLY, A. and SYLVA, K. (Eds) (1976). *Play – Its Role in Development and Evolution*. Harmondsworth: Penguin.

BUNCE, B.H. (1991). Referential communication skills: guidelines for therapy. *Lang. Speech Hear. in Schools* **22**, 296–301.

BUNCH, G. (1987). Designing an integration rating guide. *Volta Rev.* **89**, 35–47.

BUNCH, G.O. (1979). Degree and manner of acquisition of written English language rules by the deaf. *Am. Ann. Deaf* **124**, 10–15.

BURCH, E. and HYDE, M. (1984). Deaf adults and total communication: a questionnaire survey of knowledge, attitudes and use. *Aust. Teacher of the Deaf* **25**, 34–38.

BURKE, L.E. and NERBONNE, M.A. (1978). The influence of the guess factor on the speech reception threshold. *J. Am. Audit. Soc.* **4**, 87–90.

BUSBY, P.A., TONG, Y.C. and CLARK, G.M. (1984). Underlying dimensions and individual differences in auditory, visual and auditory–visual vowel perception by hearing-impaired children. *J. Acoust. Soc. Am.* **75**, 1858–1865.

BUSBY, P.A., TONG, Y.C. and CLARK, G.M. (1988). Underlying structure of auditory–visual consonant perception by hearing-impaired children and the influences of syllabic compression. *J. Speech Hear. Res.* **31**, 156–165.

BUSBY, P.A., ROBERTS, S.A., TONG, Y.C. and CLARK, G.M. (1991). Results of speech perception and speech production training for three prelingually deaf patients using a multiple-electrode cochlear implant. *Br. J. Audiol.* **25**, 291–302.

BUTLER, K.G. (1981). Language processing disorders: factors in diagnosis and remediation. In: Keith (1981b).

BUTTERWORTH, B. (Ed.) (1980). *Language Production, Vol. I, Speech and Talk*. New York: Academic Press.

BYRNE, B. and SHEA, P. (1979). Semantic and phonetic memory codes in beginning readers. *Mem. Cognit.* **7**, 333–338.

BYRNE, D. (1983). Word familiarity in speech perception testing of children. *Aust. J. Audiol.* **5**, 77–80.

BYRNE, D. and COTTON, S. (1987). Preferred listening levels of sensorineurally hearing-impaired listeners. *Aust. J. Audiol.* **9**, 7–14.

BYRNE, D. and COTTON, S. (1988). Evaluation of the national acoustic laboratories' new hearing aid selection procedure. *J. Speech Hear. Res.* **31**, 178–186.

BYRNE, D.J. and TONISSON, W. (1976). Selecting the gain of hearing aids for persons with sensorineural hearing impairments. *Scand. Audiol.* **5**, 51–59.

BYRNE, D. and WALKER, G. (1982). The effects of multichannel compression and expansion amplification on perceived quality of speech. *Aust. J. Audiol.* **4**, 1–8.

BZOCH, K.R. and LEAGUE, R. (1971). *Assessing Language Skills in Infancy: A Handbook for the Multidimensional Analysis of Emergent Language*. Baltimore, MD: University Park Press.

CACCAMISE, F., BREWER, L. and MEATH-LANG, B. (1983). Selection of signs and sign languages for use in clinical and academic settings. *Audiology* **8**, 31–44.

CACCAMISE, F., UPDEGRAFF, D. and NEWELL, W. (1990). Staff sign skills assessment – development at the Michigan School for the Deaf: achieving an important need. *J. Aud. Rehab. Assoc.* **23**, 27–41.

California Achievement Test (1977). Monterey, CA: CTB/McGraw-Hill.

CALVERT, D.R. (1986). Speech in perspective. In: Luterman (1986).

CALVERT, D.R. and SILVERMAN, S.R. (1975). Speech and Deafness. Washington, DC: Alexander Graham Bell Association.

CAMPBELL, R. and WRIGHT, H. (1989). Immediate memory in the orally trained deaf: effects of 'lipreadability' in the recall of written syllables. Br. J. Psychol. 80, 299–312.

CAMPBELL, R. and WRIGHT, H. (1990). Deafness and immediate memory for pictures: dissociatons between 'inner speech' and the 'inner ear'. J. Exp. Child Psychol. 50, 259–286.

CANTWELL, D.P., BARTAK, L. and RUTTER, M. (1978). A comparative study of infantile autism and specific developmental receptive language disorder IV: analysis of syntax and language function. J. Child Psychol. Psychiat. 19, 351–362.

CARNEY, A.E. (1986). Understanding speech intelligibility in the hearing-impaired. Topics Lang. Disord. 6, 47–59.

CARROW, E. (1974). The Carrow Elicited Language Inventory. Boston, MA: Teaching Resources Corporation.

CASELLI, M.C. (1983). Communication to language: deaf children's and hearing children's development compared. Sign Lang. Stud. 39, 113–144.

CASTLE, D. (1984). Telephone Training for Hearing Impaired Persons: Amplified Telephones, TTD, Codes. Rochester, New York: NTID/RIT Press.

CATES, D.S. and SHONTZ, F.C. (1990). Role-taking ability and social behavior in deaf school children. Am. Ann. Deaf 135, 217–221.

CATES, J.A. (1991). Comparison of human figure drawings by hearing and hearing-impaired children. Volta Rev. 93, 31–39.

CAZALS, Y. and PALIS, L. (1991). Effect of silence duration in intervocalic velar plosive on voicing perception for normal and hearing-impaired subjects. J. Acoust. Soc. Am. 89, 2916–2921.

CAZDEN, C. (1976). Play with language and metalinguistic awareness. In: Bruner et al. (1976).

CHALIFOUX, L.M. (1991). The implications of congenital deafness for working memory. Am. Ann. Deaf 136, 292–299.

CHAMPIE, J. (1984). Is total communication enough? The hidden curriculum. Am. Ann. Deaf 129, 317–318.

CHAPIN, P.G. (1988). American sign language and the liberal education. Sign Lang. Stud. 59, 109–113.

CHARROW, V.R. (1975). A psycholinguistic analysis of 'deaf English'. Sign Lang. Stud. 7, 139–150.

CHAZAN, D., MEDAN, Y. and SHAUDRON, U. (1987). Evaluation of adaptive multimicrophone algorithms for hearing aids. J. Rehab. Res. Devel. 24, 111–118.

CHEN, K. (1976). Acoustic image in visual detection for deaf and hearing college students. J. Gen. Psychol. 94, 243–246.

CHEROW, E. (Ed.) (1985). Hearing-Impaired Children and Youth with Developmental Disabilities. Washington DC: Gallaudet College Press.

CHI, M.T.H. and CECI, S.J. (1987). Content knowledge: its role, representation, and restructuring in memory development. Adv. Child Dev. Behav. 20, 91–142.

CHILD, D. (1991). A survey of communication approaches used in schools for the deaf in the UK. J. Br. Assn. Teachers of the Deaf 15, 20–24.

CHIPMAN, S.F, SEGAL, J.W., and GLASER, R. (Eds) (1985). Thinking and Learning Skills: Current Research and Open Questions. Hillsdale, NJ: Erlbaum.

CHOMSKY,C. (1986). Analytic study of the Tadoma Method: language abilities of three deaf–blind subjects. J. Speech Hear. Res., 29, 332–347.

CHOMSKY, N. (1957). Syntactic Structures. The Hague: Mouton.

CHOMSKY, N. (1965). Aspects of the Theory of Syntax. Cambridge, MA: MIT Press.

CHOMSKY, N. (1968). Language and Mind. New York: Harcourt, Brace and World.

CHOMSKY, N. (1971). Deep structure, surface structure and semantic interpretation. In: Steinberg and Jakobovits (1971).

CHOROST, S. (1988). The hearing-impaired child in the mainstream: a survey of the attitudes of regular classroom teachers. Volta Rev. 90, 7–12.

CHOUARD, C.H., MEYER, B., JOSSET, P. and BUCHE, J.F. (1983). The effect of the acoustic nerve electrical stimulation upon the guinea pig cochlear nucleus development. *Acta Otolaryngol.* **95**, 639–645.

CHRISTENSEN, K.M. (1988). I see what you mean: nonverbal communication strategies of young deaf children. *Am. Ann. Deaf* **133**, 270–275.

CHRISTENSEN, K.M. (1990). Thinking about thinking: a discussion of the development of cognition and language in deaf children. *Am. Ann. Deaf,* **135**, 222–226.

CLARK, G.M. and TONG, Y.C. (1982). A multiple-channel cochlear implant: a survey of results for two patients. *Arch. Otolaryngol.* **108**, 214–217.

CLARK, T. (Ed.) (1975). *Programming for Hearing Impaired Infants through Amplification and Home Intervention.* Logan, UT: Utah State University.

CLARKE, A.D.B. (1958). The abilities and trainability of imbeciles. In: Clarke and Clarke (1958).

CLARKE, A.D.B. (1972). Commentary on Kulochova's 'Severe deprivation in twins: a case study'. *J. Child Psychol. Psychiat.* **13**, 103–106.

CLARKE, A.M. and CLARKE, A.D.B. (Eds) (1958). *Mental Deficiency: The Changing Outlook.* London: Methuen.

CLARKE, A.M. and CLARKE, A.D.B. (1976). *Early Experience: Myth and Evidence.* London: Open Books.

CLARKE, B.R. and KENDALL, D.C. (1976). Communication for hearing-handicapped people in Canada. In: Oyer (1976).

CLARKE, B.R. and LING, D. (1976). The effects of using cued speech: a follow-up study. *Volta Rev.* **78**, 23–34.

CLARKE, B.R., ROGERS, W.T. and BOOTH, J.A. (1982). How hearing-impaired children learn to read: theoretical and practical issues. *Volta Rev.* **84**, 57–69.

CLAY, M.M. (1979). *Reading: The Patterning of Complex Behavior,* 2nd Edn. Exeter, NH: Heinemann educational Books.

COCHRANE, J. (1991). Some necessary skills for entering mainstream schooling. *Taralye Bull., Melbourne* **9**, 22–23.

COHEN, E., NAMIR, L. and SCHLESINGER, I.M. (Eds) (1977). *A New Dictionary of Sign Language Employing the Eshkol-Wachmann Movement Notation System.* The Hague: Mouton.

COHEN, G. (1977). *Psychology of Cognition.* London: Academic Press.

COHEN, N.L., WALTZMAN, S.B. and SHAPIRO, W.H. (1989). Telephone speech comprehension with use of the Nucleus cochlear implant. *Ann. Otol. Rhinol. Laryngol. Suppl.* **142**, 8–11.

COHEN, O.P., FISCHGRUND, J.E. and REDDING, R. (1990). Deaf children from ethnic, linguistic and racial minority backgrounds: an overview. *Am. Ann. Deaf* **135**, 67–73.

COKELY, D. (1990). The effectiveness of three means of communication in the classroom. *Sign Lang. Stud.* **69**, 415–422.

COLE, E.B. and MISCHOOK, M. (1985). Survey and annotated bibliography of curricula used by oral preschool programs. *Volta Rev.* **87**, 139–154.

COLE, E.B. and ST CLAIR-STOKES, J. (1984). Caregiver–child interactive behaviors: a videotape analysis procedure. *Volta Rev.* **86**, 200–216.

COLE, S.H. and EDELMANN, R.J. (1991). Self perception of deaf adolescents from three school settings. *J. Br. Assn. Teachers of the Deaf* **15**, 86–89.

COLLINS, B.E. and RAVEN, B.H. (1969). Group structure: attraction, coalitions, communication and power. In: Lindzey and Aronson (1969).

COLLINS, M.J. and HURTIG, R.R. (1985). Categorical perception of speech sounds via the tactile mode. *J. Speech Hear. Res.* **28**, 594–598.

COLLINS-AHLGREN, M. (1975). Language development of two deaf children. *Am. Ann. Deaf* **120**, 524–539.

COMMISSION ON EDUCATION OF THE DEAF (1988). Commission on Education of the Deaf Recommendations. *Am. Ann. Deaf* **133**, 79–84.

CONNARD, P. and KANTOR, R. (1988). A partnership perspective viewing normal-hearing parent/hearing-impaired child communication. *Volta Rev.* **90**, 133–148.

CONNOR, L.E. (Ed.) (1971). *Speech for the Deaf Child: Knowledge and Use*. Washington, DC: Alexander Graham Bell Association.

CONRAD, R. (1970). Short term memory processes in the deaf. *Br. J. Psychol.* **61**, 179–195.

CONRAD, R. (1972a). Profound deafness as a psycholinguistic problem. In: Fant (1972).

CONRAD, R. (1972b). Speech and reading. In: Kavanagh and Mattingly (1972).

CONRAD, R. (1972c). Short-term memory in the deaf: a test for speech coding. *Br. J. Psychol.* **63**, 173–180.

CONRAD, R. (1976). Matters arising. In: Henderson (1976).

CONRAD, R. (1977a). The reading ability of deaf school leavers. *Br. J. Educ. Psychol.* **47**, 138–148.

CONRAD, R. (1977b). Lipreading by deaf and hearing children. *Br. J. Educ. Psychol.* **47**, 60–65.

CONRAD, R. (1979). *The Deaf School Child*. London: Harper and Row.

CONRAD, R. (1980). Let the children choose. *Internat. J. Pediat. Otorhinolaryngol.* **1**, 317–329.

CONRAD, R. (1981). Sign language in education: some consequent problems. In: Woll et al. (1981).

CONRAD, R. and RUSH, M.L. (1965). On the nature of short-term memory encoding by the deaf. *J. Speech Hear. Disord.* **30**, 336–343.

CONRAD, R. and WEISKRANTZ, B.C. (1981). On the cognitive ability of deaf children with deaf parents. *Am. Ann. Deaf* **126**, 995–1003.

CONWAY, D. (1985). Children (re)creating writing: a preliminary look at the functions of free-choice writing of hearing-impaired kindergarteners. *Volta Rev.* **87**, 91–107.

CONWAY, D.F. (1990). Semantic relationships in the word meanings of hearing-impaired children. *Volta Rev.* **92**, 339–349.

COOPER, A.F. (1976). Deafness and psychiatric illness. *Br. J. Psychiat.* **129**, 216–226.

COOPER, C. and ARNOLD, P. (1981). Hearing impairment and visual perceptual processes in reading. *Br. J. Disord. Commun.* **16**, 43–49.

CORINA, D.P. (1989). Recognition of affective and noncanonical linguistic facial expressions in hearing and deaf subjects. *Brain Cognit.* **9**, 227–237.

CORNELIUS, G. and HORNETT, D. (1990). The play behavior of hearing-impaired kindergarten children. *Am. Ann. Deaf* **135**, 316–321.

CORNETT, O. (1967). Cued speech. *Am. Ann. Deaf* **112**, 3–13.

CORNETT, O. (1972). Cued speech. In: Fant (1972).

CORNETT, R.O. (1985). Diagnostic factors bearing on the use of cued speech with hearing-impaired children. *Ear Hear.* **6**, 33–35.

CORRIGAN, R. (1978). Language development as related to stage 6 object permanence development. *J. Child Lang.* **5**, 173–189.

COSSU, G. and MARSHALL, J.C. (1990). Are cognitive skills a prerequisite for learning to read and write? *Cognit. Neuropsychol.* **7**, 21–40.

COSTELLO, M.R. (1957). *A Study of Speech-Reading as a Developing Language Process in Deaf and in Hard of Hearing Children*. Northwestern University: unpublished Doctoral Thesis.

COWAN, R.S.C., BLAMEY, P.J., ALCANTARA, J.I., CLARK, G.M. and WHITFORD, L.A. (1989). Speech feature recognition with an electrotactile speech processor. *Aust. J. Audiol.* **11**, 57–72.

CRAIG, W.N. (1964). Effects of pre-school training on the development of reading and lipreading skills of deaf children. *Am. Ann. Deaf* **109**, 280–296.

CRAIG, W.N. and COLLINS, J.L. (1969). *Communication Patterns in Classes for Deaf Students*. Research Report: US Office of Education, Project No. 70640.

CRAIG, W.N. and COLLINS, J.L. (1970). Analysis of communicative interaction in classes for deaf children. *Am. Ann. Deaf* **115**, 79–85.

CRAWFORD, J., DANCER, J. and PITTENGER, J. (1986). Initial performance level on a speechreading task as related to subsequent improvement after shortterm training. *Volta Rev.* **88**, 101–105.

CRICKMORE, B.L. (1988). Working with families of hearing impaired children as a cultural subgroup. *Proc. Nat. Conf. Aust. Early Childhood Assoc.* **88**, 1–6.

CRITCHLEY, E., DENMARK, J., WARREN, F. and WILSON, K. (1981). Hallucinatory experiences of prelingually profoundly deaf schizophrenics. *Br. J. Psychiat.* **138**, 30–32.

CRITTENDEN, J.B. (1974). Categorization of cheremic errors in sign language reception. *Sign Lang. Stud.* **5**, 64–71.

CRITTENDEN, J.B. (1986). Attitudes toward sign communication mode: a survey of hearing and hearing-impaired educators of the deaf. *Am. Ann. Deaf* **131**, 275–280.

CRITTENDEN, J.B., RITTERMAN, S.I. and WILCOX, E.W. (1986). Communication mode as a factor in the performance of hearing-impaired children on a standardized receptive vocabulary test. *Am. Ann. Deaf* **131**, 356–360.

CROSS, T.G. (1977). Mothers' speech adjustments: the contribution of selected child listener variables. In: Snow and Ferguson (1977).

CROSS, T.G. and MORRIS, J.E. (1980). Linguistic feedback and maternal speech: comparisons of mothers addressing infants, one-year-olds, and two-year-olds. *First Lang.* **1**, 98–121.

CRYSTAL, D. (Ed.) (1979). *Working with LARSP*. London: Edward Arnold.

CRYSTAL, D. and CRAIG, E. (1978). Contrived sign language. In: Schlesinger and Namir (1978).

CRYSTAL, D., FLETCHER, P. and GARMAN, M. (1976). *The Grammatical Analysis of Language Disability*. London: Edward Arnold.

CUNNINGHAM, J.K. (1990). Parents' evaluations of the effects of the 3M/House cochlear implant on children. *Ear Hear.* **11**, 375–381.

CURTISS, S. (1977). *Genie: A Psycholinguistic Study of a Modern-Day 'Wild Child'*. New York: Academic Press.

CURTISS, S., PRUTTING, C.A. and LOWELL, E.L. (1979). Pragmatic and semantic development in young children with impaired hearing. *J. Speech Hear. Res.* **22**, 534–552.

DALBY, J.T., GIBSON, D., GROSSI, V. and SCHNEIDER, R.D. (1980). Lateralized hand gesture during speech. *J. Mot. Behav.* **12**, 292–297.

DAMICO, J.S., OLLER, J.W. and STOREY, M.E. (1984). The diagnosis of language disorders in bilingual children: surface-oriented and pragmatic criteria. *J. Speech Hear. Disord.* **48**, 385–394.

DAMPER, R.I. (1982). Speech technology – implications for biomedical engineering. *J. Eng. Technol.* **6**, 135–149.

DANEMAN, M. (1988). Word knowledge and reading skill. In: Daneman et al. (1988).

DANEMAN, M., MACKINNON, G.E. and WALLER, T.G. (Eds) (1988). *Reading Research: Advances in Theory and Practice*. New York: Academic Press.

DARROW, A.A. (1984). A comparison of rhythmic responsiveness in normal and hearing-impaired children and an investigation of the relationship of rhythmic responsiveness to the suprasegmental aspects of speech perception. *J. Music Ther.* **21**, 48–66.

DATO, D.F. (Ed.) (1975). *Development Linguistics: Theory and Applications*. Washington DC: Georgetown University Press.

DAVEY, B. and KING, S. (1990). Acquisition of word meanings from context by deaf readers. *Am. Ann. Deaf* **135**, 227–234.

DAVEY, B., LaSASSO, C. and MACREADY, G. (1983). A comparison of reading comprehension task performance for deaf and hearing subjects. *J. Speech Hear. Res.* **26**, 622–628.

DAVIES, D.G. (1984). Utilization of creative drama with hearing-impaired youth. *Volta Rev.* **86**, 106–113.

DAVIES, S.N. (1991). The transition toward bilingual education of deaf children in Sweden and Denmark: perspectives on language. *Sign Lang. Stud.* **71**, 169–195.

DAVIS, C. (1976) (Untitled). In: Henderson (1976).

DAVIS, C. and BULLIS, M. (1990). The school-to-community transition of hearing-impaired persons with developmental disabilities. *Am. Ann. Deaf* **135**, 352–363.

DAVIS, H. and SILVERMAN, S.R. (1964). *Hearing and Deafness*. New York: Holt, Rinehart and Winston.

DAVIS, H., STEVENS, S.S., NICHOLS, R.H., HUDGINS, C.V., MARQUIS, R.J., PETERSON, G.F. and ROSS, D.A. (1947). *Hearing Aids – An Experimental Study of Design Objectives*. Cambridge, MA: Harvard University Press.

DAVIS, J.M. (1977). Reliability of hearing impaired children's responses to oral and total presentations of the test of auditory comprehension of language. *J. Speech Hear. Disord.* **52**, 520–527.

DAVIS, J.M. and HARDICK, E.J. (1981). *Rehabilitative Audiology for Children and Adults.* New York: Wiley.

DAVIS, K. (1947). Final note on a case of extreme social isolation. *Am. J. Sociol.* **52**, 432–437.

DAVIS, S.M. and RAMPP, D.L. (1983). Normal and disordered auditory processing skills: a developmental approach. *Audiology* **8**, 45–58.

DAWSON, E. (1981). Psycholinguistic processes in prelingually deaf adolescents. In: Woll et al. (1981).

DAWSON, P. (1990). A music program to improve prosodic production and perception by profoundly deaf children. *Taralye Bull., Melbourne* **8**, 13–16.

DAWSON, P.W., BLAMEY, P.J., ROWLAND, L.C., DETTMAN, S.J., ALTIDIS, P.M., CLARK, G.M., BUSBY, P.A., BROWN, A.M. and DOWELL, R.C. (1990). Speech perception results in children using the 22-electrode cochlear implant. *Aust. J. Audiol. Suppl.* **4**, 9.

DAY, P.S. (1986). Deaf children's expression of communicative intentions. *J. Commun. Disord.* **19**, 367–385.

DEAN, M. and NETTLES, J. (1987). Reverse mainstreaming: a successful model for interaction. *Volta Rev.* **89**, 27–34.

DE FILIPPO, C.L. (1982). Memory for articulated sequences and lipreading performance of hearing-impaired observers. *Volta Rev.* **31**, 134–146.

DE FILIPPO, C.L. (1984). Laboratory projects in tactile aids to lipreading. *Ear Hear.* **5**, 211–227.

DE FILIPPO, C.L. (1990). Speechreading training: believe it or not! *ASHA* April, 46–48.

DE FILIPPO, C.L. and SCOTT, B.L. (1978). A method for training and evaluating the reception of ongoing speech. *J. Acoust. Soc. Am.* **63**, 1186–1192.

DE FILIPPO, C.L. and SIMS, D.G. (Eds) (1988). New reflections on speechreading. *Volta Rev.* **90**, No. 5.

DE l'EPÉE, l'ABBÉ, C.M. (1784). *La Veritable Manière d'Instruire les Sourds et les Muets.* Paris: Nyon l'Aire.

DELGADO, G.L. (1982). Beyond the norm – social maturity and deafness. *Am. Ann. Deaf* **127**, 356–360.

DENCKLA, M.B. (1983). Learning for language and language for learning. In: Kirk (1983).

DENCKLA, M.B., RUDEL, R.G. and BROMAN, M. (1981). Tests that discriminate between dyslexic and other learning-disabled boys. *Brain Lang.* **13**, 118–129.

DENGERINK, J.E. and PORTER, J.B. (1984). Children's attitudes toward peers wearing hearing aids. *Lang. Speech Hear. Services in Schools* **15**, 205–209.

DENNIS, R., REICHLE, J., WILLIAMS, W. and VOGELSBERG, R.T. (1982). Motoric factors influencing the selection of vocabulary for sign production programs. *J. Assn. Severely Handicapped* **7**, 20–32.

DEPARTMENT OF EDUCATION AND SCIENCE (1964). *The Health of the School Child, 1962 and 1963.* London: HMSO.

DEPARTMENT OF EDUCATION AND SCIENCE (1972). *The Health of the School Child, 1969 and 1970.* London: HMSO.

DERMODY, P. and MACKIE, K. (1987). Speech tests in audiological assessment at the National Acoustics Laboratories. In: Martin (1987).

DEUCHAR, M. (1983). Is British sign language an SVO language? In: Kyle and Woll (1983).

DEVENS, J., HOYER, E. and MCGROSKEY, R. (1978). Dynamic auditory localization by normal and by learning disability children. *J. Am. Audiol. Soc.* **3**, 172–178.

DICKSON, W.P. (Ed.) (1981). *Children's Oral Communication Skills.* New York: Academic Press.

DICKSON, W.P. and MIOSKOFF, M.A. (1980). *A Computer Readable Literature Review of Studies of Referential Communication: A Meta-analysis.* Madison, WS: Research and Development Center for Individualized Schooling.

DIEFENDORF, A. and ARTHUR, D. (1987). Monitoring children's hearing aids: re-examining the problem. *Volta Rev.* **89**, 17–26.

DIEHL, R., WALSH, M. and KLUENDER, K. (1991). On the interpretability of speech/nonspeech comparisons. *J. Acoust. Soc. Am.* **89**, 2905–2909.

DI FRANCESCA, S. (1972). *Academic Achievement Test Results of a National Testing Program for Hearing Impaired Students, United States, Spring 1971.* Series D, No. 9, Washington, DC: Gallaudet College, Office of Demographic Studies.

DI PIETRO, L.J., KNIGHT, C.H. and SAMS, J.S. (1981). Health care delivery for deaf patients: the provider's role. *Am. Ann. Deaf* **126**, 106–112.

DITTMAN A.T. (1972). The body movement – speech rhythm relationship as a cue to speech encoding. In: Siegman and Pope (1972).

DI VESTA, F.J. (1966). A developmental study of the semantic structures of children. *J. Verb. Learn. Verb. Behav.* **5**, 249–259.

DIXON, R.F. and NEWBY, H.A. (1959). Children with non-organic problems. *Arch. Otolaryn.* **70**, 619–623.

DJOURNO, A. and EYRIES, C. (1957). Prothèse auditive par excitation électrique à distance du nerf sonoriel à l'aide d'un bobinage inclus à demeure. *Presse Med.* **35**, 14–17.

DODD, B. (1972). Effects of social and vocal stimulation on infant babbling. *Devel. Psychol.* **7**, 80–83.

DODD, B. (1976). The phonological systems of deaf children. *J. Speech Hear. Disord.* **41**, 185–198.

DODD, B. (1979). Lip-reading in infants: attention to speech presented in- and out-of synchrony. *Cognit. Psychol.* **11**, 478–484.

DODD, B. (1987). The acquisition of lip-reading skills by normally hearing children. In: Dodd and Campbell (1987).

DODD, B. and CAMPBELL, R. (1987). *Hearing by Eye: The Psychology of Lip-Reading.* Hillsdale, NJ: Erlbaum.

DODD, B. and HERMELIN, B. (1977). Phonological coding by the prelinguistically deaf. *Percept. Psychophys.* **21**, 413–417.

DODD, B., HOBSON, P., BRASHER, J. and CAMPBELL, R. (1983). Short-term memory in deaf children. *Br. J. Devel. Psychol.* **1**, 354–364.

DODD, B., PLANT, G. and GREGORY, M. (1989). Teaching lip-reading: the efficacy of lessons on video. *Br. J. Audiol.* **23**, 229–238.

DONALDSON, M. (1978). *Children's Minds.* London: Fontana.

DONOGHUE, R.J. (1968). The deaf personality – a study in contrasts. *J. Rehab. Deaf.* **2**, 37–51.

DORE, J. (1974). A pragmatic description of early language development. *J. Psycholing. Res.* **3**, 343–350.

DORMAN, M.F., DANKOWSKI, K., MCCANDLESS, G., PARKIN, J.L. and SMITH, L. (1991). Vowel and consonant recognition with the aid of a multichannel cochlear implant. *Q. J. Exp. Psychol.* **43A**, 585–601.

DORMAN, M.F., DANKOWSKI, K., MCCANDLESS, G. and SMITH, L. (1989). Identification of synthetic vowels by patients using the Symbion multichannel cochlear implant. *Ear Hear.* **10**, 40–43.

DORMAN, M.F., LINDHOLM, J.M. and HANNLEY, M.T. (1985). Influence of the first formant on the recognition of voiced stop consonants by hearing-impaired listeners. *J. Speech Hear. Res.* **28**, 377–380.

DOUGLAS, J.E. and SUTTON, A. (1978). The development of speech and mental processes in a pair of twins: a case study. *J. Child Psychol. Psychiat.* **19**, 49–56.

DOWELL, R.C., BROWN, A.M., SELIGMAN, P.M. and CLARK, G.M. (1985a). Patient results for a multiple-channel cochlear prosthesis. In: Schindler and Merzenich (1985).

DOWELL, R.C., SELIGMAN, P.M., BLAMEY, P.J. and CLARK, G.M. (1987). Speech perception using a two-formant 22-electrode cochlear prosthesis in quiet and in noise. *Acta Otolaryngol. (Stockh.)* **104**, 439–446.

DOWELL, R.C., TONG, Y.C., BLAMEY, P.J. and CLARK, G.M. (1985b). Psychophysics of multiple-channel stimulation. In: Schindler and Merzenich (1985).

DOWNS, M. (1966). *The Establishment of Hearing Aid Use: A Program for Parents.* Minneapolis, MN: MAICO Audiological Library Series 4.

DOWNS, M.P. (1967). Testing hearing in infancy and early childhood. In: Freeman and Ward (1967).

DOWNS, M.P. (1974). The Deafness Management Quotient. *Hear. Speech News* Jan–Feb.

DOWNS, M.P. (1976). Early identification of hearing loss: Where are we? where do we go from here? In: Mencher (1976).

DOYLE, J. (1987). Audiologists, the audiogram and the perception of hearing-impaired children's speech. *Aust. J. Audiol.* 9, 1–6.

DREVER, J. and COLLINS, M. (1944). *Performance Tests of Intelligence,* 3rd Edn. Edinburgh: Oliver and Boyd.

DUBNO, J.R. and DIRKS, D.D. (1983). Suggestions for optimizing reliability with the Synthetic Sentence Identification Test. *J. Speech Hear. Disord.* 48, 98–103.

DUBNO, J.R., DIRKS, D.D. and SCHAEFER, A.B. (1987). Effects of hearing loss on utilization of short-duration spectral cues in stop consonant recognition. *J. Acoust. Soc. Am.* 81, 1940–1947.

DUCKWORTH, E. (1979). Either we're too early and they can't learn it or we're too late and they know it already: the dilemma of applying Piaget. *Harvard Educ. Rev.* 49, 297–312.

DUFFY, A. (1984). Discourse in the classroom. *Aust. Teacher of the Deaf* 25, 4–10.

DUNLAP, W.R. and ICEMAN SANDS, D. (1990). Classification of the hearing impaired for independent living using the Vineland Adaptive Behavior Scale. *Am. Ann. Deaf* 135, 384–388.

DUNN, L.M. (1965). *Peabody Picture Vocabulary Test.* Circle Pines, MN: American Guidance Service.

DUNN, L. and DUNN, L. (1981). *Peabody Picture Vocabulary Test – Revised.* Circle Pines, MN: American Guidance Service.

DUNN, L.M. and MARKWARDT, F.C. (1970). *Peabody Individual Achievement Test Revised.* Circle Pines, MN: American Guidance Service.

EAGNEY, P. (1987). ASL? English? Which? Comparing comprehension. *Am. Ann. Deaf* 132, 272–275.

EDITORIAL (1981). Hearing loss and perceptual dysfunction in schizophrenia. *Lancet* ii, 848–849.

EFRON, R. (1990). *The Decline and Fall of Hemispheric Specialization.* Hillsdale, NJ: Erlbaum.

EHRI, L. (1975). Word consciousness in readers and prereaders. *J. Educ. Psychol.* 67, 204–212.

EILERS, R.E., OZDAMAR, O., OLLER, D.K., MISKIEL, E. and URBANO, R. (1988a). Similarities between tactual and auditory speech perception. *J. Speech Hear. Res.* 31, 124–131.

EILERS, R.E., WIDEN, J.E. and OLLER, D.K. (1988b). Assessment techniques to evaluate tactual aids for hearing-impaired subjects. *J. Rehab. Res. Devel.* 25, 33–46.

EIMAS, P.D., SIQUELAND, E.R., JUSCYK, P.W. and VIGORITO, J. (1971). Speech perception in infants. *Science* 171, 303–306.

EISENBERG, L.S. (1982). Use of the cochlear implant by the prelingually deaf. In: House and Berliner (1982).

EISENBERG, L.S. (1985). Training strategies for the post-implant patient. In: Schindler and Merzenich (1985).

EKMAN, P. and FRIESEN, W. (1978). *Facial Action Coding System.* Palo Alto, CA: Consulting Psychologists Press.

ELLENBERGER, R. and STEYAERT, M. (1978). A child's representation of action in American Sign Language. In: Siple (1978b).

ELLER, R.G., PAPPAS, C.C. and BROWN, E. (1988). The lexical development of kindergarteners: learning from written context. *J. Read. Behav.* 20, 5–23.

ELLIOTT, H., GLASS, L. and EVANS, J.W. (Eds) (1987). *Mental Health Assessment of Deaf Clients: A Practical Manual.* Boston, MA: Little, Brown and Co.

ELLIOTT, L.L. and HAMMER, M.A. (1988). Longitudinal changes in auditory discrimination in normal children and children with language-learning problems. *J. Speech Hear. Disord.* **53**, 467–474.

ELLIOTT, R. and POWERS, A. (1988). Preparing teachers to serve the learning disabled hearing impaired. *Volta Rev.* **90**, 13–18.

ELLIS, D. (Ed.) (1986). *Sensory Impairments in Mentally Handicapped People*. San Diego, CA: College Hill Press.

ELLIS, R.A.F. and WHITTINGTON, D. (1981). *A Guide to Social Skill Training*. London: Croom Helm.

EMMOREY, K. and CORINA, D. (1990). Lexical recognition in sign language: effects of phonetic structure and morphology. *Percept. Mot. Skills* **71**, 1227–1252.

ENGLISH, K. (1991). Best practice in educational audiology. *Lang. Speech Hear. Serv. Schools* **22**, 283–286.

EPSTEIN, J. (1980). *No Music by Request*. Sydney: Collins.

ERBER, N.P. (1972). Auditory, visual and auditory–visual recognition of consonants by children with normal and impaired hearing. *J. Speech Hear. Res.* **15**, 413–422.

ERBER, N.P. (1974). Pure-tone thresholds and word-recognition abilities of hearing-impaired children. *J. Speech Hear. Res.* **17**, 194–202.

ERBER, N.P. (1978). Vibratory perception by deaf children. *Internat. J. Rehab. Res.* **1**, 27–37.

ERBER, N.P. (1979). Auditory–visual perception of speech with reduced optical clarity. *J. Speech Hear. Res.* **22**, 212–223.

ERBER, N.P. (1980). Use of the Auditory Numbers Test to evaluate speech perception abilities of hearing-impaired children. *J. Speech Hear. Disord.* **45**, 527–532.

ERBER, N.P. (1983). Speech perception and speech development in hearing-impaired children. In: Hochberg et al. (1983).

ERBER, N.P. (1985). *Telephone Communication and Hearing Impairment*. London and Philadelphia: Taylor and Francis.

ERBER, N.P. (1988). *Communication Therapy for Hearing Impaired Adults*. Victoria, Australia: Clavis.

ERBER, N.P. and ALENCEWICZ, C.M. (1976). Audiological evaluation of deaf children. *J. Speech Hear. Disord.* **41**, 256–267.

ERICKSON, F. (1981). Timing and context in everyday discourse. In: Dickson (1981).

ERICKSON, F. and SCHULTZ, J. (1980). When is a context? In: Green and Wallat (1980).

ERLBAUM, S.J. (1990). A comprehensive PEL-IEP speech curriculum overview and related carryover and summary forms designed for speech therapy services for the hearing-impaired. *Lang. Speech Hear. Serv. Schools* **21**, 196–199.

ERTING, C. (1980). Sign language and communication between adults and children. In: Baker and Battison (1980).

EVANS, A.D. and FALK, W.W. (1986). *Learning to Be Deaf*. Berlin: Mouton de Gruyter.

EVANS, J. and ELLIOTT, H. (1987). The mental status examination. In: Elliot et al. (1987).

EVANS, J.W. (1989). Thoughts on the psychosocial implications of cochlear implantation in children. In: Owens and Kessler (1989).

EVANS, L. (1981). Psycholinguistic perspectives on visual communication. In: Woll et al. (1981).

EVANS, P.I.P. (1987). Speech audiometry for differential diagnosis. In: Martin (1987).

EVANS, T. (Ed.) (1977). *Psychophysics and Physiology of Hearing*. London: Academic Press.

EVERHART, V.S. and MARSCHARK, M. (1988). Linguistic flexibility in signed and written language productions of deaf children. *J. Exp. Child Psychol.* **46**, 174–193.

EWING, A.W.G. (Ed.) (1957). *Educational Guidance and the Deaf Child*. Manchester: Manchester University Press.

EWOLDT, C. (1985). A descriptive study of the developing literacy of young hearing-impaired children. *Volta Rev.* **87**, 109–126.

EWOLDT, C. and HAMMERMEISTER, F. (1986). The language–experience approach to facilitating reading and writing for hearing-impaired students. *Am. Ann. Deaf* **131**, 271–274.

EXLEY, S. and ARNOLD, D.P. (1987). Partially hearing and hearing children's speaking, writing and comprehension of sentences. *J. Commun. Disord.* **20**, 403–411.

FAIRBANK, D., POWERS, A. and MONAGHAN, C. (1986). Stimulus overselectivity in hearing-impaired children. *Volta Rev.* **88**, 269–278.

FAIRBANKS, G. (1958). Test of phonemic differentiation: the rhyme test. *J. Acoust. Soc. Am.* **30**, 596–600.

FANT, G. (1962). Descriptive analysis of the acoustics of speech. *Logos* **5**, 3–17.

FANT, G. (Ed.) (1972). *Speech Communication Ability and Profound Deafness*. Washington, DC: Alexander Graham Bell Association.

FANT, G. (Ed.) (1974). *Speech Communication*. New York: Halstead Press.

FANT, G. and TATHAM, M.A.A. (Eds) (1975). *Auditory Analysis and Perception of Speech*. London: Academic Press.

FARB, P. (1973). *Word Play: What Happens when People Talk*. New York: Bantam.

FARWELL, R.M. (1976). Speechreading: a research review. *Am. Ann. Deaf* **121**, 19–30.

FASOLD, R. (1984). *The Sociolinguistics of Society*. Oxford: Blackwell.

FAULKNER, A., BALL, V. and FOURCIN, A. (1990). Compound speech pattern information as an aid to lipreading. *Speech Hear. Lang. Work in Progress, No. 3*. London: University College.

FEINSTEIN, C.B. (1983). Early adolescent deaf boys: a biosocial approach. *Adolesc. Psychiat.* **11**, 147–162.

FENN, G. and ROWE, J.A. (1975). An experiment in manual communication. *Br. J. Disord. Commun.* **10**, 3–16.

FENN, G. and SMITH, B.Z. (1987). The assessment of lipreading ability: some practical considerations in the use of tracking procedures. *Br. J. Audiol.* **21**, 253–258.

FERGUSON, J.B., BERNSTEIN, L.E. and GOLDSTEIN, M.H. (1988). Speech training aids for hearing-impaired individuals: II. Configuration of the Johns Hopkins aids. *J. Rehab. Res. Devel.* **25**, 63–68.

FERGUSON, N. and WATT, J. (1980). Professionals and the parents of mentally handicapped children. *Bull. Br. Psychol. Soc.* **33**, 59–60.

FESHBACH, S. (1970). Aggression. In: Mussen (1970).

FESTEN, J.M. and PLOMP, R. (1990). Effects of fluctuating noise and interfering speech on the speech reception threshold for impaired and normal hearing. *J. Acoust. Soc. Am.* **88**, 1725–1736.

FEYEREISEN, P. (1983). Manual activity during speaking in aphasic subjects. *Internat. J. Psychol.* **18**, 545–556.

FISCH, L. (1983). Integrated development and maturation of the hearing system. *Br. J. Audiol.* **17**, 137–154.

FISCH, L. (1990). Letter to the editor: the significance of early auditory stimulation. *Br. J. Audiol.* **24**, 141–142.

FISCHER, S.D. (1978). Sign language and Creoles. In: Siple (1978b).

FISHER, E. and SCHNEIDER, K. (1986). Integrating auditory learning at the preschool level. *Volta Rev.* **88**, 83–91.

FLANDERS, N. (1965). *Analyzing Teacher Behaviour*. Reading, MA: Addison-Wesley.

FLAVELL, J.H. (1968). *The Development of Role-taking and Communication Skills in Children*. New York: Wiley.

FLAVELL, J.H. (1977). *Cognitive Development*. Englewood Cliffs, NJ: Prentice-Hall.

FLAVELL, J.H. (1985). *Cognitive Development*, 2nd Edn. Englewood Cliffs, NJ: Prentice-Hall.

FLAVELL, J.H. and WELLMAN, H.M. (1977). Metamemory. In: Kail and Hagen (1977).

FLETCHER, H. (1953). *Speech and Hearing in Communication*. New York: Kreiger Publishing Corp.

FLETCHER, P. and GARMAN, M. (Eds) (1979). *Language Acquisition*. Cambridge: Cambridge University Press.

FLETCHER, S.G. (1986). Visual feedback and lip-positioning skills of children with and without impaired hearing. *J. Speech Hear. Res.* **29**, 231–239.

FLETCHER, S.G., SMITH, S.C. and HASEGAWA, A. (1985). Vocal/verbal response times of normal-hearing and hearing-impaired children. *J. Speech Hear. Res.* **28**, 548–555.

FLEXER, C. and WOOD, L.A. (1984). The hearing aid: facilitator or inhibitor of auditory interaction? *Volta Rev.* **86**, 354–361.

FLEXER, C., WRAY, D. and BLACK, T. (1986). Support group for moderately hearing-impaired college students: an expanding awareness. *Volta Rev.* **88**, 223–229.

FLORES d'ARCAIS, G.B. (Ed.) (1973). *Advances in Psycholinguistics*. Amsterdam: North Holland Press.

FONTANA, J.M. (1990). Is ASL like Digueno or Digueno like ASL? A study of internally headed relative clauses in ASL. In: Lucas (1990).

FORCHHAMMER, G. (1903). *Om Nodvendigheden af Sikre Meddelelsesmidler i Dovstume Under Evisningen*. Copenhagen: J. Frimodts, Fortag.

FORNER, L.L. and HIXON, T.J. (1977). Respiratory kinematics in profoundly hearing-impaired speakers. *J. Speech. Hear. Res.* **20**, 373–408.

FOSTER, J.R. and HAGGARD, M.P. (1979). (FAAF) An efficient analytical test of speech perception. *Proc. Inst. Acoust.*, IA 3, 9–12.

FOSTER, J.R. and HAGGARD, M.P. (1984). *Introduction and Test Manual for FAAF II*. Nottingham: MRC Institute of Hearing Research.

FOSTER, S., BAREFOOT, S.M. and DeCARO, P.M. (1989). The meaning of communication to a group of deaf college students: a multidimensional perspective. *J. Speech Hear. Disord.* **54**, 558–569.

FOSTER, S. and BROWN, P. (1989). Factors influencing the academic and social integration of hearing-impaired college students. *J. Postsec. Educ. Disabil.* **7**, 78–96.

FOURCIN, A.J. (1976). Speech pattern tests for deaf children. In: Stephens (1976).

FOURCIN, A.J. and ABBERTON, E. (1975). First applications of a new laryngograph. *Med. Biol.* **21**, No. 3.

FOURCIN, A.J., ROSEN, S.M., MOORE, B.C., DOUEK, E.E., CLARKE, G.P., DODSON, H. and BANNISTER, L.H. (1979). External electrical stimulation of the cochlea: clinical, psychophysical, speech-perceptual and histological findings. *Br. J. Audiol.* **13**, 85–107.

FOWLER, C.A. (1991). Auditory perception is not special: we see the world, we feel the world, we hear the world. *J. Acoust. Soc. Am.* **89**, 2910–2915.

FRAISSE, P. (1964). *The Psychology of Time*. London: Eyre and Spottiswoode.

FRANKS, J.R. (1979). The influence of exaggerated mouth movement on lipreading. *Audiol. Hear. Educn.* **5**, 12–16.

FREEDMAN, D.A. (1981). Speech, language, and the vocal–auditory connection. *Psychoanalyt. Study of the Child*. **36**, 105–127.

FREEMAN, M. and WARD, P.H. (Eds) (1967). *Deafness in Childhood*. Nashville, TN: Vanderbilt University Press.

FREEMAN, R., CARBIN, C. and BOESA, R. (1981). *Can't Your Child Hear? A Guide for Those Who Care about Deaf Children*. Baltimore, MD: University Park Press.

FREEMAN, S.T. (1989). Cultural and linguistic bias in mental health evaluations of deaf people. *Rehab. Psychol.* **34**, 51–63.

FREUD, S. (1915). Instincts and their vicissitudes. In: Institute of Psychoanalysis (1957).

FRIEDMAN, L. A. (1976). The manifestation of subject, object and topic in American Sign Language. In: Li (1976).

FRISHBERG, N. (1975). Arbitrariness and iconicity: historical change in American Sign Language. *Language* **51**, 696–719.

FRISHBERG, N. (1988). Signers of tales: the case for literary status of an unwritten language. *Sign Lang. Stud.* **59**, 149–170.

FROMKIN, V. A. (1988). Sign languages: evidence for language universals and the linguistic capacity of the human brain. *Sign Lang. Stud.* **59**, 115–127.

FROMKIN, V., KRASHEN, S., CURTISS, S., RIGLER, D. and RIGLER, M. (1974). The development of language in Genie: a case of language acquisition beyond the critical period. *Brain Lang* **1**, 81–107.

FROST, B. and BROOKS, P. (1983). Identification of novel words and sentences using a tactile vocoder. *J. Acoust. Soc. Am.* **74**, Suppl. 104(A).

FRUCHTER, A., WILBUR, R.B. and FRASER, J.B. (1984). Comprehension of idioms by hearing-impaired students. *Volta Rev.* **86**, 7–19.

FRY, D.B. (1961). Word and sentence tests for use in speech audiometry. *Lancet* ii, 197–199.

FRY, D.B. (1966). The development of the phonological system in the normal and the deaf child. In: Smith and Miller (1966).

FUCCI, D. (1972). Oral vibrotactile sensation: an evaluation of normal and defective speakers. *J. Speech Hear. Res.* **15**, 179–183.

FUCCI, D. and ROBERTSON, J.H. (1971). Functional defective articulation: an oral sensory disturbance. *Percept. Mot. Skills* **33**, 711–714.

FUGAIN, C., MEYER, B. and CHOUARD, C.H. (1985). Speech processing strategies and clinical results of the French multichannel cochlear implant. In: Schindler and Merzenich (1985).

FULLER, D.R. and WILBUR, R.B. (1987). The effect of visual metaphor cueing on recall of phonologically similar signs. *Sign Lang. Stud.* **54**, 59–80.

FURTH, H.G. (1961). Influence of language on the development of concept formation in deaf children. *J. Abnorm. Soc. Psychol.* **63**, 386–389.

FURTH, H.G. (1963). Conceptual discovery and control on a pictorial part–whole task as a function of age, intelligence, and language. *J. Educ. Psychol.* **54**, 191–196.

FURTH, H.G. (1964a). Research with the deaf: implications for language and cognition. *Psychol. Bull.* **62**, 145–164.

FURTH, H.G. (1964b). Conservation of weight in deaf and hearing children. *Child Devel.* **35**, 143–150.

FURTH, H.G. (1966a). *Thinking without Language: Psychological Implications of Deafness*. New York: Free Press.

FURTH, H.G. (1966b). A comparison of reading test norms of deaf and hearing children. *Am. Ann. Deaf* **111**, 461–462.

FURTH, H.G. (1970). A review and perspective on the thinking of deaf people. In: Helmuth (1970).

FURTH, H.G. (1971). Linguistic deficiency and thinking: research with deaf subjects 1964–1969. *Psychol. Bull.*, **74**, 58–72.

FURTH, H.G. (1973). *Deafness and Learning: A Psychosocial Approach*. Belmont, CA: Wadsworth.

FURTH, H.G. and YOUNISS, J. (1975). Congenital deafness and the development of thinking. In: Lenneberg and Lenneberg (1975).

FUSFELD, I.S. (1955). The academic programme of schools for the deaf. *Volta Rev.* **57**, 63–70.

GAINES, R., MANDLER, J. and BRYANT, P. (1981). Immediate and delayed story recall by hearing and deaf children. *J. Speech Hear. Res.* **24**, 463–469.

GALLAGHER, T.M. and MEADOR, H.E. (1989). Communication mode use of two hearing-impaired adolescents in conversation. *J. Speech Hear. Disord.* **54**, 570–575.

GALLAGHER, T.M. and PRUTTING, C.A. (Eds) (1983). *Pragmatic Assessment and Intervention Issues in Language*. San Diego, CA: College Hill Press.

GALLAWAY, C., APLIN, D.Y., NEWTON, V.W. and HOSTLER, M.E. (1990). The GMC project: some linguistic and cognitive characteristics of a population of hearing-impaired children. *Br. J. Audiol.* **24**, 17–27.

GANNON, J.R. (1981). *Deaf Heritage: A Narrative History of Deaf America*. Silver Spring. MD: National Association of the Deaf.

GANTZ, B.J., TYLER, R.S., KNUTSON, J.F., WOODWORTH, G., ABBAS, P., MCCABE, B.F., HINRICHS, J., TYE-MURRAY, N., LANSING, C., KUK, F. and BROWN, C. (1988). Evaluation of five different cochlear implant designs: audiologic assessment and predictors of performance. *Laryngoscope* **98**, 1100–1106.

GARDNER, E.F., RUDMAN, H.C., KARLSEN, G. and MERWIN, J.C. (1982). *Stanford Achievement Test*, 17th Edn. Cleveland, OH: Psychological Corporation.

GARMAN, M. (1990). *Psycholinguistics*. Cambridge: Cambridge University Press.

GARRETT, M.F. (1980). Levels of processing in sentence production. In: Butterworth (1980).

GARRISON, W.M. and TESCH, S. (1978). Self-concept and deafness: a review of research literature. *Volta Rev.* **80**, 457–466.

GATES, A.J. and MCGINITIE, W.H. (1965). *Gates–McGinitie Reading Test*. Chicago, IL: Riverside.

GATHERCOLE, S.E. (1990). Working memory and language development: how close is the link? *The Psychologist* **2**, 57–60.

GAULT, R.H. (1924). Progress in experiments on tactual interpretation of oral speech. *J. Abnorm. Soc. Psychol.* **14**, 155–159.

GAY, T. (1978). Effect of speaking rate on vowel formant movements. *J. Acoust. Soc. Am.* **63**, 223–230.

GAZZANIGA, M.S. (Ed.) (1979). *Handbook of Behavioral Neurobiology* Vol. 2, New York: Plenum.

GEERS, A. and MOOG, J. (1989). Factors predictive of the development of literacy in profoundly hearing-impaired adolescents. *Volta Rev.* **91**, 69–86.

GEERS, A., MOOG, J. and SCHICK, B. (1984). Acquisition of spoken and signed English by profoundly deaf children. *J. Speech Hear. Disord.* **49**, 378–388.

GEERS, A.E. and MOOG, J.S. (1987). Predicting spoken language acquisition of profoundly hearing-impaired children. *J. Speech Hear. Disord.* **52**, 84–94.

GEFFNER, D. and DONOVAN, N. (1974). Intelligibility functions of normal and sensorineural loss subjects on the W-22 lists. *J. Aud. Res.* **14**, 82–86.

GEFFNER, D.S. and FREEMAN, L.R. (1980). Speech assessment at the primary level: interpretation relative to speech training. In: Subtelny (1980).

GELDARD, F.A. (1972). *The Human Senses,* 2nd Edn. New York: Wiley.

GENTILE, A. and DI FRANCESCA, S. (1969). *Academic Achievement Test Performances of Hearing Impaired Students*. Washington, DC: Gallaudet College, Office of Demographic Studies.

GEOFFRION, L. (1982). An analysis of teletype conversations. *Am. Ann. Deaf* **127**, 747–752.

GEOFFRION, L.D. and GEOFFRION, O.P. (1983). *Computers and Reading Instruction*. Reading, MA: Addison-Wesley.

GEOFFRION, L.D. and GOLDENBERG, E.P. (1981). Computer–based exploratory learning systems for communication-handicapped children. *J. Spec. Educ.* **15**, 325–332.

GERBER, S.E. and MENCHER, G.T. (Eds) (1978). *Early Diagnosis of Hearing Loss*. New York: Grune and Stratton.

GETTY, D.J. and HOWARD, J.H. (Eds) (1981). *Auditory and Visual Pattern Recognition*. Hillsdale, NJ: Erlbaum.

GIBSON, E.J. (1972). Reading for some purpose. In: Kavanagh and Mattingly (1972).

GIORCELLI, L. (1985). Communication: the essential ingredient. *Aust. Teacher of the Deaf* **26**, 19–20.

GLASER, R. (Ed.) (1978). *Advances in Instructional Psychology*. Hillsdale, NJ: Erlbaum.

GLASER, R. and BASSOK, M. (1989). Learning theory and the study of instruction. *Ann. Rev. Psychol.* **40**, 631–666.

GLEASON, J.B. (1975). Fathers and other strangers: men's speech to young children. In: Dato (1975).

GODA, S. (1964). Spoken syntax of normal, deaf and retarded adolescents. *J. Verb. Learn. Verb. Behav.* **3**, 401–405.

GODFREY, J. and MILLAY, K. (1978). Perception of rapid spectral change in speech by listeners with mild and moderate sensorineural hearing loss. *J. Am. Audiol. Soc.* **3**, 200–208.

GOFFMAN, E. (1967). *Interaction Ritual: Essays on Face to Face Behavior*. Garden City, NY: Doubleday.

GOLD, T. (1980). Speech production in hearing-impaired children. *J. Commun. Disord.* **13**, 397–418.

GOLDBERG, D., NIEHL, P. and METROPOULOS, T. (1989). Parent checklist for placement of a hearing-impaired child in a mainstreamed classroom. *Volta Rev.* **91**, 327–332.

GOLDIN-MEADOW, S. and MYLANDER, C. (1984). Gestural communication in deaf children: the effects and noneffects of parental input on early language development. *Monogr. Soc. Res. Child Devel.* **49**, 1–151.

GOLDMAN, R., FRISTOE, M. and WOODCOCK, R.W. (1970). *Test of Auditory Discrimination*. Circle Pines, MN: American Guidance Service.

GOLINKOFF, R.M. and AMES, G.J. (1979). A comparison of fathers' and mothers' speech with their young children. *Child Devel.* **50**, 28–32.

GONZALEZ, K.A. (1984). The content of practicum observation and supervized interaction. In: Northcott (1984).

GOODMAN, Y. and BURKE, C. (1980). *Reading Strategies: Focus on Comprehension*. New York: Holt, Rinehart and Winston.

GOODY, E.N. (1978). *Questions and Politeness: Strategies in Social Interaction*. Cambridge: Cambridge University Press.

GORELICK, P.B. and ROSS, E.D. (1987). The aprosodias: further functional–anatomical evidence for the organization of affective language in the right hemisphere. *J. Neurol. Neurosurg. Psychiat.* **50**, 553–560.

GORGA, M.P. and THORNTON, A.R. (1989). The choice of stimuli for ABR measurements. *Ear Hear.* **10**, 217–230.

GORMLEY, K. and SARACHAN-DEILY, A.B. (1987). Evaluating hearing-impaired students' writing: a practical approach. *Volta Rev.* **89**, 157–169.

GORMLEY, K.A. (1981). On the influence of familiarity on deaf students' text recall. *Am. Ann. Deaf* **126**, 1024–1030.

GORMLEY, K.A. (1982). The importance of familiarity in hearing-impaired readers' comprehension of text. *Volta Rev.* **84**, 71–80.

GORMLEY, K.A. and FRANZEN, A.M. (1978). Why can't the deaf read? Comments on asking the wrong question. *Am Ann. Deaf* **123**, 542–547.

GOTTLIEB, D.D. and ALLEN, W. (1985). Visual disorders in a selected population of hearing-impaired students. *Volta Rev.* **87**, 165–170.

GOTTMAN, J.M. (1981). *Time Series Analysis*. Cambridge: Cambridge University Press.

GRANT, K.W. (1987a). Encoding voice pitch for profoundly hearing-impaired listeners. *J. Acoust. Soc. Am.* **82**, 423–432.

GRANT, K.W. (1987b). Identification of intonation contours by normally hearing and profoundly hearing-impaired listeners. *J. Acoust. Soc. Am.* **82**, 1172–1178.

GRAVES, D. (1983). *Writing: Teachers and Children at Work*. Portsmouth, NH: Heinemann.

GRAY, C., FYFE, R. and BANKS, J. (1991). Some approaches to the study of story-schematic inference in deaf readers: a review of picture arrangement tests. *J. Br. Assn. Teachers of the Deaf* **15**, 1–8.

GREEN, J. and WALLAT, C. (Eds) (1980). *Ethnographic Approaches to Face to Face Interaction in Educational Settings*. Norwood, NJ: Ablex.

GREEN, W.B. (1974). The development of semantic differential scales for deaf children. *Am. Ann. Deaf* **119**, 361–364.

GREEN, W.B. and GREEN, K.W. (1984). The process of speechreading. In: Northcott (1984).

GREEN, W.B. and SHEPHERD, D.C. (1975). The semantic structure in deaf children. *J. Commun. Disord.* **8**, 357–365.

GREENBERG, M.T. and CALDERON, R. (1984). Early intervention: outcomes and issues. *Topics Early Child. Spec. Educ.* **3**, 1–9.

GREENBERG, M.T., CALDERON, R. and KUSCHÉ, C. (1984). Early intervention using Simultaneous Communication with deaf infants: the effect on communication development. *Child Devel.* **55**, 607–616.

GREENFIELD, P.M. and SMITH, J. H. (1976). *The Structure of Communication in Early Language Development*. New York: Academic Press.

GREENO, J.G. and SIMON, H.A. (1988). Problem solving and reasoning. In: Atkinson et al. (1988).

GREENSTEIN, J.M., GREENSTEIN, B.B., MCCONVILLE, K. and STELLINI, L. (1975). *Mother–Infant Communication and Language Acquisition in Deaf Infants*. New York: Lexington School for the Deaf.

GREGG, N. (1991). Disorders of written expression. In: Bain et al. (1991).

GREGORY, J.F. (1987). An investigation of speechreading with and without child speech. *Am. Ann. Deaf* **132**, 393–398.

GREGORY, R.L. (1974). Perceptions as hypotheses. In: Brown (1974).

GREGORY, S. and HARTLEY, G.M. (Eds) (1991). *Constructing Deafness*. London: Pinter.

GREGORY, S. and MOGFORD, K. (1981). Early language development in deaf children. In: Woll et al. (1981).

GREVILLE, K.A., KEITH, W.J. and LAVEN, J.W. (1985). Performance of children with previous OME on central auditory measures. *Aust. J. Audiol.* **7**, 69–78.

GRIFFITHS, C. (1967). *Conquering Childhood Deafness*. New York: Exposition Press.

GRIFFITHS, C. (1988). The importance of the critical age of hearing and its implications. In: Taylor (1988).

GRIMWADE, J.C., WALKER, D.W., BARTLETT, M., GORDON, S. and WOOD, C. (1971). Human fetal heart rate change and movement in response to sound and vibration. *Am. J. Obstet. Gynec.* **109**, 86–90.

GRONER, R. and FRAISSE, P. (Eds) (1982). *Cognition and Eye Movements*. Amsterdam: North-Holland Publishing Co.

GROSJEAN, F. and GEE, J.P. (1987). Prosodic structure and spoken word recognition. *Cognition* **25**, 135–156.

GROVE, C., O'SULLIVAN, F.D. and RODDA, M. (1979). Communication and language in severely deaf adolescents. *Br. J. Psychol.* **70**, 531–540.

GROVE, C. and RODDA, M. (1984). Receptive communication skills of hearing-impaired students: a comparison of four methods of communication. *Am. Ann. Deaf* **129**, 378–385.

GRUNEBERG, M.M., MORRIS, P.E. and SYKES, R.N. (Eds) (1988). *Practical Aspects of Memory*, Vol. 2. Chichester: Wiley.

GUBERINA, P. and ASP, C.W. (1981). *The Verbo-Tonal Method for Rehabilitating People with Communication Problems*. New York: World Rehabilitation Fund.

GUELKE, R.W. (1985). The performance of hearing aids in relation to their frequency response. *Volta Rev.* **87**, 171–176.

GULIAN, E., HINDS, P. and NIMMO-SMITH, I. (1986). Modifications in deaf children's vowel production: perceptual evidence. *Br. J. Audiol.* **20**, 181–194.

GURALNICK, M.J. and BENNETT, F.C. (1987a). A framework for early intervention. In: Guralnick and Bennett (1987b).

GURALNICK, M.J. and BENNETT, F.C. (Eds) (1987b). *The Effectiveness of Early Intervention for At-Risk and Handicapped Children*. Orlando, FL: Academic Press.

GUSTASON, G. (1981). Does Signing Exact English work? *Teaching English To The Deaf* **7**, 16–20.

GUSTASON, G. (1983). Where do we go from here? In: Kyle and Woll (1983).

GUSTASON, G., PFETZING, D. and ZAWOLKOW, E. (1972). *Signing Exact English*. Rossmoor, CA: Modern Signs Press.

HADADIAN, A. and ROSE, S. (1991). An investigation of parents' attitudes and the communication skills of their deaf children. *Am. Ann. Deaf* **136**, 273–277.

HAGBORG, W. (1987). Hearing-impaired students and sociometric ratings: an exploratory study. *Volta Rev.* **89**, 221–228.

HAKES, D. (1980). *The Development of Metalinguistic Abilities in Children*. New York: Springer-Verlag.

HALL, E.T. (1989). Deaf culture, tacit culture and ethnic relations. *Sign Lang. Stud.* **65**, 291–304.

HAMILTON, H. (1985). Development of sign-based perception by deaf children. *Percept. Mot. Skills* **60**, 699–704.

HAMILTON, H. and HOLZMAN, T.G. (1989). Linguistic encoding in short-term memory as a function of stimulus type. *Mem. Cognit.* **17**, 541–550.

HAMILTON, H. and LILLO-MARTIN, D. (1986). Imitative production of ASL verbs of movement and location: a comparative study. *Sign Lang. Stud.* **50**, 29–57.

HAMMERMEISTER, F.K. (1971). Reading achievements in deaf adults. *Am. Ann. Deaf* **116**, 25–28.

HAMP, N.W. (1972). Reading attainment and some associated factors in deaf and partially hearing children. *Teacher of the Deaf* 70, 203–215.

HANEY, W.V. (1973). *Communication and Organizatioal Behavior*, 3rd Edn. Homewood, IL: Irwin.

HANNLEY, M. and JERGER, J. (1985). Patterns of phoneme identification error in cochlear and eighth nerve disorders. *Audiology* 24, 157–166.

HANSEN, B. (1975). Varieties in Danish sign language and grammatical features of the original sign language. *Sign Lang. Stud.* 8, 249–256.

HANSON, V.L. (1982). Short-term recall by deaf signers of American Sign Language: implications of encoding strategy for order recall. *J. Exp. Psychol.: Learn. Mem. Cognit.* 8, 572–583.

HANSON, V.L. (1986). Access to spoken language and the acquisition of orthographic structure: evidence from deaf readers. *Q. J. Exp. Psychol.* 38A, 193–212.

HANSON, V.L. and FELDMAN, L.B. (1989). Language specificity in lexical organization: evidence from deaf signers' lexical organisation of American Sign Language and English. *Mem. Cognit.* 17, 292–301.

HANSON, V.L., GOODELL, E.W. and PERFETTI, C.A. (1991). Tongue-twister effects in the silent reading of hearing and deaf college students. *J. Mem. Lang.* 30, 319–330.

HANSON, V.L., SHANKWEILER, D. and FISCHER, F.W. (1983). Determinants of spelling ability in deaf and hearing adults: access to linguistic structure. *Cognition* 14, 323–344.

HARGIE, O., SAUNDERS, C. and DICKSON, D. (1981). *Social Skills in Interpersonal Communication*. London: Croom Helm.

HARNAD, S. (Ed.) (1976). *The Origins and Evolution of Language and Speech*. New York: New York Academy of Sciences.

HARRIS, L.J. (1989). Hand preference and gestures and signs in the deaf and hearing: some notes on early evidence and theory. *Brain Cognit.* 10, 189–221.

HARRIS, P.L., KRUITHOF, A., TERGWOGT, M.M. and VISSER, T. (1981). Children's detection and awareness of textual anomaly. *J. Exp. Child Psychol.* 31, 212–231.

HARRIS, R.I. (1978). The relationship of impulse control to parent hearing status, manual communication, and academic achievement in deaf children. *Am. Ann. Deaf* 123, 52–67.

HARRIS, R.W., BREY, R.H., ROBINETTE, M.S., CHABRIES, D.M., CHRISTIANSEN, R.W. and COLLEY, R.G. (1988). Use of adaptive digital signal processing to improve speech communication for normally hearing and hearing-impaired subjects. *J. Speech Hear. Res.* 31, 265–271.

HARRISON, D.R., SIMPSON, P.A. and STUART, A. (1991). The development of written language in a population of hearing impaired children. *J. Br. Assn. Teachers of the Deaf* 15, 76–85.

HARRISON, M.F., LAYTON, T.L. and TAYLOR, T.D. (1987). Antecedent and consequent stimuli in teacher–child dyads. *Am. Ann. Deaf* 132, 227–231.

HARTUP, W.W. (1976). Peer relations and the behavioral development of the individual child. In: Schopler and Reichler (1976).

HARTVIG JENSEN, J., BORRE, S. and ANGAARD JOHANSEN, P. (1989). Unilateral sensorineural hearing loss in children and auditory performance with respect to right/left ear differences. *Br. J. Audiol.* 23, 207–213.

HARVEY, M.A. (1984a). Family therapy with deaf persons: the systemic utilization of an interpreter. *Family Process.* 23, 205–213.

HARVEY, M.A. (1984b). Rejoinder to Scott. *Family Process.* 23, 216–221.

HARVEY, M.A. (1989). *Psychotherapy with Deaf and Hard-of-hearing Persons: A Systematic Model*. Hillsdale, NJ: Erlbaum.

HARVEY, N. (1991). British research into skill: what is going on? *The Psychologist* 4, 443–448.

HASS, E.J. and SAMS, K.M. (1987). A method for examining gestural language structure. *Percept. Mot. Skills* 64, 391–397.

HAWKINS, J.E. and STEVENS, S.S. (1950). The masking of pure tones of speech by white noise. *J. Acoust. Soc. Am.* 22, 6–13.

HAY, J. (1978). Courtesy, humour and adjustment to a mad world. In: Montgomery (1978).

HAYCOCK, G.S. (1933). *The Teaching of Speech*. Washington, DC: Alexander Graham Bell Association.

HAYES, J.R. (Ed.) (1970). *Cognition and the Development of Language*. New York: Wiley.

HAZAN, V., FOURCIN, A. and ABBERTON, E. (1991). Development of phonetic labeling in hearing-impaired children. *Ear Hear.* **12**, 71–84.

HEFFERNAN, C. (1990). A Kodaly-based music programme for hearing-impaired children. *Tarolye Bull., Melbourne* **8**, 12–18.

HEIDER, F. and HEIDER, G.M. (1940). A comparison of sentence structure of deaf and hearing children. *Psychol. Monogr.* **52**, 42–103.

HEIDER, F. and HEIDER, G.M. (1941). Studies in the psychology of the deaf. *Psychol. Monogr.* **53**, 1–56.

HEIDINGER, V.A. (1972). *An Exploratory Study of Procedures for Improving Temporal Features in the Speech of Deaf Children*. Columbia University: unpublished Doctoral Thesis.

HELLIGE, J.B. (1980). Visual laterality and cerebral hemisphere specialization: methodological and theoretical considerations. In: Sidowski (1980).

HELLMAN, S.A., CHUTE, P.M., KRETSCHMER, R.E., NEVINS, M.E., PARISIER, S.C. and THURSTON, L.C. (1991). The development of a children's implant profile. *Am. Ann. Deaf* **136**, 77–81.

HELMUTH, J. (Ed.) (1970). *Cognitive Studies*, Vol 1. New York: Brunner.

HENDERSON, L. (1982). *Orthography and Word Recognition in Reading*. London: Academic Press.

HENDERSON, P. (Ed.) (1976). *Methods of Communication Currently Used in the Education of Deaf Children*. London: Royal National Institute for the Deaf.

HENSHALL, W.R. (1972). Intrauterine sound levels. *Am. J. Obstet. Gynec.* **112**, 576–578.

HERMELIN, B. and O'CONNOR, N. (1975). The recall of digits by normal, deaf and autistic children. *Br. J. Psychol.* **66**, 203–209.

HESS, D.W. (1969). Evaluation of the young deaf adult. *J. Rehab. Deaf* **3**, 6–21.

HIDI, A. and HILDYARD, A. (1983). The comparison of oral and written productions in two discourse types. *Discourse Processes* **6**, 91–105.

HIGGINS, E.T., FONDACARO, R. and MCCANN, C.D. (1981). Rules and Roles. In: Dickson (1981).

HIRSH, I.J. (1952). *The Measurement of Hearing*. New York: McGraw-Hill.

HIRSH, I.J., DAVIS, H., SILVERMAN, S.R., REYNOLDS, E.G., ELDERT, E. and BENSON, R.W. (1952). Development of materials for speech audiometry. *J. Speech Hear. Disord.* **17**, 321–337.

HIRSH-PASEK, K. (1987). The metalinguistics of fingerspelling: an alternate way to increase reading vocabulary in congenitally deaf readers. *Read. Res. Q.* **22**, 455–474.

HIRSH-PASEK, K. and TREIMAN, R. (1982). Recoding in silent reading: can the deaf child translate print into a more manageable form? *Volta Rev.* **84**, 71–82.

HOCHBERG, I., LEVITT, H. and OSBERGER, M.J. (1983). *Speech of the Hearing-Impaired: Research, Training, and Personnel Preparation*, Baltimore, MD: University Park Press.

HOEMANN, H.W. (1972). The development of communication skills in deaf and hearing children. *Child Devel.* **43**, 990–1003.

HOEMANN, H.W. (1975). The transparency of meaning of sign language gestures. *Sign. Lang. Stud.* **7**, 151–161.

HOEMANN, H.W. (1976). *The American Sign Language: Lexical and Grammatical Notes with Translation Exercises*. Silver Spring, MD: National Association of the Deaf.

HOEMANN, H.W. (1978a). *Communicating with Deaf People: A Resource Manual for Teachers and Students of American Sign Language*. Baltimore, MD: University Park Press.

HOEMANN, H.W. (1978b). Categorical coding of sign and English in short-term memory by deaf and hearing subjects. In: Siple (1978b).

HOEMANN, H.W. (1988). Communication skills in deaf and hearing children: a theoretical model. In: Taylor (1988).

HOEMANN, H.W. and KOENIG, T.J. (1990). Categorical coding of manual and English alphabet characters by beginning students of American Sign Language. *Sign Lang. Stud.* **67**, 175–181.

HOFFMEISTER, R. and MOORES, D.F. (1987). Code switching in deaf adults. *Am. Ann. Deaf* **132**, 31–34.

HOLLAND, J.H., HOLYOAK, K.J., NISBETT, R.E. and THAGARD, P.R. (1986). *Induction*. Cambridge, MA: MIT Press.

HOLLINGSHEAD, A. (1982). Issues raised by some recent research for the teaching of language to hearing-impaired pupils. In: Power and Hollingshead (1982).

HOLTON, S.A. (1978). Not so different: spatial and distancing behavior of deaf adults. *Am. Ann. Deaf* **123**, 920–924.

HORII, Y. (1982). Some voice fundamental frequency characteristics of oral reading and spontaneous speech by hard of hearing young women. *J. Speech Hear. Res.* **25**, 608–610.

HORTON, K.B. (1975). Early intervention through parent training. *Otolaryngol. Clin. North Am.* **8**, 144–157.

HORTON, K.B. (1976). Early intervention for hearing-impaired infants and young children. In: Tjossem (1976).

HOUDE, R.A. (1980). Evaluation of independent drill with visual aids for speech training. In: Subtelny (1980).

HOUSE, W.F. (1976). Cochlear implants. *Ann. Otol. Rhinol. Laryngol.* (Suppl. 27) **85**, 1–93.

HOUSE, W.F. and BERLINER, K.I. (1982). Cochlear implants: progress and perspectives. *Ann. Otol. Rhinol. Laryngol.* (Suppl.91), **91**, 1–124.

HOUSE, W.F. and BERLINER, K.I. (1986). Safety and efficacy of the House/37 cochlear implant in profoundly deaf adults. *Otolaryngol. Clin. North Am* **19**, 275–286.

HOUSTON, S. (1972). *A Survey of Psycholinguistics*. The Hague: Mouton.

HOWARTH, C. and WOOD, D. (1977). Research into the intellectual abilities of deaf children. *J. Br. Assoc. Teachers of the Deaf* **1**, 5–12.

HOYT, M.F., SIEGELMAN, E.Y. and SCHLESINGER, H.S. (1981). Special issues regarding psychotherapy with the deaf. *Am. J. Psychiat.* **138**, 807–811.

HUDGINS, C.V. and NUMBERS, F. (1942). An investigation of the intelligibility of the speech of the deaf. *Genet. Psychol. Monogr.* **25**, 289–392.

HUGHES, M.C. and JAMES, S.L. (1985). Deaf children's revision behaviors in conversations. *J. Commun. Disord.* **18**, 227–243.

HULL, R.H. (Ed.) (1982). *Rehabilitative Audiology*. New York: Grune and Stratton.

HULL, R.H. and ALPINER, J.G. (1976). The effect of syntactic word variations on the predictability of sentence content in speechreading. *J. Acad. Rehab. Audiol.* **9**, 42–56.

HULL, R.H. and DILKA, K.L. (1984). *The Hearing-impaired Child in School*. Orlando, FL: Grune and Stratton.

HULME, C. (1988). Short-term memory development and learning to read. In: Gruneberg et al. (1988).

HUMMEL, J.W. (1982). Description of a successful inservice program. *Teacher Educ. Spec. Educ.* **5**, 7–14.

HUMMEL, J.W. and SCHIRMER, B.E. (1984). Review of research and description of programs for the social development of hearing-impaired students. *Volta Rev.* **86**, 259–266.

HUMPHRIES, T. (1991). An introduction to the culture of deaf people in the United States: content notes & reference material for teachers. *Sign Lang. Stud.* **72**, 209–240.

HUMPHREY, G. (1948). *Directed Thinking*. New York: Dodd and Mead.

HUNG, D.L., TZENG, O.J.L. and WARREN, D.H. (1981). A chronometric study of sentence processing in deaf children. *Cognit. Psychol.* **113**, 583–610.

HUNTINGTON, A. and WHATTON, F. (1981). Language and interaction in the classroom (Part 1): Teacher Talk. *J. Br. Assn. Teachers of the Deaf* **5**, 162–173.

HUNTINGTON, A. and WHATTON, F. (1984). Language and interaction in the education of hearing-impaired children (Part 2). *J. Br. Assn. Teachers of the Deaf* **8**, 137–144.

HUNTINGTON, A. and WHATTON, F. (1986). The spoken language of teachers and pupils in the education of hearing-impaired children. *Volta Rev.* **88**, 5–19.

HURFORD, D.P. (1988). *Assessment and Remediation of a Phonemic Discrimination Deficit in Reading Disabled Second- and Fourth-Graders*. University of Akron: unpublished Doctoral Thesis.

HURST, J. (1988). Metaphors of communication in the dreams of deaf people. *Psychiat. J. Univ. Ottawa.* **13**, 75–78.

HUTCHINSON, J.M. and SMITH, L.L. (1976). Aerodynamic functioning in consonant production by hearing-impaired adults. *Audiol. Hear. Educ.* **2**, 16–25.

HUTCHINSON, K. (1990). An analytic distinctive feature approach to auditory training. *Volta Rev.* **92**, 5–12.

INSTITUTE OF PSYCHOANALYSIS (1957). *The Standard Edition of the Complete Psychological Works of Sigmund Freud* (1957). London: Hogarth Press and the Institute of Psychoanalysis.

IRAN-NEJAD, A., ORTONY, A. and RITTENHOUSE, R. (1981). The comprehension of metaphorical uses of English by deaf children. *J. Speech Hear. Res.* **24**, 551–556.

ISRAELITE, N., SCHLOSS, P. and SMITH, M. (1986). Teaching proverb use through a modified table game. *Volta Rev.* **88**, 195–207.

ISRAELITE, N.K. (1986). Hearing-impaired children and the psychological functioning of their normal-hearing siblings. *Volta Rev.* **88**, 47–54.

IVIMEY, G.P. (1976). The written syntax of an English deaf child: an exploration in method. *Br. J. Disord. Commun.* **11**, 103–120.

IVIMEY, G.P. (1977a). The perception of speech: an information-processing approach. Part 1 – The acoustic nature of spoken utterances. *J. Br. Assn. Teachers of the Deaf* **1**, 40–48.

IVIMEY, G.P. (1977b). The perception of speech: an information-processing approach. Part 2 – perceptual and cognitive processes. *J. Br. Assn. Teachers of the Deaf* **1**, 64–73.

IVIMEY, G.P. (1977c). The perception of speech: an information-processing approach. Part 3 – lipreading and the deaf. *J. Br. Assn. Teachers of the Deaf* **1**, 90–100.

IVIMEY, G.P. (1981). The production and perception by profoundly deaf children of syntactic time cues in English. *Br. J. Educ. Psychol.* **51**, 58–65.

JACKSON, C.A. (1989). Language acquistion in two modalities: the role of nonlinguistic cues in linguistic mastery. *Sign Lang. Stud.* **62**, 1–22.

JACKSON, P.L. and KELLY-BALLWEBER, D. (1979). Auditory stress pattern recognition in sentences. *Proc. ASHA Convention*, November.

JEFFERS, J. and BARLEY, M. (1971). *Speechreading (Lipreading)*. Springfield, IL: Charles C. Thomas.

JENSEMA, C.J., KARCHMER, M. and TRYBUS, R.J. (1978). *The Rated Speech Intelligibility of Hearing-Impaired Children*. Washington, DC: Gallaudet College, Office of Demographic Studies.

JENSEMA, C.J. and TRYBUS, R.J. (1978). *Communication Patterns and Educational Achievements*. Washington, DC: Gallaudet College.

JERGER, J., SPEAKS, C. and TRAMMELL, J.L. (1968). A new approach to speech audiometry. *J. Speech Hear. Disord.* **33**, 318–328.

JERGER, S. and JERGER, J. (1984). *Pediatric Speech Intelligibility Test*. St Louis, MS: Auditec.

JERGER, S., JERGER, J. and ABRAMS, S. (1983). Speech audiometry in the young child. *Ear Hear.* **4**, 56–66.

JERGER, S., JERGER, J. and LEWIS, S. (1981). Pediatric speech intelligibility test. II: Effect of receptive language age and chronological age. *Int. J. Pediat. Otorhinolaryngol.* **3**, 101–118.

JERGER, S., MARTIN, R.C. and JERGER, J. (1987). Specific auditory perceptual dysfunction in a learning disabled child. *Ear Hear.* **8**, 78–86.

JOHANSSON, B., WEDENBERG, E. and WESTIN, B. (1964). Measurement of tone response by the human foetus. *Acta Otolaryngol.* **57**, 188–192.

JOHN, J.E.J., GEMMILL, J., HOWARTH, J., KITZINGER, M. and SYKES, M. (1976). Some factors affecting the intelligibility of deaf children's speech. In: Stephens (1976).

JOHN, J.E.J. and HOWARTH, J.N. (1965). The effect of time distortions on the intelligibility of deaf children's speech. *Lang. Speech* **8**, 127–134.

JOHNSON, D., WHALEY, P. and DORMAN, M.F. (1984). Processing cues for stop consonant voicing by young hearing-impaired listeners. *J. Speech Hear. Res.* **27**, 112–118.

JOHNSON, D.D., CACCAMISE, F., ROTHBLUM, A.M., HAMILTON, L.F. and HOWARD, M. (1981). Identification and follow-up of visual impairments in hearing-impaired populations. *Am. Ann. Deaf.* **126**, 321–360.

JOHNSON, D.D., TOMS-BRONOWSKI, S. and PITTELMAN, S.D. (1982). Vocabulary development. *Volta Rev.* **84**, 11–24.

JOHNSON, F.L. (1977). Role-taking and referential communication abilities in first- and third-grade children. *Hum. Commun. Res.* **3**, 135–145.

JOHNSON, H. and GRIFFITH, P. (1985). The behavioral structure of an eighth-grade science class: a mainstreaming preparation strategy. *Volta Rev.* **87**, 291–303.

JOHNSON, H.A. (1988). A sociolinguistic aassessment scheme for the total communication student. *J. Acad. Rehab. Audiol. Monogr. Suppl.* **21**, 101–127.

JOHNSTON, T.A. (1987a). *A Preliminary Signing Dictionary of Australian Sign Language (Auslan)*. Payneham, South Australia: TAFE National Centre for Research and Development.

JOHNSTON, T.A. (1987b). *A General Introduction to Australian Sign Language (Auslan)*. Adelaide: TAFE National Centre for Research and Development.

JONES, E.E. (1985). Interpersonal distancing behavior of hearing-impaired vs. normal-hearing children. *Volta Rev.* **87**, 223–230.

JONES, T.W. (1984). A framework of identification, classification, and placement of multihandicapped hearing-impaired students. *Volta Rev.* **86**, 142–151.

JORDAN, I.K. (1983). Referential communication amongst Scottish deaf school pupils. In: Kyle and Woll (1983).

JOY, C.B. (1989). Features of discourse in an American Sign Language lecture. In: Lucas (1989).

KAGAN, J. and LEWIS, M. (1965). Studies in attention in the human infant. *Merrill–Palmer Q. Behav. Devel.* **11**, 101–119.

KAIL, R.V. and HAGEN, J.W. (Eds) (1977). *Perspectives on the Development of Memory and Cognition*. Hillsdale, NJ: Erlbaum.

KALIKOW, D.N., STEVENS, K.N. and ELIOTT, L.L. (1977). Development of a test of speech intelligibility in noise using sentence materials with controlled word predictability. *J. Acoust. Soc. Am.* **61**, 1337–1351.

KALLMAN, F. (1963). Main findings and some projections. In: Rainer et al. (1963).

KAMPFE, C.M. (1989). Reading comprehension of deaf adolescent residential school students and its relationship to hearing mothers' communication strategies and skills. *Am. Ann. Deaf* **134**, 317–322.

KAMPFE, C.M. and TURECHECK, A.G. (1987). Reading achievement of prelingually deaf students and its relationship to parental method of communication: a review of the literature. *Am. Ann. Deaf* **132**, 11–15.

KANGAS, K.A. and ALLEN, G.D. (1990). Intelligibility of synthetic speech for normal hearing and hearing-impaired listeners. *J. Speech Hear. Disord.* **55**, 751–755.

KANTOR, R. (1980). The acquisition of classifiers in ASL. *Sign Lang. Stud.* **8**, 193–208.

KAPLAN, H. and PICKETT, J.M. (1982). Differences in speech discrimination in the elderly as a function of type of competing noise: speech-babble or cafeteria. *Audiology* **21**, 325–333.

KATZ, J. (Ed.) (1985). *Handbook of Clinical Audiology*, 3rd Edn. Baltimore, MD: Williams and Wilkins.

KATZ, J. and HARMON, C.H. (1981). Phonemic synthesis: testing and training. In: Keith (1981b).

KAUTZKY-BOWDEN, S.M. and GONZALES, B.R. (1987). Attitudes of deaf adults regarding preferred sign language systems used in the classroom with deaf students. *Am. Ann. Deaf.* **132**, 251–255.

KAVANAGH, J.F. and CUTTING, J.E. (Eds) (1975). *The Role of Speech in Language*. Cambridge, MA: MIT Press.

KAVANAGH, J.F. and MATTINGLY, I.G. (Eds) (1972). *Language by Ear and by Eye: The Relationships between Speech and Reading*. Cambridge, MA: MIT Press.

KEENAN, P.A., WHITMAN, R.D. and PEPE, J. (1989). Hemispheric asymmetry in the processing of high and low spatial frequencies: a facial recognition task. *Brain Cognit.* **11**, 229–237.

KEITH, R.W. (1981a). Audiological and auditory language tests of central auditory function. In: Keith (1981b).

KEITH, R.W. (Ed.) (1981b). *Central Auditory and Language Disorders in Children*. Houston, TX: College Hill Press.

KEITH, R.W. (1984). The basic audiologic evaluation. In: Northern (1984).

KELLY, M.S., BEST, C.T. and KIRK, U. (1989). Cognitive processing deficits in reading disabilities: a prefrontal cortical hypothesis. *Brain Cognit.* **11**, 275–293.

KEMP, D.T., BRAY, P., ALEXANDER, L. and BROWN, A.M. (1986). Acoustic emission cochleography – practical aspects. *Scand. Audiol. Suppl.* **25**, 71–95.

KENDALL, M. and ORD, J.K. (1990). *Time series.* London: Edward Arnold.

KENDON, A. (1981a). Introduction: current issues in the study of 'nonverbal communication'. In: Kendon (1981b).

KENDON, A. (1981b). *Nonverbal Communication, Interaction, and Gesture: Selections from Semiotica.* The Hague: Mouton.

KENWORTHY, O.T. (1986). Caregiver–child interaction and language acquisition of hearing-impaired children. *Topics Lang. Disord.* **6**, 1–11.

KIERNAN, C., REID, B. and JONES, L. (1979). Signs and symbols: who uses what? *Spec. Educ. Forward Trends* **6**, 32–35.

KIERNAN, C., REID, B. and JONES, L. (1982). *Signs and Symbols: Use of Non-Vocal Communication Systems.* London: Heinemann.

KIMURA, D. (1973a). Manual activity during speaking. I. Right handers. *Neuropsychologia* **11**, 45–50.

KIMURA, D. (1973b). Manual activity during speaking. II. Left handers. *Neuropsychologia* **11**, 51–55.

KIMURA, D. (1983). Speech representation in an unbiased sample of left-handers. *Hum. Neurobiol.* **2**, 147–154.

KIMURA, D. (1990). How special is language? *Sign Lang. Stud.* **66**, 79–84.

KIMURA, D. and HUMPHRYS, C.A. (1981). A comparison of left- and right-arm movements during speaking. *Neuropsychologia* **19**, 807–812.

KING, A.B. (1987). Speech perception tests for the profoundly deaf. In: Martin (1987).

KING, C.M. and QUIGLEY, S.P. (1985). *Reading and Deafness.* Basingstoke: Taylor and Francis.

KING, F. (1989). Assessment of pragmatic skills. *Child Lang. Teaching Ther.* **5**, 191–201.

KINGSLEY, P.R. and HAGEN, J.W. (1969). Induced versus spontaneous rehearsal in short-term memory in nursery school children. *Devel. Psychol.* **1**, 40–46.

KIRK, S., MCCARTHY, J. and KIRK, W. (1968). *Illinois Test of Psycholinguistic Abilities.* Urbana, IL: University of Illinois Press.

KIRK, U. (1983). *Neuropsychology of Language, Reading, and Spelling.* New York: Academic Press.

KISILEVSKY, B.S. and MUIR, D.W. (1991). Human fetal and subsequent newborn responses to sound and vibration. *Infant Behav. Devel.* **14**, 1–26.

KITSON, H.D. (1915). Psychological tests for lip-reading ability. *Volta Rev.* **17**, 471–476.

KITSON, N. and FRY, R. (1990). Prelingual deafness and psychiatry. *Br. J. Hosp. Med.* **44**, 353–356.

KLAHR, D. and KOTOVSKY, K. (Eds) (1989). *Complex Information Processing: The Impact of Herbert A. Simon.* Hillsdale, NJ: Erlbaum.

KLECAN-AKER, J. and BLONDEAU, R. (1990). An examination of the written stories of hearing-impaired school-age children. *Volta Rev.* **92**, 275–282.

KLIMA, E.S. and BELLUGI, U. (1979). *The Signs of Language.* Cambridge, MA: Harvard University Press.

KLUWIN, T. (1981). The grammaticality of manual representations of English in classroom settings. *Am. Ann. Deaf* **126**, 417–421.

KLUWIN, T. (1983). Discourse in deaf classrooms: the structure of teaching episodes. *Discourse Processes* **6**, 275–293.

KLUWIN, T.N. and GAUSTAD, M.G. (1991). Predicting family communication choices. *Am. Ann Deaf* **136**, 28–34.

KLUWIN, T.N. and KELLY, A.B. (1991). The effectiveness of dialogue journal writing in improving the writing skills of young deaf writers. *Am. Ann. Deaf* **136**, 284–291.

KNELL, S.M. and KLONOFF, E.A. (1983). Language sampling in deaf children: a comparison of oral and signed communication modes. *J. Commun. Disord.* **16**, 435–447.

KNIGHT, T.K. (1989). The use of cumulative cloze to investigate contextual build-up in deaf and hearing readers. *Am. Ann Deaf* **134**, 268–272.

KNIGHTS, R.M. and BAKKER, K.K. (Eds) (1976). *Neuropsychology of Learning Disorders: Theoretical Approaches*. Baltimore, MD: University Park Press.

KNUDSEN, V.O. (1928). 'Hearing' with the sense of touch. *J. Gen. Psychol.* **1**, 320–351.

KNUTSON, J.F. and LANSING, C.R., (1990). The relationship between communication problems and psychological difficulties in persons with profound acquired hearing loss. *J. Speech Hear. Disord.* **55**, 656–664.

KOH, S.D., VERNON, M. and BAILEY, W. (1971). Free-recall learning of word lists by prelingually deaf subjects. *J. Verb. Learn. Verb. Behav.* **10**, 542–547.

KOLERS, P.A., WROLSTAD, N.E. and BOUMA, H. (Eds) (1979). *The Processing of Visible Language I*. New York: Plenum.

KOLUCHOVA, J. (1972). Severe deprivation in twins: a case study. *J. Child Psychol. Psychiat.* **13**, 107–114.

KOLUCHOVA, J. (1976). The further development of twins after severe and prolonged deprivation: a second report. *J. Child Psychol. Psychiat.* **17**, 181–188.

KRAKOW, R.A. and HANSON, V.L. (1985). Deaf signers and serial recall in the visual modality: memory for signs, fingerspelling and print. *Mem. Cognit.* **13**, 265–272.

KRASHEN, S.D. (1973). Lateralisation, language learning and the critical period: some new evidence. *Lang. Learning* **23**, 63–74.

KRASHEN, S.D. (1982). *Principles and Practice in Second Language Acquisition*. Oxford: Pergamon Press.

KREIMEYER, K. and ANTIA, S. (1988). The development and generalization of social interaction skills in preschool hearing-impaired children. *Volta Rev.* **90**, 219–231.

KRETSCHMER, R. (Ed.)(1985). *Writing to Learn and Learning to Write: Implications for the Hearing-Impaired* Washington, DC: Alexander Graham Bell Association.

KRETSCHMER, R.E. (1982). Reading and the hearing-impaired individual: summation and application. *Volta Rev.* **84**, 107–122.

KRETSCHMER, R. and KRETSCHMER, L. (1980). Pragmatics: development in normal-hearing and hearing-impaired children. In: Subtelny (1980).

KRETSCHMER, R.R. and KRETSCHMER, L.W. (1978). *Language Development and Intervention with the Hearing Impaired*. Baltimore, MD: University Park Press.

KRETSCHMER, R.R. and KRETSCHMER, L.W. (1986). Language in perspective. In: Luterman (1986).

KRETSCHMER, R.R. and KRETSCHMER, L.W. (1990). Language. *Volta Rev.* **92**, 56–71.

KRICOS, P.B. and LESNER, S.A. (1985). Effect of talker differences on the speechreading of hearing-impaired teenagers. *Volta Rev.* **87**, 5–14.

KRICOS, P., LESNER, S. and LAZARUS, G. (1990). Influence of visual information on speech assessment with hearing-impaired children. *Volta Rev.* **92**, 213–222.

KRINSKY, S. (1990). The feeling of knowing in deaf adolescents. *Am. Ann. Deaf* **135**, 389–395.

KRYTER, K.D. (1970). *The Effects of Noise on Man*. New York: Academic Press.

KUHL, P.K. (1980). Perceptual constancy for speech sound categories in early infancy. In: Yeni-Komishian et al. (1980).

KUSCHÉ, C.A., GREENBERG, M.T., CALDERON, R. and GUSTAFSON, R.N. (1987). Generalization strategies from the PATHS project for the prevention of substance use disorders. In: Anderson and Watson (1987).

KUSCHÉ, C.A., GREENBERG, M.T. and GARFIELD, T.S. (1983). Nonverbal intelligence and verbal achievement in deaf adolescents: an examination of heredity and environment. *Am. Ann. Deaf* **128**, 458–466.

KYLE, J. (Ed.) (1987). *Sign and School: Using Signs in Deaf Children's Development*. Clevedon, PA: Multilingual Matters Ltd.

KYLE, J.G. (1977). Audiometric analysis as a predictor of speech intelligibility. *Br. J. Audiol.* **11**, 51–58.

KYLE, J.G. (1978). The study of auditory deprivation from birth. *Br. J. Audiol.* **12**, 37–39.

KYLE, J.G. (1980a). Auditory deprivation from birth – clarification of some issues. *Br. J. Audiol.* **14**, 30–32.

KYLE, J.G. (1980b). Reading development of deaf children. *J. Res. Read.* **3**, 86–97.

KYLE, J.G. (1981). Signs of speech. *Spec. Educ. Forward Trends* **8**, 19–23.

KYLE, J.G. (1983a). Looking for meaning in sign language sentences. In: Kyle and Woll (1983).

KYLE, J.G. (1983b). Meaning in sign: reading events in BSL and English. In: Rogers and Sloboda (1983).

KYLE, J.G. and ALLSOP, L. (1982). Communicating with young deaf people: some issues. *J. Br. Assn. Teachers of the Deaf* **6**, 71–79.

KYLE, J.G. and WOLL, B. (Eds) (1983). *Language in Sign: An International Perspective on Sign Language.* London: Croom Helm.

KYLE, J.G. and WOLL, B. (1985). *Sign Language: The Study of Deaf People and Their Language.* Cambridge: Cambridge University Press.

LADD, G., MUNSON, H. and MILLER, J. (1984). Social integration of deaf adolescents in secondary-level mainstream programs. *Except. Child.* **50**, 420–428.

LADEFOGED, P. (1962). *Elements of Acoustic Phonetics.* Chicago, IL: University of Chicago Press.

LADEFOGED, P. (1967). *Three Areas of Experimental Phonetics.* London: Oxford University Press.

LA GRECA, A.M. and MESIBOV, G.B. (1979). Social skills intervention with learning disabled children: selecting skills and implementing training. *J. Clin. Child Psychol.* **8**, 234–241.

LAKOFF, G. (1987). *Women, Fire and Dangerous Things: What Categories Reveal About the Mind.* Chicago, IL: University of Chicago Press.

LAMBERT, N. and BOWER, E. (1979). *A Picture Game.* Monterey, CA: Publishers Test Service.

LANE, H. (1988). Educating the American Sign Language speaking minority of the United States: a paper prepared for the Commission on the Education of the Deaf. *Sign Lang. Stud.* **59**, 221–230.

LANE, H. (1990). Cultural and infirmity models of deaf Americans. *J. Aural Rehab. Assoc.* **23**, 11–26.

LANE, H. and BAKER, D. (1974). Reading achievement of the deaf: another look. *Volta Rev.* **76**, 489–499.

LANE, H., BOYES-BRAEM, P. and BELLUGI, U. (1976). Preliminaries to a distinctive feature analysis of American Sign Language. *Cognit. Psychol.* **8**, 263–289.

LANE, H.S. (1948). Some psychological problems involved in working with the deaf and the hard-of-hearing. *J. Rehabil.* **24–29** and **36**.

LARSON, C.O., DANSEREAU, D.F., O'DONNELL, A., HYTHECKER, V., LAMBIOTTE, J.G. and ROCKLIN, T. (1984). Verbal ability and cooperative learning. *J. Read. Behav.* **16**, 289–295.

LARTZ, M.N. and MCCOLLUM, J. (1990). Maternal questions while reading to deaf and hearing twins: a case study. *Am. Ann. Deaf* **135**, 235–240.

LaSASSO, C. (1980). The validity and reliability of the cloze procedure as a measure of readability for prelingually, profoundly deaf students. *Am. Ann. Deaf* **125**, 559–563.

LaSASSO, C. (1985). Visual matching test-taking strategies used by deaf readers. *J. Speech Hear. Res.* **28**, 2–7.

LaSASSO, C. (1986). A comparison of visual matching test-taking strategies of comparably-aged normal-hearing and hearing-impaired subjects with comparable reading levels. *Volta Rev.* **88**, 231–241.

LaSASSO, C. (1987). Survey of reading instruction for hearing-impaired students in the United States. *Volta Rev.* **89**, 85–98.

LaSASSO, C.J. (1990). Developing the ability of hearing impaired students to comprehend and generate question forms. *Am. Ann. Deaf* **135**, 409–412.

LaSASSO, C. and DAVEY, B. (1987). The relationship between lexical knowledge and reading comprehension for prelingually, profoundly hearing-impaired students. *Volta Rev.* **89**, 211–220.

LASS, N.J. (Ed.) (1983). *Speech and Language: Advances in Basic Research and Practice*, Vol. 9. New York: Academic Press.

LAWSON, R. (1978). Patterns of communication in intermediate level classrooms of the deaf. *Audiol. Hear. Educ.* 4, 19–23.

LECOURS, A.R. (1975). Myelogenetic correlates of the development of speech and language. In: Lenneberg and Lenneberg (1975).

LEDER, S.B., SPITZER, J.B. and KIRCHNER, J.C. (1987). Speaking fundamental frequency of postlingually profoundly deaf adult men. *Ann. Otol. Rhinol. Laryngol.* 96, 322–324.

LEDERBERG, A.R. (1984). Interaction between deaf preschoolers and unfamiliar hearing adults. *Child Devel.* 55, 598–606.

LEDERBERG, A.R. (1991). Social interaction among deaf preschoolers. *Am. Ann. Deaf* 136, 53–59.

LEDERBERG, A.R. and MOBLEY, C.E. (1990). The effect of hearing impairment on the quality of attachment and mother–toddler interaction. *Child Devel.* 61, 1596–1604.

LEE, L.L. (1966). Developmental Sentence Types: a method for comparing normal and deviant syntactic development. *J. Speech Hear. Disord.* 31, 311–330.

LEE, L.L. (1969). *The Northwestern Syntax Screening Test*. Evanston, IL: Northwestern University Press.

LEE, L.L. and CANTER, S.M. (1971). Developmental Sentence Scoring: a clinical procedure for estimating syntax development in children's spontaneous speech. *J. Speech Hear. Disord.* 36, 315–340.

LEINHARDT, G. and GREENO, J.G. (1986). The cognitive skills of teaching. *J. Educ. Psychol.* 78, 75–95.

LEMANEK, K.L., WILLIAMSON, D.A., GRESHAM, F.M. and JENSEN, B.J. (1986). Social skills training with hearing-impaired children and adolescents. *Behav. Modif.* 10, 55–71.

LENNEBERG, E.H. (1967). *Biological Foundations of Language*. New York: Wiley.

LENNEBERG, E.H. and LENNEBERG, E. (Eds) (1975). *Foundations of Language Development: A Multidisciplinary Approach*. New York: Academic Press.

LEOTTA, D.F., RABINOWITZ, W.M., REED, C.M. and DURLACH, N.I. (1988). Preliminary results of speech-reception tests obtained with the synthetic Tadoma system. *J. Rehab. Res. Devel.* 25, 45–52.

LESLIE, P.T. and CLARKE, B.R. (1977). A study of selected syntactic structures in the language of young deaf children. *J. Br. Assn. Teachers of the Deaf* 1, 128–133.

LESNER, S.A. (1988). The talker. In: De Filippo and Sims (1988).

LESNER, S., SANDRIDGE, S. and KRICOS, P. (1987). Training influences on visual consonant and sentence recognition. *Ear Hear.* 8, 283–287.

LEVELT, W.J.M. (1989). *Speaking: From Intention to Articulation*. Cambridge, MA: MIT Press.

LEVINE, E.S. (1960). *The Psychology of Deafness: Techniques of Appraisal for Rehabilitation*. New York: Columbia University Press.

LEVINE, S. (1986). Hemispheric specialization and implications for the education of the hearing impaired. *Am. Ann. Deaf* 131, 238–242.

LEVINSON, P.J. and SLOAN, C. (Eds) (1980). *Auditory Processing and Language*. New York: Grune and Stratton.

LEVITT, H. (1971). Speech production for the deaf child. In: Connor (1971).

LEVITT, H., MCGARR, N.S. and GEFFNER, D. (Eds) (1987). *Development of Language and Communication Skills in Hearing-Impaired Children*. Washington, DC: ASHA.

LEVITT, H., SMITH, C. and STROMBERT, H. (1974). Acoustic, perceptual and articulatory characteristics of the speech of deaf children. In: Fant (1974).

LEVITT, H., STARK, R.E., MCGARR, N., CARP, J., STROMBERT, M., GAFFNEY, R.H., BARRY, C., VILEZ, A., OSBERGER, M.J., LEITER, E. and FREEMAN, L. (1976). Language communication skills of deaf children. 1973/1975. *Proc. Language Assessment for the Hearing Impaired – A Work Study Institute*. New York: New York State Education Department.

LEWIS, M.M. (1968). *Language and Personality in Deaf Children*. Slough, Buckinghamshire: National Foundation for Educational Research in England and Wales.

LEWIS, T.K. and WILCOX, J.C. (1978). The perceptual use of semantic rules by normal-hearing and hard-of-hearing children. *J. Commun. Disord.* **11**, 107–118.

LI, C.N. (Ed.) (1976). *Subject and Topic.* New York: Academic Press.

LIBEN, L.S. (Ed.) (1978). *Deaf Children: Developmental Perspectives.* New York: Academic Press.

LIBEN, L.S. (1979). Free recall by deaf and hearing children: semantic clustering and recall in trained and untrained groups. *J. Exp. Child Psychol.* **27**, 105–119.

LIBERMAN, A.M., COOPER, F.S., SHANKWEILER, D.P. and STUDDERT-KENNEDY, M. (1967). Perception of the speech code. *Psychol. Rev.* **74**, 431–461.

LIBERMAN, I.Y., MANN, V.A., SHANKWEILER, D. and WERFELMAN, M. (1982). Children's memory for recurring linguistic and non-linguistic material in relation to reading ability. *Cortex* **18**, 367–375.

LIBERMAN, I.Y., SHANKWEILER, D., LIBERMAN, A.M., FOWLER, C. and FISCHER, F.W. (1977). Phonetic segmentation and recoding in the beginning reader. In: Reber and Scarborough (1977).

LIDDELL, S. (1978a). Nonmanual signals and relative clauses in American Sign Language. In: Siple (1978b).

LIDDELL, S. (1978b). An introduction to relative clauses in ASL. In: Siple (1978b).

LIDDELL, S. (1980). *American Sign Langauge Syntax.* The Hague: Mouton.

LIDEN, G. and KANKKUNEN, A. (1973). Hearing aid procedures in young deaf and hard of hearing children. *Scand. Audiol. Suppl.* **3**, 47–54.

LIEBERTH, A.K. (1982). Functional speech therapy for the deaf child. In: Sims et al. (1982).

LIEBERTH, A.K. (1990). Rehabilitative issues in the bilingual education of deaf children. *J. Aural. Rehab. Assn.* **23**, 53–61.

LIEBERTH, A.K. and GAMBLE, M.E.B. (1991). The role of iconicity in sign language learning by hearing adults. *J. Commun. Disord.* **24**, 89–99.

LIEBERTH, A.K. and WHITEHEAD, R.L. (1987). Orosensory perception and articulatory proficiency in hearing-impaired adults. *Percept. Mot. Skills* **64**, 611–617.

LIEMOHN, W., HARGIS, C., WRISBERG, C. and WINTER, T. (1990). Rhythm production/perception by hearing-impaired students. *Volta Rev.* **92**, 13–24.

LILES, B., SCHULMAN, M. and BARTLETT, S. (1977). Judgments of grammar by normal and language-disorded children. *J. Speech Hear. Disord.* **42**, 199–209.

LILLO-MARTIN, D. (1990). Parameters for questions: evidence from wh-movement in ASL. In: Lucas (1990).

LINDZEY, G. and ARONSON, E. (Eds) (1969). *Handbook of Social Psychology.* Reading, MA: Addison-Wesley.

LING, D. (1976). *Speech and the Hearing-Impaired Child: Theory and Practice.* Washington DC: Alexander Graham Bell Association.

LING, D. (1979). Principles underlying the development of speech communication skills among hearing-impaired children. *Volta Rev.* **81**, 211–223.

LING, D. (Ed.) (1984a). *Early Intervention for Hearing-Impaired Children: Total Communication Options.* San Diego, CA: College Hill Press.

LING, D. (Ed.) (1984b). *Early Intervention for Hearing-Impaired Children: Oral Options.* San Diego, CA: College Hill Press.

LING, D. (1989). *The Foundations of Spoken Language for Hearing-impaired Children.* Washington DC: Alexander Graham Bell Association.

LING, D. (1991). *Phonetic–Phonologic Speech Evaluation Form: A Manual.* Washington DC: Alexander Graham Bell Association.

LING, D. and LING, A.H. (1978). *Aural Habilitation: The Foundations of Verbal Learning in Hearing-Impaired Children.* Washington DC: Alexander Graham Bell Association.

LING, D. and NIENHUYS, T.G. (1983). The deaf child: habilitation with and without a cochlear implant. *Ann. Otol. Rhinol. Laryngol.* **92**, 593–598.

LIVINGSTON, S. (1989). Revision strategies of deaf student writers. *Am. Ann. Deaf* **134**, 21–26.

LIVINGSTON, S. (1991). Comprehension strategies of two deaf readers. *Sign Lang. Stud.* **71**, 115–130.

LLOYD, L.L. and DOHERTY, J. (1983). The influence of production mode on the recall of signs in normal adult subjects. *J. Speech Hear. Res.* **26**, 595–600.

LOCKE, J.L. (1978). Phonemic effects in the silent reading of hearing and deaf children. *Cognition* **6**, 175–187.

LOCKE, J.L. and LOCKE, V.L. (1971). Deaf children's phonetic, visual, and dactylic coding in a grapheme recall task. *J. Exp. Psychol.* **89**, 142–146.

LOEB, R.C., HORST, L. and HORTON, P. (1980). Family interaction patterns associated with self-esteem in preadolescent girls and boys. *Merrill-Palmer Q. Behav. Devel.* **26**, 205–217.

LOEB, R. and SARIGIANI, P. (1986). The impact of hearing impairment on self-perceptions of children. *Volta Rev.* **88**, 89–100.

LOTT, B.E. and LEVY, J. (1960). The influence of certain communicator characteristics on lip reading efficiency. *J. Soc. Psychol.* **51**, 419–425.

LOU, M.W. (1988). The history of language use in the education of the deaf in the United States. In: Strong (1988).

LOU, M.W., FISCHER, S. and WOODWARD, J. (1987). A language-independent measure of communicative competence for deaf adolescents and adults. *Sign Lang. Stud.* **57**, 353–370.

LUCAS, C. (Ed.) (1989). *The Sociolinguistics of the Deaf Community*. San Diego, CA: Academic Press.

LUCAS, C. (Ed.) (1990). *Sign Language Research: Theoretical Issues*. Washington, DC: Gallaudet University Press.

LUCAS, C. and VALLI, C. (1989). Language contact in the American deaf community. In: Lucas (1989).

LUCKNER, J. (1991a). The competencies needed for teaching hearing-impaired students. *Am. Ann. Deaf* **136**, 17–20.

LUCKNER, J.L. (1991b). Mainstreaming hearing-impaired students: perceptions of regular educators. *Lang. Speech Hear. in Schools* **22**, 302–307.

LUDDERS, B.B. (1987). Communication between health care professionals and deaf patients. *Health Soc. Work.* **4**, 303–310.

LUETKE-STAHLMAN, B, (1984). Replicating single-subject assessment of language in deaf elementary-age children. *Am. Ann. Deaf* **129**, 40–44.

LUETKE-STAHLMAN, B. and MOELLER, M.P. (1990). Enhancing parents' use of SEE-2: progress and retention. *Am. Ann. Deaf* **135**, 371–378.

LUFTIG, R.L. and LLOYD, L.L. (1981). Manual sign translucency and referential concreteness in the learning of signs. *Sign Lang. Stud.* **30**, 49–60.

LUFTIG, R.L., PAGE, J.L. and LLOYD, L.L. (1983). Ratings of translucency in manual signs as a predictor of sign learnability. *J. Child. Commun. Disord.* **6**, 117–134.

LUPTON, L.K. and ZELAZNIK, H.N. (1990). Motor learning in sign language students. *Sign Lang. Stud.* **67**, 153–173.

LUTERMAN, D. (1979). *Counselling Parents of Hearing-Impaired Children*. Boston, MA: Little, Brown and Co.

LUTERMAN, D.M. (Ed.) (1986). *Deafness in Perspective*. San Diego, CA: College-Hill Press.

LYON, R. (1977). Auditory perceptual training: the state of the art. *J. Learn. Disabil.* **10**, 564–572.

LYREGAARD, P.E., ROBINSON, D.W. and HINCHCLIFFE, R. (1976). *A Feasibility Study of Speech Audiometry, N.P.L., Acoustics Report Ac73*. Teddington, Middlesex: National Physical Laboratory.

LYXELL, B. and RONNBERG, J. (1987). Guessing and speechreading. *Br. J. Audiol.* **21**, 13–20.

LYXELL, B. and RONNBERG, J. (1989). Information-processing skill and speech-reading. *Br. J. Audiol.* **23**, 339–347.

LYXELL, B. and RONNBERG, J. (1991). Word discrimination and chronological age related to sentence-based speech-reading skill. *Br. J. Audiol.* **25**, 3–10.

MAASSEN, B. (1986). Marking word boundaries to improve the intelligibility of the speech of the deaf. *J. Speech Hear. Res.* **29**, 227–230.

MAASSEN, B. and POVEL, D.J. (1984). The effect of segmental and suprasegmental corrections on the intelligibility of deaf speech. *J. Acoust. Soc. Am.* **78**, 877–886.

McAFEE, M.C., KELLY, J.F. and SAMAR, V.J. (1990). Spoken and written English errors of postsecondary students with severe hearing impairment. *J. Speech Hear. Disord.* **55**, 528–634.

McALISTER, P.V. (1990). The effects of hearing aids on speech discrimination in noise by normal-hearing listeners. *J. Rehab. Res. Devel.* **27**, 33–42.

McANNALLY, P.L., ROSE, S. and QUIGLEY, S.P. (1987). *Language Learning Practices with Deaf Children*. Boston, MA: College-Hill Press.

McCANE, N.P. (1980). Responding to classroom behavior problems among deaf children. *Am. Ann. Deaf* **125**, 902–905.

McCARTNEY, B. (1984). Education in the mainstream. *Volta Rev.* **86**, 41–52.

McCARTNEY, B.D. (1986). An investigation of the factors contributing to the ability of hearing-impaired children to communicate orally as perceived by oral deaf adults and teachers of the hearing-impaired. *Volta Rev.* **88**, 133–143.

McCAULEY, R.W., BRUININKS, R.H. and KENNEDY, P. (1976). Behavioral interactions of hearing-impaired children in regular classrooms. *J. Spec. Educ.* **10**, 277–284.

McCONKEY ROBBINS, M.S. (1986). Facilitating language comprehension in young hearing-impaired children. *Topics Lang. Disord.* **6**, 12–24.

McCORMICK, B., CURNOCK, D.A. and SPAVINS, F. (1984). Auditory screening of special care neonates using the auditory response cradle. *Arch. Dis. Childhood* **59**, 1168–1172.

McDEVITT, T.M., SPIVEY, N., SHEEHAN, E.P., LENNON, R. and STORY, R. (1990). Children's beliefs about listening: is it enough to be still and quiet? *Child Devel.* **61**, 713–721.

McDONALD, E.T. (1980). Disorders of articulation. In: Van Hattum (1980).

MacDONALD, J. and McGURK, H. (1978). Visual influences on speech perception processes. *Percept. Psychophys.* **24**, 253–257.

McDONALD, J.L. and MacWHINNEY, B. (1991). Levels of learning: a comparison of concept formation and language acquisition. *J. Mem. Lang.* **30**, 407–430.

McGARR, N.S. and HARRIS, K.S. (1983). Articulatory control in a deaf speaker. In: Hochberg et al. (1983).

McGINNIS, M.D., ORR, C.D. and FREUTEL, J.M. (1980). Becoming a social being. *Volta Rev.* **82**, 370–379.

MacGREGOR, S.K. and THOMAS, L.B. (1988). A computer-mediated text system to develop communication skills for hearing-impaired students. *Am. Ann. Deaf* **133**, 280–284.

McGROSKEY, R. and KIDDER, A. (1980). Auditory fusion among learning-disabled, reading-disabled and normal children. *J. Learn. Disabil.* **13**, 18–25.

McGUIGAN, F.J. (1970). Covert oral behavior during the silent performance of language tasks. *Psychol. Bull.* **74**, 309–326.

McGURK, H. and MacDONALD, J. (1976). Hearing lips and seeing voices. *Nature* **264**, 746–748.

McINTIRE, M.L. (1977). The acquisition of American Sign Language hand configurations. *Sign Lang. Stud.* **16**, 247–266.

MacKAY, D.G. (1981). The problem of rehearsal or mental practice. *J. Motor Behav.* **13**, 274–285.

MacKAY, D.G. (1987). *The Organization of Perception and Action: A Theory of Language and other Cognitive Skills*. New York: Springer-Verlag.

MacKAY-SOROTA, S., TREHUB, S.E. and THORPE, L.A. (1987). Deaf children's referential messages to mother. *Child Devel.* **58**, 385–394.

McKEE, B.G. and DOWALIBY, F.J. (1985). The relationship between student, course, and instructor characteristics and hearing-impaired students' ratings of instruction. *Volta Rev.* **87**, 77–86.

McKEEVER, W.F., HOEMANN, H.W., FLORIAN, V.A. and VAN DEVENTER, A.D. (1976). Evidence of minimal cerebral asymmetries for the processing of English words and American Sign Language in the congenitally deaf. *Neuropsychologia* **14**, 413–423.

McKEOWN, M. and CURTIS, M. (Eds) (1987). *The Nature of Vocabulary Acquisition*. Hillsdale, NJ: Erlbaum.

MacKINNON, G.E. and WALLER, T.G. (Eds) (1981). *Reading Research: Advances in Theory and Practice. Vol. 3.* New York: Academic Press.

McKIRDY, L.S. and BLANK, M. (1982). Dialogue in deaf and hearing pre-schoolers. *J. Speech Hear. Res.* **25**, 487–499.

MacLEOD, A. and SUMMERFIELD, Q. (1987). Quantifying the contribution of vision to speech perception in noise. *Br. J. Audiol.* **21**, 131–141.

MacLEOD, A. and SUMMERFIELD, Q. (1990). A procedure for measuring auditory and audio-visual speech-reception thresholds for sentences in noise: rationale, evaluation and recommendations for use. *Br. J. Audiol.* **24**, 29–43.

McPHERSON, D.L. and DAVIS, M.S. (Eds) (1978). *Advances in Prosthetic Devices for the Deaf: A Technical Workshop.* Rochester, NY: National Technical Institute for the Deaf.

MAGEN, Z. (1990). Positive experiences and life aspirations among adolescents with and without hearing impairments. *Int. J. Disabil. Devel. Educ.* **37**, 57–69.

MAKI, J. (1980). Visual feedback as an aid to speech therapy. In: Subtelny (1980).

MAKI, J.D. (1983). Application of the speech spectrographic display in developing articulatory skills in hearing-impaired adults. In: Hochberg et al. (1983).

MANDELBAUM, D. (Ed.) (1949). *Selected Writings of Edward Sapir in Language, Culture, and Personality.* Berkeley, CA: University of California Press.

MANION, I.G. and BUCHER, B. (1986). Generalization of a sign language rehearsal strategy in mentally retarded and hearing deficient children. *Appl. Res. Ment. Retard.* **7**, 133–148.

MANN, V.A., LIBERMAN, I.Y. and SHANKWEILER, D. (1980). Children's memory for sentences and work strings in relation to reading ability. *Mem. Cognit.* **8**, 329–335.

MANNING, A.A., GOBLE, W., MARKMAN, R. and LABRECHE, T. (1977). Lateral cerebral differences in the deaf response to linguistic and nonlinguistic stimuli. *Brain Lang.* **4**, 309–321.

MARCEL, A.J., KATZ, L. and SMITH, M. (1974). Laterality and reading proficiency. *Neuropsychologia* **12**, 131–139.

MARCOTTE, A.C. and LA BARBA, R.C. (1985). Cerebral lateralization for speech in deaf and normal children. *Brain Lang.* **26**, 244–258.

MARGOLIS, H. (1986). Patterns, thinking, and cognition. In: Mason and Au (1986).

MARKIDES, A. (1967). *The Speech of Deaf and Partially-Hearing Children with Special Reference to Factors Affecting Intelligibility.* University of Manchester: unpublished Doctoral Thesis.

MARKIDES, A. (1970). The speech of deaf and partially-hearing children with special reference to factors affecting intelligibility. *Br. J. Disord. Commun.* **5**, 126–140.

MARKIDES, A. (1983). *The Speech of Hearing-Impaired Children.* Manchester: Manchester University Press.

MARKIDES, A. (1987). Speech tests of hearing for children. In: Martin (1987).

MARKIDES, A. (1988). Speech intelligibility: auditory–oral approach versus total communication. *J. Br. Assn. Teachers of the Deaf* **12**, 136–141.

MARKIDES, A. (1989a). Background noise and lipreading ability. *Br. J. Audiol.* **23**, 251–253.

MARKIDES, A. (1989b). Lipreading: theory and practice. *J. Br. Assn. Teachers of the Deaf* **13**, 29–47.

MARMOR, G. and PETITTO, L. (1979). Simultaneous communication in the classroom: how well is English grammar represented? In: Stokoe (1979).

MARSCHARK, M. and WEST, S.A. (1985). Creative language abilities of deaf children. *J. Speech Hear. Res.* **28**, 73–78.

MARSCHARK, M., WEST, S.A., NALL, L. and EVERHART, V. (1986). Development of creative language devices in signed and oral production. *J. Exp. Child Psychol.* **41**, 534–550.

MARSHALL, W.A. (1970). Contextual constraints on deaf and hearing children. *Am. Ann. Deaf* **115**, 682–689.

MARTELLO, A. (1981). The Ling approach to teaching speech as adapted in a day program for the hearing impaired. *Volta Rev.* **83**, 458–465.

MARTIN, D.S. (Ed.) (1984). *International Symposium on Cognition, Education and Deafness.* Washington DC: Gallaudet College Press.

MARTIN, D.S. (Ed.) (1985). *Cognition, Education and Deafness: Directions for Research and Instruction.* Washington DC: Gallaudet University Press.

MARTIN, E.S., PICKETT, J.M. and COLTEN, S. (1972). Discrimination of vowel formant transitions by listeners with severe sensorineural hearing loss. In: Fant (1972).

MARTIN, F.N., ABADIE, K.T. and DESCOUZIS, D. (1989). Counseling families of hearing-impaired children: comparisons of the attitudes of Australian and US parents and audiologists. *Aust. J. Audiol.* 11, 41–54.

MARTIN, F.N., BERNSTEIN, M.E., DALY, J.A. and CODY, J.P. (1988). Classroom teachers' knowledge of hearing disorders and attitudes about mainstreaming hard-of-hearing children. *Lang. Speech Hear. Services in Schools* 19, 83–95.

MARTIN, F.N. and FORBIS, N.R. (1978). The present status of audiometric practice: a follow-up study. *ASHA* 20, 531–541.

MARTIN, M. (Ed.) (1987). *Speech Audiometry.* London: Taylor and Francis.

MARTINEK, T.J. (1980). Students' expectations as related to a teacher's expectations and self-concepts of elementary age children. *Percept. Mot. Skills* 50, 555–561.

MARTONY, J. (1968). On the correction of the voice pitch level for severely hard of hearing subjects. *Am. Ann. Deaf* 113, 195–202.

MARTONY, J. (1972). Visual aids for speech correction: summary of three years' experiences. In: Fant (1972).

MASHIE, J.J., VARI-ALQUIST, D., WADDY-SMITH, B. and BERNSTEIN, L.F. (1988). Speech training aids for hearing-impaired individuals: III. Preliminary observations in the clinic and children's homes. *J. Rehab. Res. Devel.* 25, 69–82.

MASON, J.M. (1980). When do children begin to read: an exploration of four-year-old children's letter and word reading competencies. *Read. Res. Q.* 2, 203–227.

MASON, J.M. and AU, K.H. (1986). *Reading Instruction for Today.* Glenview, IL: Scott, Foresman and Co.

MASON, M.K. (1942). Learning to speak after six and one-half years of silence. *J. Speech Disord.* 7, 295–304.

MATEY, C. and KRETSCHMER, R. (1985). A comparison of mother speech to Down's syndrome, hearing-impaired, and normal-hearing children. *Volta Rev.* 87, 205–213.

MATHER, S.A. (1989). Visually oriented teaching strategies with deaf preschool children. In: Lucas (1989).

MATKIN, N.D. (1981). Amplification for children: current status and future priorities. In: Bess et al. (1981).

MATZKER, V.J. (1960). Schizophrenie und Taubheit. *Z. Laryngol. Rhinol. Otol.* 39, 43–52.

MAXON, A.B., BRACKETT, D. and VAN DEN BERG, S.A. (1991). Self perception of socialization: the effects of hearing status, age and gender. *Volta Rev.* 93, 7–18.

MAXWELL, M. (1980). Language acquisition in a deaf child of deaf parents: speech, sign variations, and print variations. In: Nelson (1980).

MAXWELL, M.M. (1986). Beginning reading and deaf children. *Am. Ann. Deaf* 131, 14–20.

MAXWELL, M.M. (1988). The alphabetic principle and fingerspelling. *Sign Lang. Stud.* 61, 377–404.

MAXWELL, M.M. (1989). A signing deaf child's use of speech. *Sign Lang. Stud.* 62, 23–42.

MAXWELL, M.M. (1990). Simultaneous Communication: the state of the art and proposals for change. *Sign Lang. Stud.* 69, 333–389.

MAXWELL, M. and BERNSTEIN, M. (1985). The synergy of sign and speech in Simultaneous Communication. *Appl. Psycholing.* 6, 63–81.

MAYBERRY, R.I. and EICHEN, E.B. (1991). The long-lasting advantage of learning sign language in childhood: another look at the critical period for language acquisition. *J. Mem. Lang.* 30, 486–512.

MAYBERRY, R.I. and FISCHER, S.D. (1989). Looking through phonological shape to lexical meaning: the bottleneck of non-native sign language processing. *Mem. Cognit.* 17, 740–754.

MAYER, P. and LOWENBRAUN, S. (1990). Total communication use among elementary teachers of hearing-impaired children. *Am. Ann. Deaf* 135, 257–263.

MEAD, R.A. and LAPIDUS, L.B. (1989). Psychological differential, arousal, and lipreading efficiency in hearing-impaired and normal children. *J. Clin. Psychol.* 45, 851–859.

MEADOW, K.P. (1968). Early manual communication in relation to the deaf child's intellectual, social and communicative functioning. *Am. Ann. Deaf* 113, 29–41.

MEADOW, K.P. (1980). *Deafness and Child Development.* London: Arnold.

MEADOW, K. (1981). Studies of behavior problems of deaf children. In: Stein et al. (1981).

MEADOW-ORLANS, K.P. (1987). An analysis of the effectiveness of early intervention programs for hearing-impaired children. In: Guralnick and Bennett (1987b).

MEDICAL RESEARCH COUNCIL (1947). *Committee on Electroacoustics, Hearing Aids and Audiometers, MRC Special Report Series No. 261.* London: HMSO.

MEISELS, S.J. and SHONKOFF, J.P. (Eds) (1990). *Handbook of Early Childhood Intervention.* Cambridge: Cambridge University Press.

MENCHER, G.T. (Ed.) (1976). *Early Identification of Hearing Loss.* Basel: S. Karger.

MENCKE, E.O., OCHSNER, G.J. and TESTUT, E.W. (1984). Speech intelligibility of deaf speakers and distinctive feature usage. *J. Aud. Res.* 24, 63–68.

MENCKE, E.O., OCHSNER, G.J. and TESTUT, E.W. (1985). Distinctive-feature analyses of the speech of deaf children. *J. Aud. Res.* 25, 191–200.

MENDELSON, J.H., SIGER, L. and SOLOMON, P. (1960). Psychiatric observations on congenital and acquired deafness: symbolic and perceptual processes in dreams. *Am. J. Psychiat.* 116, 883–888.

MERKLEIN, R.A. (1981). A short speech perception test for severely and profoundly deaf children. *Volta Rev.* 83, 36–45.

MERTENS, D.M. (1989). Social experiences of hearing-impaired high school youth. *Am. Ann. Deaf* 134, 15–19.

MERTENS, D.M. (1991). Teachers working with interpreters: the deaf student's educational experience. *Am. Ann. Deaf* 136, 48–52.

METZ, D.E., SAMAR, V.J., SCHIAVETTI, N., SITLER, R.W. and WHITEHEAD, R.L. (1985). Acoustic dimensions of hearing-impaired speakers' intelligibility. *J. Speech Hear. Res.* 28, 345–355.

METZ, D.E., SCHIAVETTI, N., SAMAR, V.J. and SITLER, R.W. (1990a). Acoustic dimensions of hearing-impaired speakers' intelligibility: segmental and suprasegmental characteristics. *J. Speech Hear. Res.* 33, 476–487.

METZ, D.E., SCHIAVETTI, N., SITLER, R.W. and SAMAR, V.J. (1990b). Speech production stability characteristics of hearing-impaired speakers. *Volta Rev.* 92, 223–235.

MEYER, A.S. (1990). The time course of phonological encoding of successive syllables of a word. *J. Mem. Lang.* 29, 524–545.

MICHELSON, R.P. (1971). Electrical stimulation of the human cochlea. *Arch. Otolaryngol.* 93, 317–323.

MILLER, G.A. (1947). The masking of speech. *Psychol. Bull.* 44, 105–129.

MILLER, G.A., HEISE, G.A. and LICHTEN, W. (1951). The intelligibility of speech as a function of the context of the test materials. *J. Exp. Psychol.* 41, 329–335.

MILLER, G.A. and NICELY, P.E. (1955). An analysis of perceptual confusions among some English consonants. *J. Acoust. Soc. Am.* 27, 338–352.

MILLER, G.A. and TAYLOR, W.G. (1948). Perception of repeated bursts of noise. *J. Acoust. Soc. Am.* 20, 171–182.

MILLER, L. (1981). Remediation of auditory language learning disorders. In: Roeser and Downs (1981).

MILLER, M.S. (1987). Sign iconicity: single-sign receptive vocabulary skills of nonsigning hearing preschoolers. *J. Commun. Disord.* 20, 359–365.

MILLS, C. and WELDON, L. (1983). Effects of semantic and cheremic context on acquisition of manual signs. *Mem. Cognit.* 11, 93–100.

MILLS, J.H. (1975). Noise and children: a review of literature. *J. Acoust. Soc. Am.* 58, 767–779.

MINDESS, A. (1990). What name signs can tell us about deaf culture. *Sign Lang. Stud.* 66, 1–23.

MISCHOOK, M. and COLE, E. (1986). Auditory learning and teaching of hearing-impaired infants. *Volta Rev.* **88**, 67–81.

MISHKIN, M. and FORGAYS, D.G. (1952). Word recognition as a function of retinal locus. *J. Exp. Psychol.* **43**, 43–48.

MITCHELL, G. (1978). Stigma, stereotype and rehabilitation. In: Montgomery (1978).

MOELLER, M.P. (1985). Developmental approaches to communication assessment and enhancement. In: Cherow (1985).

MOELLER, M.P. and LUETKE-STAHLMAN, B. (1990). Parents' use of Signing Exact English: a descriptive analysis. *J. Speech Hear. Disord.* **55**, 327–338.

MOELLER, M.P., MCCONKEY, A.J. and OSBERGER, M.J. (1983). Evaluation of the communicative skills of hearing-impaired children. *Audiology* **8**, 113–127.

MOERK, E.L. (1977). *Pragmatic and Semantic Aspects of Early Language Development.* Baltimore, MD: University Park Press.

MOHAY, H. (1982). A preliminary description of the communication systems evolved by two deaf children in the absence of a sign language model. *Sign Lang. Stud.* **34**, 73–91.

MOHAY, H. (1983). The effects of cued speech on the language development of three deaf children. *Sign Lang. Stud.* **38**, 25–49.

MONSEN, R. (1981). A usable test for the speech intelligibility of deaf talkers. *Am. Ann. Deaf* **126**, 845–852.

MONSEN, R.B. (1976). Normal and reduced phonological space: the production of English vowels by deaf adolescents. *J. Phonet.* **4**, 189–198.

MONSEN, R.B. (1978). Toward measuring how well hearing-impaired children speak. *J. Speech Hear. Res.* **21**, 197–219.

MONSEN, R.B. (1979). Acoustic qualities of phonation in young hearing-impaired children. *J. Speech Hear. Res.* **22**, 270–288.

MONTGOMERY, A.A. and EDGE, R.A. (1988). Evaluation of two speech enhancement techniques to improve intelligibility for hearing-impaired adults. *J. Speech, Hear. Res.* **31**, 386–393.

MONTGOMERY, A.A., WALDEN, B.E. and PROSEK, R.A. (1987). Effects of consonantal context on vowel lipreading. *J. Speech Hear. Res.* **30**, 50–59.

MONTGOMERY, G. (1976). The integration of the oral–manual language ability of profoundly deaf children. In: Henderson (1976).

MONTGOMERY, G. (Ed.) (1978). *Of Sound and Mind: Deafness, Personality and Mental Health.* Edinburgh: Papers on Scottish Workshop Publications.

MONTGOMERY, G., MITCHELL, G., MILLER, J. and MONTGOMERY, J. (1983). Open communication or catastrophe? A model for educational communication. In: Kyle and Woll (1983).

MONTGOMERY, G.W.G. (1966). The relationship of oral skills to manual communication in profoundly deaf students. *Am. Ann. Deaf* **111**, 557–565.

MONTGOMERY, G.W.G. (1968). A factorial study of communication and ability in deaf school leavers. *Br. J. Educ. Psychol.* **38**, 27–37.

MOOG, J. and GEERS, A. (1985). EPIC: a program to accelerate academic progress in profoundly hearing-impaired children. *Volta Rev.* **87**, 259–277.

MOOG, J.S. and GEERS, A.E. (1991). Educational management of children with cochlear implants. *Am. Ann. Deaf* **136**, 69–76.

MOORE, D.T. (1983). Perspectives on learning in internships. *J. Experient. Educn.* **6**, 40–44.

MOORE, N. (1981). Is paranoid illness associated with sensory defects in the elderly? *J. Psychosom. Res.* **25**, 69–74.

MOORES, D. (1970). Psycholinguistics and deafness. *Am. Ann. Deaf* **115**, 37–48.

MOORES, D.F. (1987). *Educating the Deaf: Psychology, Principles and Practices*, 3rd Edn. Boston, MA: Houghton Mifflin.

MOORES, D.F. (1991). The great debates: where, how, and what to teach deaf children. *Am. Ann. Deaf* **136**, 35–37.

MOORES, D.F. and SWEET, C.A. (1990). Reading and writing skills in deaf adolescents. *Internat. J. Rehab. Res.* **13**, 178–179.

MORARIU, J.A. and BRUNING, R.H. (1984). Cognitive processing by prelingual deaf students as a function of language context. *J. Educ. Psychol.* 76, 844–856.

MORGAN-REDSHAW, M., WILGOSH, L. and BIBBY, M.A. (1990). The parental experiences of mothers of adolescents with hearing impairments. *Am. Ann. Deaf* 135, 293–298.

MORRIS, C. (1946). *Signs, Language and Behavior.* New York: Braziller.

MORRIS, T. (1978). Some observations on the part played by oral teaching methods in perpetuating low standards of language achievement in severely and profoundly deaf pupils. *J. Br. Assn. Teachers of the Deaf* 2, 130–135.

MORTON, J. (1970). A functional model for memory. In: Norman (1970).

MORTON, J. (Ed.) (1971). *Biological and Social Factors in Psycholinguistics.* London: Logos Press.

MOSCOVITCH, M. (1979). Information processing and the cerebral hemispheres. In: Gazzaniga (1979).

MOSENTHAL, P., TAMOR, L. and WALMSLEY, S.A. (Eds) (1983). *Research on Writing: Principles and Methods.* New York: Longman.

MOUNTY, J.L. (1989). Beyond grammar: developing stylistic variation when the input is diverse. *Sign Lang. Stud.* 62, 43–62.

MURPHY, J. and HILL, J. (1989). Training communication functions in hearing-impaired adolescents. *Aust. Teacher of the Deaf* 30, 26–32.

MURPHY, J.S. and NEWLON, B.J. (1987). Loneliness and the mainstreamed hearing impaired college student. *Am. Ann. Deaf* 132, 21–25.

MURPHY, K.P. (1957). Test of abilities and attainments. In: Ewing (1957).

MURPHY-BERMAN, V., STOEFEN-FISHER, J. and MATHIAS, K. (1987). Factors affecting teachers' evaluations of hearing-impaired students' behavior. *Volta Rev.* 89, 145–156.

MUSIEK, F.E., BARAN, J.A. and PINHEIRO, M.L. (1990). Duration pattern recognition in normal subjects and patients with cerebral and cochlear lesions. *Audiology.* 29, 304–313.

MUSIEK, F.E. and PINHEIRO, M.L. (1987). Frequency patterns in cochlear, brainstem, and cerebral lesions. *Audiology* 26, 79–80.

MUSSELMAN, C. and CHURCHILL, A. (1991). Conversational control in mother–child dyads: auditory–oral versus total communication. *Am. Ann. Deaf* 136, 5–16.

MUSSEN, P.H. (Ed.) (1970). *Carmichael's Manual of Child Psychology,* 3rd Edn. New York: Wiley.

MYERS, T., BROWN, K. and MCGONIGLE, B. (1986). *Reasoning and Discourse Processes.* London: Academic Press.

MYKLEBUST, H.R. (1960). The psychological effects of deafness. *Am. Ann. Deaf* 105, 372–385.

MYKLEBUST, H.R. (1964). *The Psychology of Deafness: Sensory Deprivation, Learning and Adjustment,* 2nd Edn. New York: Grune and Stratton.

MYKLEBUST, H.R. (1966). The effect of early life deafness. *Proc. XVIIIth Internat. Congress of Psychology,* Moscow.

NAGY, W.E., ANDERSON, R.C. and HERMAN, P.A. (1987). Learning word meanings from context during normal reading. *Am. Educn. Res. J.* 24, 237–270.

NASH, J.E. and NASH, A. (1981). *Deafness in Society.* Lexington, MA: Lexington Books.

NATIONAL INSTITUTES OF HEALTH (1988). *Consensus Conference Report.* Baltimore, MD: National Institutes of Health.

NATIONAL UNION OF THE DEAF STEERING COMMITTEE (1982). *Charter of Rights of the Deaf, Part One: The Rights of the Deaf Child.* Guildford, Surrey: National Union of the Deaf.

NEISSER, U. (1976). *Cognition and Reality: Principles and Implications of Cognitive Psychology.* San Francisco: Freeman.

NELSON, K.E. (Ed.) (1980). *Children's Language.* Hillsdale, NJ: Erlbaum.

NELSON, T.O., LEONESIO, J., SIMAMURA, A., LANDWEHR, R. and NARENS, L. (1982). Overlearning and the feeling of knowing. *J. Exp. Psychol.: Learn. Mem. Cognit.* 8, 279–288.

NEWELL, A. and SIMON, H.A. (1972). *Human Problem Solving.* Englewood Cliffs, NJ: Prentice-Hall.

NEWELL, W., STINSON, M., CASTLE, D., MALLERY-RUGANIS, D. and HOLCOMB, B. (1990). Simultaneous Communication: a description by deaf professionals working in an educational setting. *Sign Lang. Stud.* **69**, 391–414.

NEWPORT, E. and BELLUGI, U. (1979). Linguistic expression of category levels. In: Klima and Bellugi (1979).

NEWPORT, E.L. and SUPALLA, T. (1980). Clues from the acquisition of signed and spoken English. In: Bellugi and Studdert-Kennedy (1980).

NEWTON, L. (1985). Linguistic environment of the deaf child: a focus on teachers' use of non-literal language. *J. Speech Hear. Res.* **28**, 336–344.

NICHOLLS, G.H. and LING, D. (1982). Cued speech and the reception of spoken language. *J. Speech Hear. Res.* **25**, 262–269.

NIEMEYER, W. (1972). Studies on speech perception in dissociated hearing loss. In: Fant (1972).

NIENHUYS, T., CROSS, T. and HORSBOROUGH, K. (1984). Child variables influencing maternal speech style: deaf and hearing children. *J. Comm. Disord.* **17**, 189–207.

NIENHUYS, T.G., HOSBOROUGH, K.M. and CROSS, T.G. (1985). A dialogic analysis of interaction between mothers and their deaf or hearing preschoolers. *Appl. Psycholing.* **6**, 121–139.

NIENHUYS, T.G. and TIKOTIN, J.A. (1985). Mother–infant interaction: prespeech communication in hearing and deaf babies. *Aust. J. Teacher of the Deaf* **26**, 4–12.

NIX, G.W. (1983). How total is total communication? *J. Br. Assn. Teachers of the Deaf* **7**, 177–181.

NOBER, E.H. (1967). Articulation of the deaf. *Except. Child.* **33**, 611–621.

NOLEN, S.B. and WILBUR, R.B. (1984). Context and comprehension: another look. In: Martin (1984).

NOOTEBOOM, S.G. (1973). The perceptual reality of some prosodic durations. *J. Phonet.* **1**, 25–45.

NORLIN, P. (1981). The development of relational arcs in the lexical semantic memory structure of young children. *J. Child Lang.* **8**, 385–402.

NORMAN, D.A. (Ed.) (1970). *Models of Human Memory.* New York: Academic Press.

NORTHCOTT, W. (1975). Normalization of the pre-school child with hearing impairment. *Otolaryngol. Clin. North Am.* **8**, 159–186.

NORTHCOTT, W.H. (Ed.) (1984). *Oral Interpreting: Principles and Practice.* Baltimore, MD: University Park Press.

NORTHERN, J.L. (Ed.) (1984). *Hearing Disorders,* 2nd Edn. Boston, MA: Little, Brown and Co.

NORTHERN, J.L. and DOWNS, M.P. (1984). *Hearing in Children,* 3rd Edn. Baltimore, MD: Williams and Wilkins.

NOVELLI-OLMSTEAD, T. and LING, D. (1984). Speech production and speech discrimination by hearing-impaired children. *Volta Rev.* **86**, 72–80.

NOWICKI, S. and STRICKLAND, B.R. (1973). A locus of control scale for children. *J. Consult. Clin. Psychol.* **40**, 148–155.

OBERKLAID, F., HARRIS, C. and KEIR, E. (1989). Auditory dysfunction in children with school problems. *Clin. Pediat.* **28**, 397–403.

OBLOWITZ, N., GREEN, L. and HEYNS, I. de V. (1991). A self-concept scale for the hearing-impaired. *Volta Rev.* **93**, 19–29.

O'BRIEN, D.H. (1987). Reflection–impulsivity in total communication and oral deaf and hearing children: a developmental study. *Am. Ann. Deaf* **132**, 213–217.

OCHS, M.T., HUMES, L.E., OHDE, R.N. and GRANTHAM, D.W. (1989). Frequency discrimination ability and stop-consonant identification in normally hearing and hearing-impaired subjects. *J. Speech Hear. Res.* **32**, 133–142.

O'CONNOR, N. and HERMELIN, B. (1973). Short term memory for the order of pictures and syllables by deaf and hearing children. *Neuropsychologia* **11**, 437–442.

O'CONNOR, N. and HERMELIN, B.M. (1976). Backward and forward recall by deaf and hearing children. *Q. J. Exp. Psychol.* **28**, 83–92.

O'CONNOR, N. and HERMELIN, B. (1986). Sensory handicap and cognitive deficits. In: Ellis (1986).

ODOM, P., BLANTON, R. and NUNNALLY, J. (1967). Cloze technique studies of language capability in the deaf. *J. Speech Hear. Res.* **10**, 816–827.

OGDEN, P. (1984). Parenting in the mainstream. *Volta Rev.* **86**, 29–39.

OGDEN, P.W. and LIPSETT, S. (1982). *The Silent Garden: Understanding the Hearing Impaired Child*. New York: St Martin's Press.

OLÉRON, P. (1978). *Le Langage Gestuel des Sourds: Syntaxe et Communication*. Paris: Éditions du Centre National de la Recherche Scientifique.

OLLER, D.K., EILERS, R.E., BULL, D.H. and CARNEY, A.E. (1985). Prespeech vocalizations of a deaf infant: a comparison with normal metaphonological development. *J. Speech Hear. Res.* **28**, 47–63.

OLLER, D.K., EILERS, R., VERGARA, K. and LA VOIE, E. (1986). Tactual vocoders in a multisensory program training speech production and reception. *Volta Rev.* **88**, 21–36.

OLSON, D. (1977). Oral and written language and the cognitive processes of children. *J. Commun.* **27**, 10–26.

OLSON, D. (Ed.) (1980). *Social Foundations of Language and Thought: Essays in Honor of J.S. Bruner*. New York: Norton.

O'NEILL, J.J. (1954). Contributions of the visual components of oral symbols to speech comprehension. *J. Speech Hear. Disord.* **19**, 429–439.

O'NEILL, J.J. and OYER, H.J. (1961). *Visual Communication for the Hard of Hearing*. Englewood Cliffs, NJ: Prentice-Hall.

ORLANSKY, M.D. and BONVILLIAN, J.D. (1984). The role of iconicity in early sign language acquisition. *J. Speech Hear. Disord.* **49**, 287–292.

OSBERGER, M.J. (1983). Development and evaluation of some speech training procedures for hearing-impaired children. In: Hochberg et al. (1983).

OSBERGER, M.J. (1987). Training effects on vowel production by two profoundly hearing-impaired speakers. *J. Speech Hear. Res.* **30**, 241–251.

OSBERGER, M.J. (1990). Audition. *Volta Rev.* **92**, 34–53.

OSBERGER, M.J. and LEVITT, H. (1979). The effect of time errors on the intelligibility of deaf children's speech. *J. Acoust. Soc. Am.* **66**, 1316–1324.

OSBERGER, M. and MCGARR, N. (1982). Speech production characteristics of the hearing-impaired. *Speech Lang.* **8**, 221–283.

OWENS, E., KESSLER, D., TELEEN, E. and SCHUBERT, E. (1985). *Minimal Auditory Capabilities Battery* (Rev. Edn). St Louis, MO: Auditec.

OWENS, E. and KESSLER, D. (Eds) (1989). *Cochlear Implants in Young Deaf Children*. Boston, MA: Little, Brown and Co.

OYER, H.J. (Ed.) (1976). *Communication for the Hearing Handicapped: An International Perspective*. Baltimore, MD: University Park Press.

PAGE, J.L. (1985a). Relative translucency of ASL signs representing three semantic classes. *J. Speech Hear. Disord.* **50**, 241–247.

PAGE, J.M. (1985b). Central auditory processing disorders in children. *Otolaryngol. Clin. North Am.* **18**, 323–335.

PAGET, G. and GORMAN, P. (1968). *A Systematic Sign Language*. London: Royal National Institute for the Deaf.

PAIVIO, A. (1971). *Imagery and Verbal Processes*. New York: Holt, Rinehart and Winston.

PAIVIO, A. and BEGG, I. (1981). *Psychology of Language*. Englewood Cliffs, NJ: Prentice-Hall.

PALMER, L., BEMENT, L. and KELLY, J. (1990). Implications of deafness and cultural diversity on communication instruction: strategies for intervention. *J. Aural Rehab. Assoc.* **23**, 43–52.

PANIAGUA, F.A. (1990). Skinner's senses of 'Guessing'. *New Ideas Psychol.* **8**, 73–79.

PANOU, L. and SEWELL, D.F. (1984). Cerebral asymmetry in congenitally deaf subjects. *Neuropsychologia* **22**, 381–383.

PARADY, S., DORMAN, M., WHALEY, P. and RAPHAEL, L. (1981). Identification and discrimination of a synthesized voicing contrast by normal and sensorineural hearing-impaired children. *J. Acoust. Soc. Am.* **69**, 783–790.

PARASNIS, I. (1983). Effects of parental deafness and early exposure to manual communication on the cognitive skills, English language skill and field independence of young deaf adults. *J. Speech Hear. Res.* **26**, 588–594.

PARKHURST, B.G. and LEVITT, H. (1978). The effect of selected prosodic errors on the intelligibility of deaf speech. *J. Commun. Disord.* **11**, 249–256.

PARKINS, C.W. and HOUDE, R.A. (1982). The cochlear (implant) prosthesis: theoretical and practical considerations. In: Sims et al. (1982).

PATERSON, M. (1986). Maximising the use of residual hearing with school-aged hearing-impaired students – a perspective. *Volta Rev.* **88**, 93–106.

PAYNE, J.A. and QUIGLEY, S. (1987). Hearing-impaired children's comprehension of verb–particle combinations. *Volta Rev.* **89**, 133–143.

PEARSON, H.R. (1984). Parenting a hearing-impaired child: a model program. *Volta Rev.* **86**, 239–243.

PEIRCE, C. (1932). *Collected Papers* (edited by C. Hartshorne and P. Weiss). Cambridge, MA: Harvard University Press.

PENDERGRASS, R.A. and HODGES, M. (1976). Deaf students in group problem solving situations: a study of the interactive process. *Am. Ann. Deaf* **121**, 327–330.

PERIGOE, C. and LING, D. (1986). Generalization of speech skills in hearing-impaired children. *Volta Rev.* **88**, 351–365.

PERKINS, W.H. (Ed.) (1984). *Hearing Disorders*. New York: Thième Stratton.

PETER, M. and BARNES, R. (Eds) (1982). *Signs, Symbols and Schools*. London: National Council for Special Education.

PETERSON, L.N. and FRENCH, L. (1988). Summarization strategies of hearing-impaired and normally hearing college students. *J. Speech Hear. Res.* **31**, 327–337.

PETERSON, C.C. and PETERSON, J.L. (1989). Positive justice reasoning in deaf and hearing children before and after exposure to cognitive conflict. *Am. Ann. Deaf* **134**, 277–282.

PETKOVSEK, M. (1961). The eyes have it. *Hearing News* **29**, 5–9.

PHIPPARD, D. (1977). Hemifield differences in visual perception in deaf and hearing subjects. *Neuropsychologia* **15**, 555–561.

PIAGET, J. (1926). *The Language and Thought of the Child*. New York: Harcourt and Brace.

PIAGET, J. (1929). *The Child's Conception of the World*. London: Routledge and Kegan Paul.

PICHENY, M.A., DURLACH, N.L. and BRAIDA, L.D. (1985). Speaking clearly for the hard of hearing I: Intelligibility differences between clear and conversational speech. *J. Speech Hear. Res.* **28**, 96–103.

PICHENY, M.A., DURLACH, N.I. and BRAIDA, L.D. (1986). Speaking clearly for the hard of hearing II: Acoustic characteristics of clear and conversational speech. *J. Speech Hear. Res.* **29**, 434–446.

PICKETT, J. and DANAHER, E. (1975). On discrimination of formant transitions by persons with severe sensorineural hearing loss. In: Fant and Tatham (1975).

PICKETT, J.M. (1980). *The Sounds of Speech Communication: A Primer of Acoustic Phonetics and Speech Perception*. Baltimore, MD: University Park Press.

PICKETT, J.M. and MCFARLAND, W. (1985). Auditory implants and tactile aids for the profoundly deaf. *J. Speech Hear. Res.* **28**, 134–150.

PICKETT, J.M., MARTIN, E., JOHNSON, D., SMITH, S., DANIEL, Z., WILLIS, D. and OTIS, W. (1972). On patterns of speech feature reception by deaf listeners. In: Fant (1972).

PICKETT, J.M., REVOILE, S.G. and DANAHER, E.M. (1983). Speech-cue measures of impaired hearing. In: Tobias and Schubert (1983).

PIEN, D. (1985). The development of communication functions in deaf infants of hearing parents. In: Martin (1985).

PIERS, E.V. and HARRIS, D.B. (1964). Age and other correlates of self-concept in children. *J. Educ. Psychol.* **55**, 91–95.

PINHEIRO, M.L. and MUSIEK, F.E. (1985a). Sequencing and temporal ordering in the auditory system. In: Pinheiro and Musiek (1985b).

PINHEIRO, M.L. and MUSIEK. F.E. (Eds) (1985b). *Assessment of Central Auditory Dysfunction*. Baltimore, MD: Williams and Wilkins.

PINTNER, R. (1941). The personality of the deaf. In: Pintner et al. (1941).

PINTNER, R., EISENSON, J. and STANTON, M. (1941). *The Psychology of the Physically Handicapped*. New York: F.S. Crofts.

PINTNER, R. and PATERSON, D.G. (1917). The ability of deaf and hearing children to follow printed directions. *Am. Ann. Deaf* 62, 448–472.

PINTNER, R. and PATERSON, D.G. (1923). *A Scale of Performance Tests*. New York: Appleton, Century, Crofts.

PINTNER, R. and REAMER, J.F. (1920). A mental and educational survey of schools for the deaf. *Am. Ann. Deaf* 65, 277–300.

PITT, M.A. and SAMUEL, A.G. (1990). Attentional allocation during speech perception: how fine is the focus? *J. Mem. Lang.* 29, 611–632.

PLANT, G. (1984). A diagnostic speech test for severely and profoundly hearing-impaired children. *Aust. J. Audiol.* 6, 1–9.

PLANT, G. (1988). A comparison of five commercially available tactile aids. *Aust. J. Audiol.* 11, 11–19.

PLANT, G. and HAMMARBERG, B. (1983). Acoustic and perceptual analysis of the speech of the deafened. *Stockholm: Speech Transmission Lab., Q. Progress and Status Report* 2–3, 85–107.

PLANT, G., MACRAE, J., DILLON, H. and PENTECOST, F. (1984a). A single-channel vibrotactile aid to lipreading: preliminary results with an experienced subject. *Aust. J. Audiol.* 6, 55–64.

PLANT, G., MACRAE, J., DILLON, H. and PENTECOST, F. (1984b). Lipreading with minimal auditory cues. *Aust. J. Audiol.* 6, 65–72.

PLAPINGER, D. and KRETSCHMER, R. (1991). The effect of context on the interaction between a normally-hearing mother and her hearing-impaired child. *Volta Rev.* 93, 75–87.

POIZNER, H., BATTISON, R. and LANE, H.H. (1979). Cerebral asymmetry for perception of American Sign Language: the effects of moving stimuli. *Brain Lang* 7, 351–362.

POIZNER, H., KAPLAN, E., BELLUGI, U. and PADDEN, C.A. (1984). Visual-spatial processing in deaf brain-damaged signers. *Brain Cognit.* 3, 281–306.

POIZNER, H., NEWKIRK, D., BELLUGI, U. and KLIMA, E.S. (1981). Representation of inflected signs from American Sign Language in short-term memory. *Mem. Cognit.* 9, 121–131.

POIZNER, H. and TALLAL, P. (1987). Temporal processing in deaf signers. *Brain Lang.* 30, 52–62.

POLLACK, D. (1967). The crucial year: a time to listen. *Internat. Audiol.* 6, 243–247.

POLLACK, M. (Ed.) (1975). *Amplification for the Hearing Impaired*. New York: Grune and Stratton.

PORTER, K.A. and DICKERSON, M.V. (1986). Syllabic complexity and its relation to speech intelligibility in a deaf population. *Am. Ann. Deaf* 131, 36–42.

POVEL, D-J., and WANSINK, M. (1986). A computer-controlled vowel corrector for the hearing impaired. *J. Speech Hear. Res.* 29, 99–105.

POWER, A. and WILGUS, S. (1983). Linguistic complexity in the written language of hearing-impaired children. *Volta Rev.* 85, 201–210.

POWER, D. and HOLLINGSHEAD, A. (Eds) (1982). *Occasional Paper No. 4*. Brisbane: Mt. Gravatt College, Centre for Human Development Studies.

POWER, D. and QUIGLEY, S.P. (1973). Deaf children's acquisition of the passive voice. *J. Speech Hear. Res.* 16, 5–11.

POWER, D.J., WOOD, D.J., WOOD, H.A. and MACDOUGALL, J. (1990). Maternal control over conversations with hearing and deaf infants. *First Lang.* 10, 19–35.

POWERS, S. (1990). A survey of secondary units for hearing-impaired children – Part 2. *J. Br. Assn. Teachers of the Deaf* 14, 114–125.

POYATOS, F. (1983). *New Perspectives in Nonverbal Communication*. Oxford: Pergamon.

PRATT, S.R. (1988). *Some Prosodic Characteristics of Maternal Speech Directed to Hearing Impaired Toddlers*. University of Iowa: unpublished Doctoral Thesis.

PREMINGER, J. and WILEY, T.L. (1985). Frequency selectivity and consonant intelligibility in sensorineural hearing loss. *J. Speech Hear. Res.* 28, 197–206.

PRESSNELL, L. MCK. (1973). Hearing-impaired children's comprehension and production of syntax in oral language. *J. Speech Hear. Res.* 16. 12–21.

PRINZ, P.M. (1985). Language and communication development, assessment and intervention in hearing-impaired individuals. In: Katz (1985).

PRINZ, P.M. and FERRIER, L.J. (1983). 'Can you give me that one?': The comprehension, production and judgment of directives in language-impaired children. *J. Speech Hear. Disord.* **48**, 44–54.

PRINZ, P.M., PEMBERTON, E. and NELSON, K.E. (1985). The ALPHA interactive microcomputer system for teaching reading, writing and communication skills to hearing-impaired children. *Am. Ann. Deaf* **130**, 444–461.

PRINZ, P.M. and PRINZ, E.A. (1985). If only you could hear what I see: discourse development in sign language. *Discourse Processes* **8**, 1–19.

PRIOR, M.R., GLAZNER, J., SANSON, A. and DEBELLE, G. (1988). Temperament and behavioural adjustment in hearing-impaired children. *J. Child Psychol. Psychiat.* **29**, 206–216.

PROCTOR, A. (1990). Oral language comprehension using hearing aids and tactile aids: three case studies. *Lang. Speech Hear. Services in Schools* **21**, 37–48.

PRUTTING, C.A. and KIRCHNER, D.M. (1983). Applied Pragmatics. In: Gallagher and Prutting (1983).

PUDLAS, K.A. (1987). Sentence reception abilities of hearing impaired students across five communication modes. *Am. Ann. Deaf* **132**, 232–236.

PUGH, G. (1946). Summaries from appraisal of the silent reading abilities of acoustically handicapped children. *Am. Ann. Deaf* **91**, 331–349.

PUMROY, D. (1966). Maryland parent attitude survey: a research instrument with social desirability controlled. *J. Psychol.* **64**, 73–78.

QUENIN, C.S. and BLOOD, I. (1989). A national survey of cued speech programs. *Volta Rev.* **91**, 283–289.

QUIGLEY, S. (1978). *Test of Syntactic Abilities.* Beaverton, OR: Dormac.

QUIGLEY, S. and KING, C. (Eds) (1984). *Reading Milestones.* Beaverton, OR: Dormac.

QUIGLEY, S.P. (1969). *The Influence of Fingerspelling on the Development of Language, Communication, and Educational Achievement in Deaf Children.* Urbana, IL: Institute for Research on Exceptional Children.

QUIGLEY, S.P. (1982). Reading achievement and special reading materials. *Volta Rev.* **84**, 95–105.

QUIGLEY, S.P. and KRETSCHMER, R.E. (1982). *The Education of Deaf Children: Issues, Theory and Practice.* London: Edward Arnold.

QUIGLEY, S.P., MONTANELLI, D.S. and WILBUR, R.B. (1976a). Some aspects of the verb system in the language of deaf students. *J. Speech Hear. Res.* **19**, 536–550.

QUIGLEY, S.P. and PAUL, P.V. (1984). *Language and Deafness.* London: Croom Helm.

QUIGLEY, S.P. and POWER, D.J. (1971). *Test of Syntactic Ability, Rationale, Test Logistics and Instructions.* Urbana, IL: Institute for Research on Exceptional Children.

QUIGLEY, S.P., STEINKAMP, M.W., POWER, D.J. and JONES, B.W. (1978). *Test of Syntactic Abilities.* Beaverton, OR: Dormac.

QUIGLEY, S.P., WILBUR, R., POWER, D., MONTANELLI, D. and STEINKAMP, M. (1976b). *Syntactic Structures in the Language of Deaf Children.* Urbana, IL: Institute for Child Behavior and Development.

QUINSLAND, L.K. and VAN GINKEL, A. (1990). Cognitive processing and the development of concepts by deaf students. *Am. Ann. Deaf* **135**, 280–284.

RAIMONDO, D. and MAXWELL, M. (1987). The modes of communication used in junior and senior high school classrooms by hearing-impaired students and their teachers and peers. *Volta Rev.* **89**, 263–275.

RAINER, J.D. (1976). Some observations on affect induction and ego development in the deaf. *Internat. Rev. Psycho-Anal.* **3**, 121–128.

RAINER, J.D. and ALTSCHULER, K.Z. (1971). A psychiatric program for the deaf: experiences and implications. *Am. J. Psychiat.* **127**, 1527–1532.

RAINER, J.D., ALTSCHULER, K.Z. and KALLMANN, F.J. (Eds) (1963). *Family and Mental Health Problems in a Deaf Population*, 2nd Edn. Springfield, IL: Charles C. Thomas.

RANEY, L., DANCER, J. and BRADLEY, R. (1984). Correlation between auditory and visual performance on two speech reception tasks. *Volta Rev.* **86**, 134–141.

REBER, A.S. and SCARBOROUGH, D. (Eds) (1977). *Toward a Psychology of Reading: The Proceedings of the CUNY Conference*. Hillsdale, NJ: Erlbaum.

REDGATE, G.W. (1972). *The Teaching of Reading to Deaf Children*. Manchester: University of Manchester Press.

REED, C. (1975). Identification and discrimination of vowel–consonant syllables in listeners with sensorineural hearing loss. *J. Speech Hear. Res.* **18**, 773–794.

REED, C.M., RABINOWITZ, W.M., DURLACH, N.I., BRAIDA, L.D., CONWAY-FITHIAN, S. and SCHULTZ, M.C. (1985). Research on the Tadoma Method of speech communication. *J. Acoust. Soc. Am.* **77**, 247–257.

REES, N.S. (1973). Auditory processing factors in language disorders: the view from Procrustes' bed. *J. Speech Hear. Disord.* **38**, 304–315.

REES, N.S. (1981). Saying more than we know: is auditory processing disorder a meaningful concept? In: Keith (1981b).

REICH, C., HAMBLETON, D. and HOULDIN, B.K. (1977). The integration of hearing-impaired children in regular classrooms. *Am. Ann. Deaf* **122**, 534–543.

REINKING, D. and SCHREINER, R. (1985). The effects of computer-mediated text on measures of reading comprehension and reading behavior. *Read. Res. Q.* **20**, 536–552.

REISBERG, D. (1978). Looking where you listen: visual cues and auditory attention. *Acta Psychol.* **42**, 331–341.

REISBERG, D., MCLEAN, J. and GOLDFIELD, A. (1987). Easy to hear but hard to understand: a lipreading advantage with intact auditory stimuli. In: Dodd and Campbell (1987).

REISBERG, D., SCHEIBER, R. and POTEMKEN, L. (1981). Eye-position and the control of auditory attention. *J. Exp. Psychol. Hum. Percept. Perform.* **7**, 318–323.

RESNICK, L.B. (Ed.) (1989). *Knowing, Learning and Instruction: Essays in Honor of Robert Glaser*. Hillsdale, NJ: Erlbaum.

REVOILE, S., PICKETT, J.M., HOLDEN-PITT, L.D., TALKIN, D. and BRANDT, F.D. (1987). Burst and transition cues to voicing perception for spoken initial stops by impaired- and normal-hearing listeners. *J. Speech Hear. Res.* **30**, 3–12.

REVOILE, S.G., KOZMA–SPYTEK, L., HOLDEN-PITT, L., PICKETT, J.M. and DROGE, J. (1991a). VCV's vs. CVC's for stop/fricative distinctions by hearing-impaired and normal-hearing listeners. *J. Acoust. Soc. Am.* **89**, 457–460.

REVOILE, S.G., PICKETT, J.M. and KOZMA-SPYTEK, L. (1991b). Spectral cues to perception of /d, n, l/ by normal- and impaired-hearing listeners. *J. Acoust. Soc. Am.* **90**, 787–798.

REYNOLDS, H.N. (1986). Performance of deaf college students on a criterion-referenced modified cloze test of reading comprehension. *Am. Ann. Deaf* **131**, 361–364.

RICHARDSON, J.E. (1981). Computer assessed instruction for the hearing impaired. *Volta Rev.* **83**, 328–335.

RIEBER, R.W. and VOYAT, G. (1983). *Dialogues on the Psychology of Language and Thought*. New York and London: Plenum.

RIESEN, A.H. (1961). Critical stimulation and optimal period. Paper presented to American Psychological Association, New York.

RIKO, K., HYDE, M.L. and ALBERT, P.W. (1985). Hearing loss in early infancy: incidence, detection and assessment. *Laryngoscope* **95**, 137–145.

RINGEL, R.L., BURK, K.W. and SCOTT, C.M. (1968). Tactile perception: form discrimination in the mouth. *Br. J. Disord. Commun.* **3**, 150–155.

RINGEL, R.L., HOUSE, A.S., BURK, K.W., DOLINSKY, J.P. and SCOTT, C.M. (1970). Some relations between orosensory discrimination and articulatory aspects of speech production. *J. Speech Hear. Disord.* **35**, 3–11.

RISBERG, A. (1976). Diagnostic rhyme test for speech audiometry with severely hard of hearing and profoundly deaf children. *Stockholm: Speech Transmission Lab., Q. Progress and Status Report* **2–3**, 40–58.

RISBERG, A. and SPENS, K.E. (1967). Teaching machine for training experiments in speech perception. *Stockholm: Speech Transmission Lab., Q. Progress and Status Report* **2–3**, 72–75.

RITTENHOUSE, R.K. and KENYON, P.L. (1987). Educational and social language in deaf adolescents: TDD and school-produced comparisons. *Am. Ann. Deaf* **132**, 210–212.

RITTENHOUSE, R., MORREAU, L. and IRAN-NEJAD, A. (1981). Metaphor and conservation in deaf and normal hearing children. *Am. Ann. Deaf* **126**, 450–453.

RITTENHOUSE, R.K. and STEARNS, K. (1990). Figurative language and reading comprehension in American deaf and hard-of-hearing children: textual interactions. *Br. J. Disord. Commun.* **25**, 369–374.

RITTENHOUSE, R.K., WHITE, K., LOWITZER, C. and SHISLER, L. (1990). The costs and benefits of providing early intervention to very young, severely hearing-impaired children in the United States: the conceptual outline of a longitudinal research study and some preliminary findings. *Br. J. Disord. Commun.* **25**, 195–208.

ROBB, M.P. and SAXMAN, J.H. (1985). Developmental trends in vocal fundamental frequency of young children. *J. Speech Hear. Res.* **28**, 421–427.

ROBBINS, A. MCC. (1990). Developing meaningful auditory integration in children with cochlear implants. *Volta Rev.* **92**, 361–370.

ROBBINS, A. MCC., OSBERGER, M.J., MIYAMOTO, R.T., KIENLE, M.L. and MYRES, W.A. (1985). Speech-tracking performance in single-channel cochlear implant subjects. *J. Speech Hear. Res.* **28**, 565–578.

ROBBINS, R.M. and GAUGER, J. (1982). Hearing aid evaluation and orientation for the severely hearing-impaired. In: Sims et al. (1982).

ROBINSON, E.J. (1981). The child's understanding of inadequate messages and communication failure: a problem of ignorance or egocentrism? In: Dickson (1981).

ROBINSON, E.J. and ROBINSON, W.P. (1983). Communication and metacommunication: quality of children's instructions in relation to judgement about the adequacy of instructions and the focus of responsibility for communication failure. *J. Exp. Child Psychol.* **36**, 305–320.

ROBINSON, J.H. and GRIFFITH, P.L. (1979). On the scientific status of iconicity. *Sign Lang. Stud.* **25**, 297–315.

RODDA, M. and GROVE, C. (1987). *Language, Cognition and Deafness*. Hillsdale, NJ: Erlbaum.

RODRIGUEZ, G.P., DISARNO, N.J. and HARDIMAN, C.J. (1990). Central auditory processing in normal-hearing elderly adults. *Audiology* **29**, 85–92.

ROESER, R.J. and DOWNS, M.P. (Eds) (1981). *Auditory Disorders in School Children*. New York: Thieme-Stratton.

ROGERS, D. and SLOBODA, J. (Eds) (1983). *The Acquisition of Symbolic Skills*. New York: Plenum.

ROMAINE, S. (1984). *The Language of Children and Adolescents*. Oxford: Basil Blackwell.

ROMMETVEIT, R. (1974). *On Message Structure: A Framework for the Study of Language and Communication*. New York: Wiley.

RONNBERG, J., ARLINGER, S., LYXELL, B. and KINNEFORS, C. (1989). Visual evoked potentials: relation to adult speechreading and cognitive function. *J. Speech Hear. Res.* **32**, 725–735.

ROSEN, S.M., FOURCIN, A.J. and MOORE, B.C.J. (1981). Voice pitch as an aid to lipreading. *Nature* **291**, 150–152.

ROSEN, S., WALLIKER, J.R., FOURCIN, A. and BALL, V. (1987). A microprocessor-based acoustic hearing aid for the profoundly impaired listener. *J. Rehab. Res. Dev.* **24**, 239–260.

ROSS, M. (1975). Hearing aid selection for pre-verbal hearing-impaired children. In: Pollack (1975).

ROSS, M. (1990). Verbal communication: the state of the art. *Volta Rev.* **78**, 324–328.

ROSS, M., BRACKETT, D. and MAXON, A. (1982). *Hard of Hearing Children in Regular Schools*. Englewood Cliffs, NJ: Prentice Hall.

ROSS, M. and GIOLAS, T.G. (Eds) (1978). *Auditory Management of Hearing-Impaired Children*. Baltimore, MD: University Park Press.

ROSS, M. and LERMAN, J. (1970). A picture identification test for hearing-impaired children. *J. Speech Hear. Res.* **13**, 44–53.

ROSS, P., PERGAMENT, L. and ANISFELD, M. (1979). Cerebral lateralisation of deaf and hearing individuals for linguistic comparison judgements. *Brain Lang.* **8**, 69–80.

ROWE, J. (1982). The Paget–Gorman Sign System. In: Peter and Barnes (1982).

RUBEN, R.J. (1986). Unsolved issues around critical periods with emphasis on clinical application. *Acta Otolaryngol. (Stockh) Suppl.* **429**, 61–64.

RUBIN, K.H. (1973). Egocentrism in childhood: a unitary construct? *Child Devel.* **44**, 102–110.

RUDEL, R.G. (1985). Hemispheric asymmetry and learning disabilities: left, right or in-between? In: Best (1985).

RUGGIERI, V., CELLI, C. and CRESCENZI, A. (1982). Gesturing and self-contact of right and left halves of the body: relationship with eye-contact. *Percept. Mot. Skills* **55**, 695–698.

RUSHMER, N. and SCHUYLER, V. (1984). The IHR model of parent–infant habilitation. In: Ling (1984a).

RUSSELL, W.K., QUIGLEY, S.P. and POWER, D.J. (1976). *Linguistics and Deaf Children: Transformational Syntax and Its Applications.* Washington, DC: Alexander Graham Bell Association.

RUTHERFORD, S.D. (1988). The culture of American deaf people. *Sign Lang. Stud.* **59**, 129–147.

RUTTER, M.L. (1981). *Maternal Deprivation Reassessed,* 2nd Edn. Harmondsworth: Penguin.

RYAN, K.M. and LEVINE, J.M. (1981). Impact of academic performance pattern on assigned grade and predicted performance. *J. Educ. Psychol.* **73**, 386–392.

SACKS, O. (1986). Mysteries of the Deaf. *New York Rev. Books* **33**, 23–33.

SACKS, O. (1989). *Seeing Voices: A Journey into the World of the Deaf.* Los Angeles, CA: University of California Press.

SAKATA, S. (1989). A study on the development of message production in referential communication. *Shinrigaku Kenkyu (Japan)* **59**, 365–368.

SALASOO, A. and PISONI, D.B. (1985). Sources of knowledge in spoken word identification. *J. Mem. Lang.* **24**, 210–231.

SALEND, S.J. and JOHNS, J. (1983). Changing teacher commitment to mainstreaming. *Teaching Except. Child.* **15**, 82–85.

SAMAR, V.J. and SIMS, D.G. (1983). Visual evoked-response correlates of speechreading performance in normal-hearing adults: a replication and a factor analytic extension. *J. Speech Hear. Res.* **26**, 2–9.

SAMAR, V.J. and SIMS, D.G. (1984). Visual evoked-response components related to speechreading and spatial skills in hearing and hearing-impaired adults. *J. Speech Hear. Res.* **27**, 162–172.

SANDERS, D.A. (1977). *Auditory Perception of Speech: An Introduction to Principles and Problems.* Englewood Cliffs, NJ: Prentice Hall.

SANDERS, G., WRIGHT, H.V. and ELLIS, C. (1989). Cerebral lateralisation of language in deaf and hearing people. *Brain Lang.* **36**, 555–579.

SANTROCK, J.W. (1986). *Life-Span Development,* 2nd Edn. Dubuque, IA: W.C. Brown.

SAPIR, E. (1949). Language and environment. In: Mandelbaum (1949).

SARACHAN-DEILY, A.B. (1982). Hearing-impaired and hearing readers' sentence processing errors. *Volta Rev.* **84**, 81–95.

SARACHAN-DEILY, A.B. (1985). Written narratives of deaf and hearing students: story recall and inference. *J. Speech Hear. Res.* **28**, 151–159.

SAUR, R., COGGIOLA, D., LONG, G.L. and SIMONSON, J. (1986). Educational mainstreaming and the career development of the hearing-impaired students: a longitudinal analysis. *Volta Rev.* **88**, 79–88.

SAUR, R., POPP-STONE, M.J. and HURLEY-LAWRENCE, E. (1987). The classroom participation of mainstreamed hearing-impaired college students. *Volta Rev.* **89**, 277–286.

SAUR, R.E. and STINSON, M.S. (1986). Characteristics of successful mainstreamed hearing-impaired students. *J. Rehab. Deaf* **20**, 15–21.

SAVAGE, R.D., EVANS, L. and SAVAGE, J.F. (1981). *Psychology and Communication in Deaf Children.* Sydney: Grune and Stratton.

SAVIN, H.B. (1972). What the child knows about speech when he starts to learn to read. In: Kavanagh and Mattingly (1972).

SCHAEFER, E.S. (1976). Scope and focus of research relevant to intervention: a socioecological perspective. In: Tjossem (1976).

SCHAEFER, R.P. (1980). *An Experimental Assessment of the Boundaries Demarcating Three Basic Semantic Categories in the Domain of Separation*. University of Kansas: unpublished Doctoral Thesis.

SCHAFFER, H.R. (Ed.) (1977). *Studies in Mother–Infant Interaction*. New York: Academic Press.

SCHICK, B.S. (1990). The effects of morphological complexity on phonological simplification in ASL. *Sign Lang. Stud.* 66, 25–41.

SCHILDROTH, A. (1988). Recent changes in the educational placement of deaf students. *Am. Ann. Deaf* 133, 61–67.

SCHILDROTH, A.N. and KARCHMER, M.A. (Eds) (1986). *Deaf Children in America*. San Diego, CA: College-Hill Press.

SCHILP, C. (1989). Correcting grammatical errors with MacWrite. *Volta Rev.* 91, 151–155.

SCHINDLER, R.A. and MERZENICH, M.M. (Eds) (1985). *Cochlear Implants*. New York: Raven Press.

SCHLESINGER, H.S. (1972). A developmental model applied to problems of deafness. In: Schlesinger and Meadow (1972).

SCHLESINGER, H.S. (1978). The effects of deafness on childhood development: an Ericksonian perspective. In: Liben (1978).

SCHLESINGER, H. (1986). Total communication in perspective. In: Luterman (1986).

SCHLESINGER, H.S. and MEADOW, K.P. (1972). *Sound and Sign: Childhood Deafness and Mental Health*. Berkeley, CA: University of California Press.

SCHLESINGER, I. (1977a). The role of cognitive development and linguistic input in language acquisition. *J. Child Lang.* 4, 153–169.

SCHLESINGER I.M. (1971). The grammar of sign language and the problems of language universals. In: Morton (1971).

SCHLESINGER, I.M. (1977b). Some aspects of sign languages. In: Cohen et al. (1977).

SCHLESINGER, I.M. and NAMIR, L. (Eds) (1978). *Sign Language of the Deaf: Psychological, Linguistic and Sociological Perspectives*. New York: Academic Press.

SCHNEIDER, W. (1985). Training high performance skills: fallacies and guidelines. *Hum. Factors* 27, 285–300.

SCHNEIDMAN, E.S. (1948). Schizophrenia and the MAPS test: a study of certain formal aspects of fantasy production in schizophrenia as revealed by performance on the Make-A-Picture Story (MAPS) test. *Genet. Psychol. Monogr.* 38, 145–223.

SCHOLES, R.J. and FISCHLER, I. (1979). Hemispheric function and linguistic skill in the deaf. *Brain Lang.* 7, 336–350.

SCHOPLER, E. and REICHLER, R.J. (Eds) (1976). *Psychopathology and Child Development: Research and Treatments*. New York: Plenum.

SCHOWE, B.M. (1979). *Identity Crisis in Deafness: A Humanistic Perspective*. Tempe, AZ: Scholars Press.

SCHOW, R.L. and NERBONNE, M.A. (1980a). Overview of aural rehabilitation. In: Schow and Nerbonne (1980b).

SCHOW, R.L. and NERBONNE, M.A. (Eds) (1980b). *Introduction to Aural Rehabilitation*. Baltimore, MD: University Park Press.

SCHUCHMAN, J.S. (1988). *Hollywood Speaks: Deafness and the Film Industry*. Chicago, IL: University of Illinois Press.

SCHULZE, G. (1965). An evaluation of vocabulary development by 32 deaf children over a 3-year period. *Am. Ann. Deaf* 110, 424–435.

SCHWARTZ, J.L., ROSS, L.J. and HOUCHINS, R.R. (1975). An investigation of the self-concept of expressive language of thirty adolescent hearing-impaired students using the Q-sort technique. *Am. Ann. Deaf* 120, 572–577.

SCOTT, B.A. (1984). Deafness in the family: will the therapist listen? *Family Process* 23, 214–216.

SCOTT, D. (1978). Stigma in and about the deaf community. In: Montgomery (1978).

SCOUTEN, E.L. (1964). The place of the Rochester Method in American education of the deaf. *Proc. Internat. Congr. Educ. Deaf* 429–433.

SCOUTEN, E.L. (1980). An instructional strategy to combat the word-matching tendencies in prelingually deaf students. *Am. Ann. Deaf* 125, 1057–1059.

SCOVEL, T. (1981). The effects of neurological age on nonprimary language acquisition. In: Anderson (1981).

SCROGGS, C.L. (1983). An examination of the communication interactions between hearing impaired infants and their parents. In: Kyle and Woll (1983).

SEAL, B.C. (1987). Working parents' dream: instructional videotapes for their signing deaf child. *Am. Ann. Deaf* 132, 386–388.

SEASHORE, R.H. (1951). Work and Motor Performance. In: Stevens (1951).

SEEWALD, R.C. and BRACKETT, D. (1984). Spoken language modifications as a function of the age and hearing ability of the listener. *Volta Rev.* 86, 20–35.

SEEWALD, R.C., ROSS, M., GIOLAS, T.G. and YONOVITZ, A. (1985). Primary modality for speech perception in children with normal and impaired hearing. *J. Speech Hear. Res.* 28, 36–46.

SELOVER, P.J. (1988). American Sign Language in the high school system. *Sign Lang. Stud.* 59, 205–212.

SERWATKA, T.S., HESSON, D. and GRAHAM, M. (1984). The effect of indirect intervention on the improvement of hearing-impaired students' reading scores. *Volta Rev.* 86, 81–88.

SHAND, M.A. (1982). Sign-based short term coding of American Sign Language signs and printed English words by congenitally deaf signers. *Cognit. Psychol.* 14, 1–12.

SHANKWEILER, D. and LIBERMAN, I.Y. (1976). Exploring the relations between reading and speech. In: Knights and Bakker (1976).

SHARP, C. (1984). Sex and deafness stereotyping by hearing and deaf adolescents – a preliminary survey. *Aust. Teacher of the Deaf* 25, 39–45.

SHATZ, M. and GELMAN, R. (1973). The development of communication skills: modifications in the speech of young children as a function of listener. *Monogr. Soc. Res. Child Devel.* 38, (Serial No. 152).

SHAW, R. and BRANSFORD, J. (Eds) (1977). *Perceiving, Acting, and Knowing: Toward an Ecological Psychology*. Hillsdale, NJ: Erlbaum.

SHEPHERD, D.C., DELAVERGNE, R.W., FRUEH, F.X. and CLOBRIDGE, C. (1977). Visual–neural correlate of speechreading ability in normal-hearing adults. *J. Speech Hear. Res.* 20, 752–765.

SHER, A.E. and OWENS, E. (1974). Consonant confusions associated with hearing loss above 2000Hz. *J. Speech Hear. Res.* 17, 669–681.

SHERIF, M. and SHERIF, C. (1964). *Reference Groups: Exploration into Conformity and Deviance in Adolescence*. New York: Harper and Row.

SHIMIZU, H. and INOUE, T. (1988). The effect of rehearsal strategies on free recall in the deaf. *Psychologia.* 31, 226–232.

SHUKLA, R.S. (1989). Phonological space in the speech of the hearing impaired. *J. Commun. Disord.* 22, 317–325.

SHULMAN, B.B. (1985). *Test of Pragmatic Skills*. Tucson, AZ: Communication Skill Builders.

SIDOWSKI, J.B. (Ed.) (1980). *Conditioning, Cognition and Methodology: Contemporary Issues in Experimental Psychology*. Hillsdale, NJ: Erlbaum.

SIEBERT, R. (1980). Speech training for the hearing impaired: principles, objectives, and strategies for preschool and elementary levels. In: Subtelny (1980).

SIEGEL, L.S. and LINDER, B.A. (1984). Short-term memory processes in children with reading and arithmetic learning disabilities. *Devel. Psychol.* 20, 200–207.

SIEGMAN, A.W. and POPE, B. (Eds) (1972). *Studies in Dyadic Communication*. New York: Pergamon.

SILVERMAN, S.R. (1983). Speech training then and now. In: Hochberg et al. (1983).

SILVERMAN, S.R. and HIRSH, I. (1955). Problems related to the use of speech in clinical audiometry. *Ann. Otol. Rhinol. Laryngol.* 64, 1234–1244.

SILVERMAN, S.R. and KRICOS, P.B. (1990). Speechreading. *Volta Rev.* **92**, 22–32.

SIMEONSSON, R.J., COOPER, D.H. and SCHEINER, A.P. (1982). A review of the effectiveness of early intervention programs. *Pediatrics* **69**, 635–641.

SIMMONS, A. (1962). A comparison of the type-token ratio of spoken and written language of deaf and hearing children. *Volta Rev.* **64**, 117–121.

SIMMONS, F.B. (1966). Electrical stimulation of the auditory nerve in man. *Arch. Otolaryngol.* **84**, 24–76.

SIMS, D.G. (1982). Hearing and speechreading evaluation for the deaf adult. In: Sims et al. (1982).

SIMS, D.G., GOTTERMEIER, J. and WALTER, C.G. (1980). Factors contributing to the development of intelligible speech among prelingually deaf persons. *Am. Ann. Deaf* **125**, 374–381.

SIMS, D.G., WALTER, G.G. and WHITEHEAD, R.L. (1982). *Deafness and Communication: Assessment and Training*. Baltimore, MD: Williams and Wilkins.

SIPLE, P. (1978a). Linguistic and psychological properties of American Sign Language: an overview. In: Siple (1978b).

SIPLE, P. (Ed.) (1978b). *Understanding Language through Sign Language Research*. New York: Academic Press.

SIPLE, P., FISCHER, S.D. and BELLUGI, U. (1977). Memory for non-semantic attributes of American Sign Language signs and English words. *J. Verb. Learn. Verb. Behav.* **16**, 561–574.

SISCO, F.H. and ANDERSON, R.J. (1980). Deaf children's performance on the WISC-R relative to hearing status of parents and child-rearing experiences. *Am. Ann. Deaf* **125**, 923–930.

SKARAKIS, E.A. and PRUTTING, C.A. (1977). Early communication: semantic functions and communicative intentions in the communication of the preschool child with impaired hearing. *Am. Ann. Deaf* **122**, 382–391.

SKINNER, M.W., BINZER, S.M., SMITH, P.G., HOLDEN, L.K., FREDRICKSON, J.M., HOLDEN, T.A., JUELICH, M.F. and TURNER, B.A. (1988). Comparison of benefit from vibrotactile and cochlear implant for postlinguistically deaf adults. *Laryngoscope* **98**, 1092–1099.

SKINNER, M.W., HOLDEN, L.K., HOLDEN, T.A., DOWELL, R.C., SELIGMAN, P.M., BRIMACOMBE, J.A. and BEITER, A.L. (1991). Performance of postlingually deaf adults with the wearable speech processor (WSPII) and mini speech processor (MSP) of the Nucleus multi-electrode cochlear implant. *Ear Hear.* **12**, 3–22.

SKUSE, D.H. (1984a). Extreme deprivation in early childhood – I. Diverse outcomes for three siblings from an extraordinary family. *J. Child Psychol. Psychiat.* **25**, 523–541.

SKUSE, D.H. (1984b). Extreme deprivation in early childhood – II. Theoretical issues and a comparative review. *J. Child Psychol. Psychiat.* **25**, 543–572.

SLIKE, S.B., CHIAVACCI, J.P. and HOBBIS, D.H. (1989). The efficiency and effectiveness of an interactive video system to teach sign language vocabulary. *Am. Ann. Deaf* **134**, 288–290.

SLOAN, C. (1980). Auditory processing disorders and language development. In: Levinson and Sloan (1980).

SLOAN, C. (1986). *Treating Auditory Processing Difficulties in Children*. San Diego, CA: College-Hill Press.

SLOBIN, D. (1979). *Psycholinguistics*, 2nd Edn. Glenview, IL: Scott, Foresman and Co.

SLOBIN, D.I. (1980). The repeated path between transparency and opacity in language. In: Bellugi and Studdert-Kennedy (1980).

SLOWIACZEK, L.M. (1990). Effects of lexical stress in auditory word recognition. *Lang. Speech* **33**, 47–68.

SLOWIACZEK, L.M., NUSBAUM, H.C. and PISONI, D.B. (1987). Phonological priming in auditory word recognition. *J. Exp. Psychol.: Learn. Mem. Cognit.* **13**, 64–75.

SMALE, A.G. (1988). The intelligibility of the speech of orally educated, prelingually deaf adolescents. In: Taylor (1988).

SMALL, L.H. and INFANTE, A.A. (1988). Effects of training and visual distance on speechreading performance. *Percept. Mot. Skills* **66**, 415–418.

SMITH, C.R. (1975a). Residual hearing and speech production in deaf children. *J. Speech Hear. Res.* **18**, 795–811.

SMITH, C.R. (1975b). Interjected sounds in deaf children's speech. *J. Commun. Disord.* **8**, 123–128.

SMITH, F. (1973). *Psycholinguistics and Reading*. New York: Holt, Rinehart and Winston.

SMITH, F. and MILLER, G. (Eds) (1966). *The Genesis of Language: A Psycholinguistic Approach*. Cambridge, MA: MIT Press.

SMITH, M. and RICHARDS, S. (1990). Some essential aspects of an effective audiological management programme for school age hearing-impaired children. *J. Br. Assn. Teachers of the Deaf* **14**, 104–113.

SNIDECOR, J.C., MALBRY, L.A. and HEARSEY, E.L. (1944). *Methods of Training Talkers for Increasing Intelligibility in Noise (ORSD Report 3178)*. New York: Psychological Corporation.

SNOW, C.E. (1972). Mothers' speech to children learning language. *Child Devel.* **43**, 549–565.

SNOW, C.E. and FERGUSON, C.A. (Eds) (1977). *Talking to Children: Language Input and Acquisition*. New York: Cambridge University Press.

SOKOLOV, A.N. (1972). *Inner Speech and Thought*. New York: Plenum Press.

SONNENSCHEIN, S. and WHITEHURST, G.W. (1984). Developing referential communication: a hierarchy of skills. *Child Devel.* **55**, 1936–1945.

SPARKS, D.W., ARDELL, L.A., BOURGEDIS, M., WEIDMER, B. and KIHL. P. (1979). Investigating the MESA (Multipoint Electrotactile Speech Aid): the transmission of connected discourse. *J. Acoust. Soc. Am.* **65**, 810–815.

SPEAKS, C. and JERGER, J. (1965). Method for measurement of speech identification. *J. Speech Hear. Res.* **8**, 185–194.

SPEAKS, C., NICCUM, N. and VAN TASELL, D. (1985). Effects of stimulus material on the dichotic listening performance of patients with sensorineural hearing loss. *J. Speech Hear. Res.* **28**, 16–25.

SPELKE, E. (1976). Infants' intermodal perception of events. *Cognit. Psychol.* **8**, 553–560.

SPENCER, P. and DELK, L. (1989). Hearing-impaired students' performance on tests of visual processing: relationships with reading performance. *Am. Ann. Deaf* **134**, 333–337.

SPENCER, P.E. and GUTFREUND, M. (1990). Characteristics of 'dialogues' between mothers and prelinguistic hearing-impaired and normally-hearing infants. *Volta Rev.* **92**, 351–360.

SPENCER, S.J., DALE, J. and KLIONS, H.L. (1989). Deaf versus hearing subjects' recall of words on a distraction task as a function of the signability of the words. *Percept. Mot. Skills* **69**, 1043–1047.

SPERLING, G. (1978). Future prospects in language and communication for the congenitally deaf. In: Liben (1978).

SPETNER, N.B. and OLSHO, L.W. (1990). Auditory frequency resolution in human infancy. *Child Devel.* **61**, 632–652.

SPILLMAN, T. and DILLIER, N. (1989). Comparison of single-channel extracochlear and multichannel intracochlear electrodes in the same patient. *Br. J. Audiol.* **23**, 25–31.

SQUIRES, S. and DANCER, J. (1986). Auditory versus visual practice effects in the intelligibility of words in everyday sentences. *J. Aud. Res.* **26**, 5–10.

STALLER, S.J., DOWELL, R.C., BEITER, A.L. and BRIMACOMBE, J.A. (1991). Perceptual abilities of children with the Nucleus 22-channel cochlear implant. *Ear Hear. Suppl.* **12**, 34–47.

STAMM, K.R. and PEARCE, W.B. (1971). Communicative Behavior and Co-Orientational States. *J. Commun.* **21**, 208–220.

STANDING, L. and CURTIS, L. (1989). Subvocalization rate versus other predictors of the memory span. *Psychol. Rep.* **65**, 487–495.

STANOVICH, K. (1986). Matthew effects in reading: some consequences of individual differences in the acquisition of literacy. *Read. Res. Q.* **21**, 360–407.

STANOVICH, K.E. (1980). Towards an interactive-compensatory model of individual differences in the development of reading fluency. *Read. Res. Q.* **16**, 32–71.

STANOVICH, K. and WEST, R. (1979). Mechanisms of sentence context effects in reading: automatic activation and conscious attention. *Mem. Cognit.* **7**, 77–85.

STATHOPOULOS, E.T., DUCHAN, J.F., SONNENMEIER, R.M. and BRUCE, N.V. (1986). Intonation and pausing in deaf speech. *Folia Phoniat.* **38**, 1–12.

STATON, J. (1985). Using dialogue journals for developing thinking, reading, and writing with hearing-impaired students. *Volta Rev.* 87, 127–154.

STEIN, L., MINDEL, E. and JABALEY, T. (Eds) (1981). *Deafness and Mental Health*. New York: Grune and Stratton.

STEINBERG, D.D. and JAKOBOVITS, L.A. (Eds) (1971). *Semantics: An Interdisciplinary Reader in Philosophy, Linguistics and Psychology*. Cambridge: Cambridge University Press.

STEPHENS, S.D.G. (Ed.) (1976). *Disorders of Auditory Function II*. London: Academic Press.

STERNBERG, M.L.A. (1981). *American Sign Language: A Comprehensive Dictionary*. New York: Harper and Rowe.

STERNBERG, R.J. (1983). Criteria for intellectual skills training. *Educ. Researcher* 12, 6–12, 26.

STERNBERG, R.J. (1987). Most vocabulary is learned from context. In: McKeown and Curtis (1987).

STEVENS, K.N., NICKERSON, R.S. and ROLLINS, A.M. (1978). On describing the suprasegmental properties of the speech of deaf children. In: McPherson and Davis (1978).

STEVENS, S.S. (Ed.) (1951). *Handbook of Experimental Psychology*. New York: Wiley. (See also Atkinson et al. (1988).)

STEWART, D.A. (1983). The use of sign by deaf children: the opinions of a deaf community. *Am. Ann. Deaf* 128, 878–883.

STOCKARD, J.E. and CURRAN, J.S. (1990). Transient elevation of threshold of the neonatal auditory brain stem response. *Ear Hear.* 11, 21–28.

STOEFEN-FISHER, J.M. (1990). Teacher judgments of student reading interests: how accurate are they? *Am. Ann. Deaf* 135, 252–256.

STOKOE, W. (Ed.) (1979). *Sign Language Studies*. Silver Spring, MD: Linstok Press.

STOKOE, W.C. (1960). *Sign Language Structure: An Outline of the Visual Communication System of the American Deaf*. Studies in Linguistics, Occasional Paper 8, Buffalo, NY: University of Buffalo.

STOKOE, W.C. (1978). *Sign Language Structure*. Silver Spring, MD: Linstok Press.

STOKOE, W.C. (Ed.) (1980). *Sign and Culture. A Reader for Students of American Sign Language*. Silver Spring, MD: Linstok Press.

STOKOE, W.C. (1983). Sign languages, linguistics and related arts. In: Kyle and Woll (1983).

STOKOE, W.C. (1987). Tell me where is grammar bred?: Critical evaluation or another chorus of 'Come Back To Milano?'. *Sign Lang. Stud.* 54, 31–58.

STOKOE, W.C. (1991). Semantic Phonology. *Sign Lang. Stud.* 71, 107–114.

STOKOE, W.C. and BATTISON, R.M. (1981). Sign language, mental health and satisfactory interaction. In: Stein et al. (1981).

STOKOE, W., CASTERLINE, D. and CRONEBERG, G. (1965). *A Dictionary of American Sign Language on Linguistic Principles*. Silver Spring, MD: Linstok Press.

STONE, P. and ADAM, A. (1986). Is your child wearing the right hearing aid? Principles for selecting and maintaining amplification. *Volta Rev.* 88, 45–54.

STRASSMAN, B.K., KRETSCHMER, R.E. and BILSKY, L.H. (1987). The instantiation of general terms by deaf adolescents/adults. *J. Commun. Disord.* 20, 1–13.

STRENG, A.H., KRETSCHMER, R.R. and KRETSCHMER, L.W. (1978). *Language, Learning, and Deafness: Theory, Application and Classroom Management*. New York: Grune and Stratton.

STROHNER, H. and NELSON, K.E. (1974). The young child's development of sentence comprehension: influence of event probability, nonverbal context, syntactic form, and their strategies. *Child Devel.* 45, 567–576.

STRONG, C.J. and SHAVER, J.P. (1991). Modifying attitudes towards persons with hearing impairments. *Am. Ann. Deaf* 136, 252–260.

STRONG, M. (Ed.) (1988). *Language Learning and Deafness*. Cambridge: Cambridge University Press.

STRONG, M. and CHARLSON, E.S. (1987). Simultaneous Communication: are teachers attempting an impossible task? *Am. Ann. Deaf* 132, 376–382.

STRONG, M., CHARLSON, E.S. and GOLD, R. (1987). Integration and segregation in mainstreaming programs for children and adolescents with hearing impairments. *Except. Child.* 34, 181–195.

STUCKLESS, E.R. (1965). *National Research Conference on Behavioral Aspects of Deafness*. Washington, DC: US Department of Health, Education and Welfare, Vocational Rehabilitation Administration.

STUCKLESS, E.R. (1991). Reflections on bilingual, bicultural education for deaf children. *Am. Ann. Deaf* **136**, 270–272.

STUDEBAKER, G.A. and SHERBECOE, R.L. (1991). Frequency-importance and transfer functions for recorded CID W-22 word lists. *J. Speech Hear. Res.* **34**, 427–438.

SUBTELNY, J.D. (Ed.) (1980). *Speech Assessment and Speech Improvement for the Hearing Impaired*. Washington, DC: Alexander Graham Bell Association.

SUBTELNY, J.D. (1982). Speech assessment of the adolescent with impaired hearing. In: Sims et al. (1982).

SUBTELNY, J.D. (1983). Integrated speech and language instruction for the hearing-impaired adolescent. In: Lass (1983).

SUBTELNY, J.D,. WHITEHEAD, R.L. and ORLANDO, N.A. (1980). Description and evaluation of an instructional program to improve speech and voice diagnosis of the hearing impaired. *Volta Rev.* **82**, 85–95.

SUMBY, W.H. and POLLACK, I. (1954). Visual contribution to speech intelligibility in noise. *J. Acoust. Soc. Am.* **26**, 212–215.

SUMMERFIELD, A.Q. (1979). Use of visual information for phonetic perception. *Phonetica* **36**, 314–331.

SUMMERFIELD, A.Q. and MCGRATH, M. (1984). Detection and resolution of audio-visual incompatibility in the perception of vowels. *Q. J. Exp. Psychol.* **36A**, 51–74.

SUTY, K. A. (1986). Individual differences in the signed communication of deaf children. *Am. Ann. Deaf* **131**, 298–304.

SVIRSKY, M.A. and TOBEY, E.A. (1991). Effect of different types of auditory stimulation on vowel formant frequencies in multichannel cochlear implant users. *J. Acoust. Soc. Am.* **89**, 2895–2904.

SWAIKO, N. (1974). The role and value of an eurhythmics program in a curriculum for deaf children. *Am. Ann. Deaf.* **119**, 321–324.

SWANSON, H.L. (1987). The effects of self-instruction training on a deaf child's semantic and pragmatic production. *J. Commun. Disord.* **20**, 425–436.

SWISHER, M.V. (1990). Developmental effects on the reception of signs in peripheral vision by deaf students. *Sign Lang. Stud.* **66**, 45–59.

SWISHER, M., CHRISTIE, K. and MILLER, S. (1989). The reception of signs in peripheral vision by deaf persons. *Sign Lang. Stud.* **63**, 99–123.

TAIT, D.M. and WOOD, D.J. (1987). From communication to speech in deaf children. *Child Lang. Teaching Ther.* **3**, 1–17.

TAIT, M. (1986). Using singing to facilitate linguistic development in hearing impaired pre-schoolers. *J. Br. Assn. Teachers of the Deaf* **10**, 103–108.

TALLAL, P. (1976). Rapid auditory processing in normal and disordered language development. *J. Speech Hear. Res.* **19**, 561–571.

TALLAL, P. (1980). Auditory processing disorders in children. In: Levinson and Sloan (1980).

TALLAL, P. (1990). Fine-grained discrimination deficits in language-learning impaired children are specific neither to the auditory modality nor to speech perception. *J. Speech Hear. Res.* **33**, 616–617.

TALLAL, P., STARK, R.E. and MELLITS, D. (1985). The relationship between auditory temporal analysis and receptive language development: evidence from studies of developmental language disorder. *Neuropsychologia.* **23**, 527–534.

TANNEN, D. (1980). Implications of the oral/literate continuum for cross-cultural communication. In: Alatis (1980).

TATE, M. (1980). A study of patterns of language development in a sample of hearing-impaired children. *J. Br. Assocn. Teachers of the Deaf* **4**, 198–204.

TAYLOR, G. and BISHOP, J. (Eds) (1991). *Being Deaf: The Experience of Deafness*. London: Pinter.

TAYLOR, I.G. (Ed.) (1988). *The Education of the Deaf: Current Perspectives*, Vol. IV. London: Croom Helm.

TELLER, H.E. and LINDSEY, J.D. (1987). Developing hearing-impaired students' writing skills: Martin Buber's mutuality in today's classroom. *Am. Ann. Deaf* **132**, 383–385.

TERNSTROM, S., SUNDBERG, J. and COLLDEN, A. (1988). Articulatory F_0 perturbations and auditory feedback. *J. Speech Hear. Res.* **31**, 187–192.

TERRIO, L. and HAAS, W. (1986). A model for evaluating tactually assistive devices. *Volta Rev.* **88**, 209–214.

TERVOORT, B. (1965). Development of language and critical period. In: Davis (1965).

TERVOORT, B.T. (1961). Esoteric symbolism in the communication behavior of young deaf children. *Am. Ann. Deaf* **106**, 436–438.

TERVOORT, B.T. (1979). What is the native language for deaf children? *Studies in Honour of Prof. B. Siertsima*. Amsterdam: Institute for General Linguistics.

THIBODEAU, L.M. (1990). Electroacoustic performance of direct-input hearing aids with FM amplification systems. *Lang. Speech Hear. Ser. in Schools* **21**, 49–56.

THOMAS-KERSTING, C. and CASTEEL, R.L. (1989). Harsh voice: vocal effort perceptual ratings and spectral noise levels of hearing-impaired children. *J. Commun. Disord.* **22**, 125–135.

THOMPSON, M.D. and SWISHER, M.V. (1985). Acquiring language through total communication. *Ear Hear.* **6**, 29–32.

TJOSSEM, T.D. (Ed.) (1976). *Intervention Strategies for High Risk Infants and Young Children*. Baltimore, MD: University Park Press.

TOBEY, E.A. and HASENSTAB, S. (1991). Effects of a Nucleus multichannel cochlear implant upon speech production in children. *Ear Hear.* **12**, 48–54.

TOBIAS, J.V. and SCHUBERT, E.D. (Eds) (1983). *Hearing Research and Theory*, Vol. 2. New York: Academic Press.

TOBIN, H. (1985). Binaural interaction tasks. In: Pinheiro and Musiek (1985b).

TOGONU-BICKERSTETH, F. (1988). Prospects and challenges of educating deaf pupils in Nigeria: teachers' perceptions. *Int. J. Rehab. Res.* **11**, 225–233.

TOLHURST, G.C. (1957). Effects of duration and articulation changes on intelligibility, word reception, and listener preference. *J. Speech Hear. Disord.* **22**, 328.

TREIMAN, R. and BARRON, J. (1981). Segmental analysis ability: development and relation to reading ability. In: MacKinnon and Waller (1981).

TREIMAN, R. and HIRSH-PASEK, K. (1983). Silent reading: insights from second generation deaf readers. *Cognit. Psychol.* **15**, 39–65.

TRELOAR, C. (1985). A survey of attitudes to the role of Auslan in the education of the deaf. *Aust. Teacher of the Deaf* **26**, 21–33.

TRINDER, J., FOSTER, J., GLYNN, C. and HAGGARD, M. (1980). Parameters of spectral shape in speech intelligibility enhancement. *J. Acoust. Soc. Am.* **68**, Suppl. 101.

TRUAX, R. (1985). Linking research to facilitate reading–writing–communication connections. *Volta Rev.* **87**, 155–169.

TRUNE, D.R. (1982). Influence of neonatal cochlear removal on the development of mouse cochlear nucleus: 1. Number, size and its neurons. *J. Comp. Neurol.* **209**, 409–424.

TRYBUS, R.J. (1980). National data on rated speech intelligibility of hearing-impaired children. In: Subtelny (1980).

TRYBUS, R.J. (1987). Century 21: Social trends and deafness. *Am. Ann. Deaf* **132**, 323–325.

TRYBUS, R.J. and KARCHMER, M.A. (1977). School achievement scores of hearing-impaired children: national data on achievement status and growth patterns. *Am. Ann. Deaf* **122**, 62–69.

TUCKER, I., HUGHES, M. and GLOVER, M. (1983). Verbal interaction with pre-school hearing-impaired children: a comparison of maternal and parental language input. *J. Br. Assn. Teachers of the Deaf* **7**, 90–98.

TUNMER, W.E. and BOWEY, J.A. (1984). Metalinguistic awareness and reading acquisition. In: Tunmer et al. (1984).

TUNMER, W.E., PRATT, C. and HERRIMAN, M.L. (Eds) (1984). *Metalinguistic Awareness in Children: Theory, Research and Implications*. New York: Springer-Verlag.

TUREK, S., DORMAN, M. FRANKS, J. and SUMMERFIELD, Q. (1980). Identification of synthetic /bdg/ by hearing-impaired listeners under monotic and dichotic formant presentation. *J. Acoust. Soc. Am.* 67, 1031–1040.

TURNER, C.W. and HENN, C.C. (1989). The relation between vowel recognition and measures of frequency resolution. *J. Speech Hear. Res.* 32, 49–58.

TURNER, C.W., HOLTE, L.A. and RELKIN, E. (1987). Auditory filtering and the discrimination of spectral shapes by normal and hearing-impaired subjects. *J. Rehab. Res. Dev.* 24, 229–238.

TURNER, C.W. and NELSON, D.A. (1982). Frequency discrimination in regions of normal and impaired sensitivity. *J. Speech Hear. Res.* 25, 34–41.

TWENEY, R.D., HOEMANN, H.W. and ANDREWS, C.E. (1975). Semantic organization in deaf and hearing subjects. *J. Psycholing. Res.* 4, 61–73.

TYE-MURRAY, N. (1987). Effects of vowel context on the articulatory closure postures of deaf speakers. *J. Speech Hear. Res.* 30, 99–104.

TYE-MURRAY, N. (1991). The establishment of open articulatory postures by deaf and hearing talkers. *J. Speech Hear. Res.* 34, 453–459.

TYE-MURRAY, N. and FOLKINS, J.W. (1990). Jaw and lip movements of deaf talkers producing utterances with known stress patterns. *J. Acoust. Soc. Am.* 87, 2675–2683.

TYE-MURRAY, N. and WOODWORTH, B. (1989). The influence of final-syllable position on the vowel and word duration of deaf talkers. *J. Acoust. Soc. Am.* 85, 313–321.

TYE-MURRAY, N., ZIMMERMAN, G.N. and FOLKINS, J.W. (1987). Movement timing in deaf and hearing speakers: comparisons of phonetically heterogeneous syllable strings. *J. Speech Hear. Res.* 30, 411–417.

TYLER, R.S., LOWDER, M.W., OTTO, S.R., PREECE, J.P., GANTZ, B.J. and MCCABE, B.F. (1984). Initial Iowa results with the multichannel implant from Melbourne. *J. Speech Hear. Res.* 27, 596–604.

TYLER, R.S., MOORE, B.C.J. and KUK, F.K. (1989). Performance of some of the better cochlear implant patients. *J. Speech Hear. Res.* 32, 887–911.

TYLER, R.S., PREECE, J.P., LANSING, C.R., OTTO, S.R. and GANTZ, B.J. (1986). Previous experience as a confounding factor in comparing cochlear-implant processing schemes. *J. Speech Hear. Res.* 29, 282–287.

UPFOLD, L.J. and ISEPY, J. (1982). Childhood deafness in Australia: incidence and maternal rubella, 1949–1980. *Med. J. Aust.* 2, 323–326.

UPFOLD, L.J. and SMITHER, M.F. (1981). Hearing-aid fitting protocol. *Br. J. Audiol.* 15, 181–188.

UTLEY, J. (1946). Factors involved in the teaching and testing of lipreading through the use of motion pictures. *Volta Rev.* 38, 657–659.

VANDELL, D.L. and GEORGE, L.B. (1981). Social interaction in hearing and deaf preschoolers: successes and failures in initiations. *Child Devel.* 52, 627–635.

VAN HATTUM, R.J. (Ed.) (1980). *Communication Disorders: An Introduction*. New York: MacMillan.

VAN KLEECK, A. (1984). Metalinguistic skills: cutting across spoken and written language and problem-solving abilities. In: Wallach and Butler (1984).

VAN RIPER, C. (1978). *Speech Correction: Principles and Methods*, 6th Edn. Englewood Cliffs, NJ: Prentice-Hall.

VAN UDEN, A. (1986). *Sign Languages Used by Deaf People, and Psycholinguistics: A Critical Evaluation*. Lisse: Swets and Zeitlinger, B.V.

VELLUMNO, F.R. (1979). *Dyslexia: Theory and Research*. Cambridge, MA: MIT Press.

VELLUTINO, F. (1983). Childhood dyslexia: a language disorder. *Prog. Learn. Disabil.* 5, 135–173.

VERBRUGGE, R.R. (1977). Resemblances in language and perception. In: Shaw and Bransford (1977).

VERNON, MCC. (1969). Sociological and psychological factors associated with hearing loss. *J. Speech Hear. Res.* 12, 541–563.

VERNON, MCC. and ANDREWS, J. (1990). *The Psychology of Deafness: Understanding Deaf and Hard-of-Hearing People*. New York: Longman.

VERNON, MCC. and OTTINGER, P.J. (1980). Psychosocial aspects of hearing impairment. In: Schow and Nerbonne (1980).

VOLTERRA, V. and CASELLI, M.C. (1986). First stage of language acquisition through two modalities in deaf and hearing children. *Ital. J. Neurol. Sci. Suppl.* **5**, 109–115.

VOLTERRA, V. and ERTING, C.J. (Eds) (1990). *From Gesture to Language in Hearing and Deaf Children*. Berlin: Springer-Verlag.

WALDEN, B., ERDMAN, S., MONTGOMERY, A., SCHWARTZ, D. and PROSEK, R. (1981). Some effects of training on speech recognition by hearing-impaired adults. *J. Speech Hear. Res.* **24**, 207–216.

WALDEN, B.W. and MONTGOMERY, A.A. (1975). Dimensions of consonant perception in normal and hearing impaired listeners. *J. Speech Hear. Res.* **18**, 444–455.

WALDRON, M.B., DIEBOLD, T.J. and ROSE, S. (1985). Hearing impaired students in regular classrooms: a cognitive model for educational services. *Except. Child.* **52**, 39–43.

WALDSTEIN, R.S. (1990). Effects of postlingual deafness on speech production: implications for the role of auditory feedback. *J. Acoust. Soc. Am.* **88**, 2099–2114.

WALKER, D.W., GRIMWADE, J.C. and WOOD, C. (1971). Intra-uterine noise: a component of the fetal environment. *Am. J. Obstet. Gynec.* **109**, 91–95.

WALKER, G., BYRNE, D. and DILLON, H. (1982). Learning effects with a closed response set nonsense syllable test. *Aust. J. Audiol.* **4**, 27–31.

WALKER, M. (1976). *The Makaton Vocabulary*. London: Royal Association for the Deaf and Dumb.

WALKER, M. and ARMFIELD, A. (1982). What is the Makaton vocabulary? In: Peter and Barnes (1982).

WALKER, M. and BUCKFIELD, P.M. (1983). The Makaton vocabulary. *New Zealand Speech Lang. Ther. J.* **38**, 26–36.

WALLACE, G. and CORBALLIS, M.C. (1973). Short-term memory and coding strategies in the deaf. *J. Exp. Psychol.* **99**, 334–348.

WALLACH, G.P. and BUTLER, K.G. (Eds.) (1984). *Language Learning Disabilities in School-Age Children*. Baltimore, MD: Williams and Wilkins.

WALMSLEY, S. (1983). Writing disability. In: Mosenthal et al. (1983).

WALTZMAN, S., COHEN, N.L., SPIVAK, L., YING, E., BRACKETT, D., SHAPIRO, W. and HOFFMAN, R. (1990). Improvement in speech perception and production abilities in children using a multichannel cochlear implant. *Laryngoscope* **100**, 240–243.

WAMPLER, D. (1971). *Linguistics of Visual English*. Santa Rosa, CA: Early Childhood Education Department, Santa Rosa Schools.

WARREN, C. and HASENSTAB, S. (1986). Self-concept of severely to profoundly hearing-impaired children. *Volta Rev.* **88**, 289–295.

WARREN, R.M. (1970). Perceptual restoration of missing speech sounds. *Science* **167**, 393–395.

WARREN, Y., DANCER, J., MONFILS, B. and PITTENGER, J. (1989). The practice effect in speechreading distributed over five days: same versus different CID sentence lists. *Volta Rev.* **91**, 321–325.

WATKINS, S. (1984). *Long-Term Effects of Home Intervention on Hearing Impaired Children*. Unpublished Doctoral Thesis, Utah State University.

WATSON, B., GOLDGAR, D., KROESE, J. and LOTZ, W. (1986). Nonverbal intelligence and academic achievement in the hearing impaired. *Volta Rev.* **88**, 151–158.

WATSON, B.U. (1991). Some relationships between intelligence and auditory discrimination. *J. Speech Hear. Res.* **34**, 621–627.

WATSON, P. (1979). The utilization of the computer with the hearing impaired and the handicapped. *Am. Ann. Deaf* **124**, 670–680.

WATSON, R. (1985). Towards a theory of definition. *J. Child Lang.* **12**, 181–197.

WATSON, T.J. (1967). *The Education of Hearing-Handicapped Children*. London: University of London Press.

WEBSTER, A. (1986). *Deafness, Development and Literacy*. London: Methuen.

WEBSTER, A. (1988). Deafness and learning to read: theoretical and research issues. *J. Br. Assn. Teachers of the Deaf* **12**, 77–83.

WEBSTER, A., BAMFORD, J.M., THYER, N.J. and AYLES, R. (1989). The psychological, educational and auditory sequelae of early, persistent secretory otitis media. *J. Child Psychol. Psychiat.* **30**, 529–546.

WEBSTER, A. and ELLWOOD, J. (1985). *The Hearing-Impaired Child in the Ordinary School*. London: Croom Helm.

WEBSTER, A., SAUNDERS, E. and BAMFORD, J.M. (1984). Fluctuating conductive hearing impairment. *J. Assn. Educ. Psychol.* **6**, 6–19.

WEBSTER, A., WOOD, D.J. and GRIFFITHS, A.J. (1981). Reading retardation or linguistic deficit? (I): Interpreting reading test performances of hearing-impaired adolescents. *J. Res. Read.* **4**, 136–147.

WEBSTER, D.B. and WEBSTER, M. (1979). Effects of neonatal conductive hearing loss on brainstem auditory nuclei. *Ann. Otol. Rhinol. Laryngol.* **88**, 684–688.

WEBSTER, J.C. (1984). Interlist equivalencies for a numeral and a vowel/consonant multiple-choice monosyllabic test for severely/profoundly deaf young adults. *J. Aud. Res.* **24**, 17–33.

WEDENBERG, E. (1954). Auditory training of severely hard of hearing preschool children. *Acta. Otolaryngol. Stockh. Suppl.* **94**, 1–129.

WEIR, R.H. (1966). Some questions on the child's learning of phonology. In: Smith and Miller (1966).

WEISEL, A. (1988). Parental hearing status, reading comprehension skills and social-emotional adjustment. *Am. Ann. Deaf.* **133**, 356–359.

WEISS, A.L. (1986). Classroom discourse and the hearing-impaired child. *Topics Lang. Disord.* **6**, 60–70.

WEISS, A.L., CARNEY, A.E. and LEONARD, L.B. (1985). Perceived contrastive stress production in hearing-impaired and normal-hearing children. *J. Speech Hear. Res.* **28**, 26–35.

WEISS, K., GOODWIN, M. and MOORES, D. (1975). *Evaluation of Programs for Hearing Impaired Children, University of Minnesota, MN: Research Report 91*. University of Minnesota, MN: Research, Development and Demonstration Center in Education of Handicapped Children.

WELLS, C.G. (1981). *Learning Through Interaction: The Study of Language Development*. Cambridge: Cambridge University Press.

WELLS, G. (1979). Variation in child language. In: Fletcher and Garman (1979).

WELSH, L.W., WELSH, J.J. and HEALY, M.P. (1983). Effect of sound deprivation on central hearing. *Laryngoscope* **93**, 1569–1575.

WELLS, G. (1984). *Language Development in the Pre-School Years*. Cambridge: Cambridge University Press.

WEPMAN, J. (1958). *Auditory Discrimination Test*. Los Angeles, CA: Western Psychological Services.

WEPMAN, J. (1960). Auditory discrimination, speech and reading. *Element. Sch. J.* **60**, 325–333.

WEPMAN, J. (1975). *Auditory Discrimination Test*. Palm Springs, FL: Language Research Associates.

WERKER, J.F. and TEES, R.C. (1984). Cross language perception: evidence for perceptual reorganisation during the first year of life. *Infant Behav. Devel.* **7**, 49–63.

WEST, J.J. and WEBER, J.L. (1973). A phonological analysis of the spontaneous language of a four-year-old hard-of-hearing child. *J. Speech Hear. Disord.* **38**, 25–35.

WEST, J.J. and WEBER, J.L. (1974). A linguistic analysis of the morphemic and syntactic structures of a hard-of-hearing child. *Lang. Speech* **17**, 68–79.

WESTBY, C.E. (1984). Development of narrative language abilities. In: Wallach and Butler (1984).

WHETNALL, E. and FRY, D.B. (1964). *The Deaf Child*. London: Heinemann.

WHITE, A. (1990). Differences in teacher expectations. *Volta Rev.* **92**, 131–144.

WHITE, A.H. and STEVENSON, V.M. (1975). The effects of total communication, manual communication, oral communication and reading on the learning of factual information in residential school deaf children. *Am. Ann. Deaf* **120**, 48–57.

WHITE, S. and WHITE, R. (1987). The effects of hearing status of the family and age of intervention on reception and expressive oral language skills in hearing-impaired infants. In: Levitt et al. (1987b).

WHITEHEAD, R. (1987). Fundamental vocal frequency characteristics of hearing-impaired young adults. *Volta Rev.* 89, 7–15.

WHITEHEAD, R. and BAREFOOT, S. (1980). Some aerodynamic characteristics of plosive consonants produced by hearing-impaired speakers. *Am. Ann. Deaf* 125, 366–373.

WHITEHEAD, R.L. (1991). Stop consonant closure durations for normal-hearing and hearing-impaired speakers. *Volta Rev.* 93, 145–153.

WHORF, B.L. (1956). *Language, Thought and Reality: Selected Writings of Benjamin Lee Whorf* (edited by J.B. Carroll). Cambridge, MA: MIT Press.

WICKHAM, C. and KYLE, J. (1987). Teachers' beliefs about BSL and their perceptions of children's signing. In: Kyle (1987).

WIEGERSMA, P.H. and VAN DER VELDE, A. (1983). Motor development of deaf children. *J. Child Psychol. Psychiat.* 24, 103–111.

WIGHTMAN, F.L. (1981). Pitch perception: an example of auditory pattern recognition. In: Getty and Howard (1981).

WIGHTMAN, F., MCGEE, T. and KRAMER, M. (1977). Factors influencing frequency selectivity in normal and hearing-impaired listeners. In: Evans (1977).

WIIG, E.H. and SEMEL, E. (1984). *Language Assessment and Intervention for the Learning Disabled.* Columbus, OH: Charles E. Merrill.

WILBERS, S. (1988). Why America needs deaf culture: cultural pluralism and the liberal arts tradition. *Sign Lang. Stud.* 59, 195–204.

WILBUR, R. (1977). An explanation of deaf children's difficulty with certain syntactic structures in English. *Volta Rev.* 79, 85–92.

WILBUR, R.B. (1979). *American Sign Language and Sign Systems.* Baltimore, MD: University Park Press.

WILBUR, R.B. (1987). *American Sign Language: Linguistics and Applied Dimensions.* Boston, MA: College Hill Press.

WILCOX, B. (1969). Visual preferences of human infants for representations of the human face. *J. Exp. Child Psychol.* 7, 10–20.

WILCOX, J. and TOBIN, H. (1974). Linguistic performance of hard-of-hearing and normal-hearing children. *J. Speech Hear. Res.* 17, 288–293.

WILCOX, S. (1988). Introduction: academic acceptance of American Sign Language. *Sign Lang. Stud.* 59, 101–108.

WILCOX, S. (1990). The structure of signed and spoken languages. *Sign Lang. Stud.* 67, 141–151.

WILLIAMS, A. (1982). The relationship between two visual communication systems: reading and lipreading. *J. Speech Hear. Res.* 25, 500–503.

WILLIAMS, C.E. (1970). Some psychiatric observations on a group of maladjusted deaf children. *J. Child Psychol. Psychiat.* 11, 1–18.

WILLIAMS, D.M.L. and DARBYSHIRE, J.O. (1982). Diagnosis of deafness: a study of family responses and needs. *Volta Rev.* 84, 24–30.

WILLIAMS, E. (1986). A use of LARSP in secondary units of hearing-impaired pupils. *Child Lang. Teach. Ther.* 2, 154–169.

WILLIAMS, J.E. and DENNIS, D. B. (1979). A partially hearing unit. In: Crystal (1979).

WILLIAMS, J.S. (1976). Bilingual experiences of a deaf child. *Sign Lang. Stud.* 15, 37–41.

WILSON, B.A., BADDELEY, A.D. and COCKBURN, J.M. (1989). How do old dogs learn new tricks: teaching a technological skill to brain injured people. *Cortex* 25, 115–119.

WILSON, B.S., FINLEY, C.C., FARMER, J.C., LAWSON, D.T., WEBER, B.A., WOLFORD, R.D., KENAN, P.D., WHITE, M.W., MERZENICH, M.M. and SCHINDLER, R.A. (1988). Comparative studies of speech processing strategies for cochlear implants. *Laryngoscope* 98, 1069–1077.

WITELSON, S.F. (1982). Hemisphere specialization from birth. *Int. J. Neurosci.* 17, 54–55.

WITELSON, S.F. (1985). On hemisphere specialization and cerebral plasticity from birth: Mark II. In: Best (1985).

WITELSON, S.F. (1987). Neurobiological aspects of language in children. *Child Devel.* 58, 653–688.

WITELSON, S. and PAILLIE, W. (1973). Left hemisphere for specialisation in the newborn. *Brain* 96, 641–646.

WOLF, M. (1984). Naming, reading and the dyslexias: a longitudinal overview. *Ann. Dyslexia* 34, 87–115.

WOLFF, A.B. (1985). Analysis. In: Martin (1985).

WOLFF, J.G. (1973). *Language, Brain and Hearing: An Introduction to the Psychology of Language with a Section on Deaf Children's Learning of Language.* London: Methuen.

WOLFF, S. (1977). Cognitive and communication patterns in classrooms for deaf students. *Am. Ann. Deaf* 122, 319–327.

WOLFLE, D. (1951). Training. In: Stevens (1951).

WOLK, S. and SCHILDROTH, A. (1984). Consistency of an associational strategy used on reading comprehension tests by hearing impaired students. *J. Res. Read.* 7, 135–142.

WOLL, B., KYLE, J. and DEUCHAR, M. (Eds) (1981). *Perspectives on British Sign Language.* London: Croom Helm.

WOOD, D. (1991). Communication and cognition: how the communication styles of hearing adults may hinder – rather than help – deaf learners. *Am. Ann. Deaf* 136, 247–251.

WOOD, D.J. (1980). Teaching the young child: some relationships between social interaction, language and thought. In: Olson (1980).

WOOD, D.J., GRIFFITHS, A.J. and WEBSTER, A. (1981). Reading retardation or linguistic deficit? (II): Test-answering strategies in hearing and hearing-impaired school children. *J. Res. Read.* 4, 148–156.

WOOD, D.J., WOOD, H.A., GRIFFITHS, A.J., HOWARTH, S.P. and HOWARTH, C.I. (1982). The structure of conversations with 6-to-10-year old deaf children. *J. Child Psychol. Psychiat.* 23, 295–308.

WOOD, D., WOOD, H., GRIFFITHS, A. and HOWARTH, I. (1986). *Teaching and Talking with Deaf Children.* Chichester, Sussex: Wiley.

WOODCOCK, R.W. (1973). *Woodcock Reading Mastery Tests.* Circle Pines, MN: American Guidance Service.

WOODS, B.T. and CAREY, S. (1979). Language deficits after apparent clinical recovery from childhood aphasia. *Ann. Neurol.* 6, 405–409.

WOODWARD, J. and ALLEN, T. (1987). Classroom use of ASL by teachers. *Sign Lang. Stud.* 54, 1–10.

WRIGHTSTONE, J.W., ARONOW, M.S. and MOSKOWITZ, S. (1963). Developing reading test norms for deaf children. *Am. Ann. Deaf* 108, 311–316.

YENI-KOMISHIAN, G.H., KAVANAGH, J.F. and FERGUSON, C.A. (Eds) (1980). *Child Phonology,* Vol. 2., *Perception.* New York: Academic Press.

YOSHINAGA-ITANO, C. (1986). Beyond the sentence level: what's in a hearing-impaired child's story? *Topics Lang. Disord.* 6, 71–83.

YOSHINAGA-ITANO, C. and SNYDER, L. (1985). Form and meaning in the written language of hearing-impaired children. *Volta Rev.* 87, 75–90.

ZAIDEL, E. (1980). Clues from hemispheric specialization. In: Bellugi and Studdert-Kennedy (1980).

ZAJONC, R.B. (1960). The process of cognitive timing communication. *J. Abnorm. Soc. Psychol.* 61, 159–167.

ZORFASS, J.M. (1981). Metalinguistic awareness in young deaf children: a preliminary study. *Appl. Psycholing.* 2, 333–352.

ZWIEBEL, A. (1987). More on the effects of early manual communication on the cognitive development of deaf children. *Am. Ann. Deaf* 132, 16–20.

Index